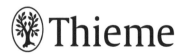

Operative Cranial Neurosurgical Anatomy

Filippo Gagliardi, MD, PhD
Neurosurgeon
Department of Neurosurgery and Gamma Knife Radiosurgery
San Raffaele Scientific Institute
Vita-Salute University
Milano, Italy

Cristian Gragnaniello, MD, PhD, MSurg, MAdvSurg, FICS
Surgical Director
Harvey H. Ammerman Microsurgical Laboratory
Department of Neurosurgery
George Washington University
Washington, DC, USA

Pietro Mortini, MD
Professor and Chairman
Department of Neurosurgery and Gamma Knife Radiosurgery
San Raffaele Scientific Institute
Vita-Salute University
Milano, Italy

Anthony J. Caputy, MD, FACS
Professor and Chairman
Hugo V. Rizzoli Professor
Department of Neurosurgery
George Washington University
Washington, DC, USA

532 illustrations

Thieme
New York • Stuttgart • Delhi • Rio de Janeiro

Executive Editor: Timothy Y. Hiscock
Managing Editor: Sarah Landis
Director, Editorial Services: Mary Jo Casey
Production Editor: Naamah Schwartz
International Production Director: Andreas Schabert
Editorial Director: Sue Hodgson
International Marketing Director: Fiona Henderson
International Sales Director: Louisa Turrell
Director of Institutional Sales: Adam Bernacki
Senior Vice President and Chief Operating Officer:
Sarah Vanderbilt
President: Brian D. Scanlan

Library of Congress Cataloging-in-Publication Data

Names: Gagliardi, Filippo, editor. | Gragnaniello, Cristian, editor.
   Mortini, Pietro, editor. | Caputy, Anthony J., editor.
Title: Operative cranial neurosurgical anatomy / Filippo Gagliardi,
   Cristian Gragnaniello, Pietro Mortini, Anthony J. Caputy.
Description: New York : Thieme, [2019] | Includes
   bibliographical references.
Identifiers: LCCN 2018041350| ISBN 9781626232167 (print) |
   ISBN 9781626232228
   (eISBN)
Subjects: | MESH: Skull—surgery | Skull—anatomy & histology |
   Neurosurgical
   Procedures—methods
Classification: LCC RD529 | NLM WL 368 | DDC 617.5/14—dc23
   LC record available at https://lccn.loc.gov/2018041350

© 2019 Thieme Medical Publishers, Inc.

Thieme Publishers New York
333 Seventh Avenue, New York, NY 10001 USA
+1 800 782 3488, customerservice@thieme.com

Thieme Publishers Stuttgart
Rüdigerstrasse 14, 70469 Stuttgart, Germany
+49 [0]711 8931 421, customerservice@thieme.de

Thieme Publishers Delhi
A-12, Second Floor, Sector-2, Noida-201301
Uttar Pradesh, India
+91 120 45 566 00, customerservice@thieme.in

Thieme Publishers Rio de Janeiro, Thieme Publicações Ltda.
Edifício Rodolpho de Paoli, 25° andar
Av. Nilo Peçanha, 50 – Sala 2508,
Rio de Janeiro 20020-906 Brasil
+55 21 3172-2297 / +55 21 3172-1896
www.thiemerevinter.com.br

Cover design: Thieme Publishing Group
Typesetting by DiTech Process Solutions

Printed in Germany by
Beltz Grafische Betriebe

ISBN 978-1-62623-216-7

Also available as an e-book:
eISBN 978-1-62623-217-4

Important note: Medicine is an ever-changing science undergoing continual development. Research and clinical experience are continually expanding our knowledge, in particular our knowledge of proper treatment and drug therapy. Insofar as this book mentions any dosage or application, readers may rest assured that the authors, editors, and publishers have made every effort to ensure that such references are in accordance with **the state of knowledge at the time of production of the book.**

Nevertheless, this does not involve, imply, or express any guarantee or responsibility on the part of the publishers in respect to any dosage instructions and forms of applications stated in the book. **Every user is requested to examine carefully** the manufacturers' leaflets accompanying each drug and to check, if necessary in consultation with a physician or specialist, whether the dosage schedules mentioned therein or the contraindications stated by the manufacturers differ from the statements made in the present book. Such examination is particularly important with drugs that are either rarely used or have been newly released on the market. Every dosage schedule or every form of application used is entirely at the user's own risk and responsibility. The authors and publishers request every user to report to the publishers any discrepancies or inaccuracies noticed. If errors in this work are found after publication, errata will be posted at www.thieme.com on the product description page.

Some of the product names, patents, and registered designs referred to in this book are in fact registered trademarks or proprietary names even though specific reference to this fact is not always made in the text. Therefore, the appearance of a name without designation as proprietary is not to be construed as a representation by the publisher that it is in the public domain.

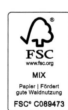

"Nothing behind of me, everything ahead of me, as is ever so on the road."
-Jack Kerouac

To my parents Cesare and Dolly with infinite love and esteem.

-F.G.

*"Controllers, abusers, and manipulative people don't
question themselves. They don't ask themselves if the problem
is them. They always say the problem is someone else."*
-Darlene Ouimet

To Katie for her unconditional love and support through these times of change and growth.

-C.G.

Contents

Contents

Part VI: Vascular Procedures

Part VII: Ventricular Shunts Procedures

Foreword

"If you can visualize it, you can actualize it."
-Dennis Conner, American Yachtsman

Progress in the field of neurosurgery over the last century has been astonishing. Much of that progress has been due to improvements in our ability to visualize that which could not previously be seen well or detected at all. Early neurosurgical procedures were performed without the assistance of any preoperative imaging studies, only a knowledge and firm conviction in the validity of cerebral localization. The progression from skull and spine x-rays to pneumoencephalography, radionuclide brain scans, CT, and MRI provided progressively improved ability to visualize the pathology neurosurgeons deal with. Likewise, advancement from the surgeon's naked eye and reflected light, to surgical loupes with a headlight, to modern operating microscopes with brilliant illumination, has steadily improved neurosurgeons' ability to visualize pathology intraoperatively, thus diversifying and expanding the breadth of our specialty.

Similarly, the improvement in surgical exposures has allowed neurosurgeons to visualize pathology that is concealed behind bone and normal anatomic structures. Early neurosurgeons utilized a relatively small number of standard surgical approaches that often required brain retraction or resection of normal tissue to provide adequate exposure of the pathology at hand. Through a better understanding of surgical anatomy and research in microsurgical anatomy, there are now an expanded number of standard surgical approaches with numerous variations to address specific challenges. The evolution of skull base exposures augmented visualization by eliminating nonessential bony structures to minimize or eliminate the need to retract brain tissue and bring the surgeon closer to the pathology.

Operative Cranial Neurosurgical Anatomy is a tour de force that includes basic as well as detailed surgical anatomy, enhanced by cadaveric dissections, options for surgical training, and methods for assessment of the ideal surgical approach, all in a standardized format that provides an exhaustive description of every imaginable neurosurgical approach to intracranial pathology, including the standard exposures as well as bespoke techniques developed for highly unique situations. It is a handbook that will be useful to all neurosurgeons, from the uninitiated to the expert.

This volume is a testament to the fact that the field of microsurgery is not static, but continues to evolve and lead us to new opportunities that actualize the dreams of our predecessors, who first developed our unique specialty and could only imagine what we now consider state-of-the-art.

Daniel L. Barrow, MD
Pamela R. Rollins Professor & Chairman
Department of Neurosurgery
Emory University School of Medicine
Atlanta, Georgia, USA

Preface

Dissection activity in anatomical laboratories is a fundamental step in the training process of each neurosurgeon. In particular, the acquisition of specific technical skills is a long and demanding task, which requires a stepwise learning of surgical anatomy and basic steps of single surgical approaches. Residents are often alone in the laboratory during this critical learning phase. Anyone who has experienced a period of tutoring activity in a lab knows the importance of reference books to learn and consequently acquire basic surgical skills. The book becomes your best friend and only companion during these times.

Conventional texts are addressed to surgeons that have already completed their training, making them less user-friendly for residents or the practicing neurosurgeon approaching a surgical technique for the first time. For this reason, trainees often must divide themselves between the preliminary phase of study in the library and the subsequent phase of practical training in the lab; this separation inevitably leads to a waste of time and energy which contributes to less effective learning.

Starting from these basic as well as fundamental considerations, we developed the idea of an innovative handbook of surgical technique that mostly referred to neurosurgery residents and practicing neurosurgeons during their training phase in the anatomical laboratories. Through this book we aim to provide an effective educational support to trainees who are approaching fundamental surgical techniques.

Operative Cranial Neurosurgical Anatomy is a systematic collection of anatomic dissections organized to illustrate and present technical principles and fundamental steps of standard neurosurgical procedures as well as related surgical anatomy. Due to its extremely user-friendly layout, the book can be kept on the dissection desk and used any time it is needed.

Leading experts in the field from all over the world have contributed with their unique expertise to chapter writing, making this book an essential tool in neurosurgical training. Contents are homogeneously organized in a highly rational fashion so they are immediately available for consultation. Each approach is discussed step-by-step through a chain of serial images, which act as a "screenshot" of each single step. Figures highlight fundamental aspects of the surgical technique with their basic variants, the surgical anatomy and landmarks, and the critical aspects which have to be taken into consideration. Relevant pitfalls, suggestions, and pearls from the major experts in the field complete each chapter. A list of references and suggested readings are also provided.

This book includes seven major sections including presurgical training techniques, patient positioning and surgical planning, cranial approaches, trans-petrosal approaches, endonasal-transoral and transmaxillary procedures, vascular procedures, and ventricular shunts procedures.

The summaries and the graphic layout make contents readily accessible for consultation during the surgical dissection. This book offers trainees both the fundamental knowledge which is necessary for critical learning as well as a graphic pathway they can easily follow to better prepare themselves to perform the surgical approach.

Operative Cranial Neurosurgical Anatomy is a unique and essential tool in understanding and learning the fundamental surgical techniques in cranial neurosurgery, designed to optimize the time and quality of practical training in the lab.

Filippo Gagliardi, MD, PhD
Cristian Gragnaniello, MD, PhD

Contributors

Saleem I. Abdulrauf, MD, FACS
Professor & Chairman
Department of Neurosurgery
Saint Louis University
St. Louis, Missouri, USA

Mohammad Abolfotoh, MD, PhD
Resident
Department of Neurosurgery
University of Louisville
Louisville, Kentucky, USA

Stefania Acerno, MD
Head of Pediatric Neurosurgery Unit
Department of Neurosurgery and
    Gamma Knife Radiosurgery
San Raffaele Scientific Institute
Vita-Salute University
Milano, Italy

Nouman Aldahak, MD
Department of Neurosurgery
Allegheny General Hospital
Pittsburgh, Pennsylvania
Drexel University College of Medicine
Philadelphia, Pennsylvania, USA

Fabiana Allevi, MD
Staff Physician and Doctoral Researcher
Department of Oral and Maxillo-Facial Surgery
San Paolo Hospital – University of Milan
Milan, Italy

João Paulo Almeida, MD
Division of Neurosurgery
Toronto Western Hospital
University of Toronto
Toronto, Ontario, Canada

Rafid Al-Mahfoudh, MBChB, FEBNS, FRCS(SN)
Consultant Neurosurgeon
Department of Neurosurgery
Brighton and Sussex University Hospital NHS Trust
Brighton, East Sussex, United Kingdom

Mohamed Arnaout, MD
Department of Neurosurgery
Allegheny General Hospital
Pittsburgh, Pennsylvania
Drexel University College of Medicine
Philadelphia, Pennsylvania, USA

Ahmed Maamoun Ashour, MD, PhD
Lecturer of Neurosurgery
Ain Shams University
Cairo, Egypt

Luca Autelitano, MD
Director of Cleft Lip and Palate Program
Department of Oral and Maxillo-Facial Surgery
San Paolo Hospital – University of Milan
Milan, Italy

Khaled M. A. Aziz, MD
Assistant Professor of Neurosurgery Drexel University
    College of Medicine
Director
Center of Complex Intracranial Surgery
Department of Neurosurgery, Allegheny General Hospital
Pittsburgh, Pennsylvania, USA

Michele Bailo, MD
Neurosurgeon
Department of Neurosurgery and
Gamma Knife Radiosurgery
San Raffaele Scientific Institute
Vita-Salute University
Milano, Italy

Luigi Beretta, MD
Associate Professor of Anesthesia and Intensive Care
General Anesthesia and Neurointensive Care
S. Raffaele University Hospital
Milan, Italy

Federico Biglioli, MD
Full Professor
Maxillo-facial Surgery Unit
San Paolo Hospital – Milan University
Milan, Italy

Nicola Boari, MD, FEBNS
Senior Staff Member
Department of Neurosurgery and Gamma Knife
Radiosurgery
San Raffaele Scientific Institute
Vita-Salute University
Milano, Italy

Phillip A. Bonney, MD
Resident
Department of Neurosurgery
University of Oklahoma
Oklahoma City, Oklahoma, USA

Luis A. B. Borba, MD, PhD, IFAANS
Professor and Chairman
Department of Neurosurgery
Federal University of Parana
Curitiba, Paraná, Brazil

Harley Brito da Silva, MD
Visiting Professor
Department of Neurological Surgery
University of Washington
Seattle, Washington, USA

Michael Buchfelder, MD, PhD
Professor and Chairman
Department of Neurosurgery
University Erlangen-Nürnberg
Erlangen, Germany

Lamia Buohliqah, MD
Consultant
Otolaryngology and Head and Neck
Ministry of Health
Dammam, Esteren Province, Saudi Arabia

Joshua D. Burks, MD
Resident
Department of Neurological Surgery
University of Miami
Miami, Florida, USA

Mario Bussi, MD
Professor
Department of Otorhinolaryngology
San Raffaele Scientific Institute
Vita-Salute University
Milan, Italy

Ricardo L. Carrau, MD
Professor and Lynne Shepard Jones Chair in Head &
Neck Oncology
Department of Otolaryngology-Head & Neck Surgery
Department of Neurological Surgery
Director of the Comprehensive Skull Base Surgery Program
The Ohio State University Wexner Medical Center
Columbus, Ohio, USA

Anthony J. Caputy, MD, FACS
Professor and Chairman
Hugo V. Rizzoli Professor
Department of Neurosurgery
George Washington University
Washington, DC, USA

Antonella Castellano, MD, PhD
Assistant Professor
Department of Neuroradiology
Vita-Salute San Raffaele University
Milan, Italy

Daniel D. Cavalcanti, MD, PhD
Director of Cerebrovascular Surgery
Department of Neurosurgery
Paulo Niemeyer State Brain Institute
Rio de Janeiro, Brazil

Nathan Cherian
Medical Student
University of Missouri—Columbia
St. Louis, Missouri, USA

Jeremy N. Ciporen, MD, FAANS
Assistant Professor
Department of Neurological Surgery
Oregon Health & Science University
Portland, Oregon, USA

Elena V. Colombo, MD
Neurosurgeon
Department of Neurosurgery
Parma University Hospital
Parma, Italy

Andrew K. Conner, MD
Resident
Department of Neurosurgery
University of Oklahoma
Oklahoma City, Oklahoma, USA

Victor Fernández Cornejo, MD, PhD
Consultant Neurosurgeon
Department of Neurosurgery
Hospital General Universitario Alicante
Alicante, Spain

Silvestre De La Rosa, MD
Doctor
Department of Neurosurgery
Hopital Nord, APHM-AMU
Marseille, France

Evandro de Oliveira, MD, PhD
Professor
Department of Neurosurgery
Instituto de Ciencias Neurologicas – ICNE
São Paulo, SP, Brazil

Jean G. de Oliveira, MD, PhD
Professor of Neurosurgery
Department of Surgery
Santa Casa de São Paulo School of Medical Sciences
(FCMSCSP)
São Paulo, SP, Brazil

Carmine Antonio Donofrio, MD
Neurosurgeon
Department of Neurosurgery and Gamma Knife
Radiosurgery
San Raffaele Scientific Institute
Vita-Salute University
Milano, Italy

Khaled El-Bahy, MD, PhD
Professor
Department of Neurosurgery
Ain Shams University
Cairo, Egypt

Samer K. Elbabaa, MD, FAANS, FAAP, FACS
Medical Director, Pediatric Neurosurgery
Director, Pediatric Neuroscience Center of Excellence
Arnold Palmer Hospital for Children
Professor of Neurosurgery
College of Medicine, University of Central Florida (UCF)
Orlando, Florida, USA
Adjunct Associate Professor of Neurosurgery
Department of Neurological Surgery
Saint Louis University School of Medicine
St. Louis, Missouri, USA

Farid M. Elhefnawi, MD
Research Fellow
Department of Neurosurgery
Ohio State University
Columbus, Ohio, USA

Jean Anderson Eloy, MD, FACS, FARS
Professor and Vice Chairman
Department of Otolaryngology – Head and Neck Surgery
Director, Rhinology and Sinus Surgery
Director, Otolaryngology Research
Co-Director, Endoscopic Skull Base Surgery Program
Professor of Neurological Surgery
Professor of Ophthalmology and Visual Science
Rutgers New Jersey Medical School
Chairman and Chief of Service
Department of Otolaryngology and Facial Plastic Surgery
Saint Barnabas Medical Center – RWJBarnabas Health
Vice President
New Jersey Academy of Otolaryngology/New Jersey
    Academy of Facial Plastic Surgery
Newark, New Jersey, USA

Nicholas J. Erickson, MD
Resident Physician
Department of Neurosurgery
The University of Alabama at Birmingham
Birmingham, Alabama, USA

Isabella Esposito, MD
Neurosurgeon
Department of Neurosurgery
Brighton and Sussex University Hospital
Brighton, Sussex, United Kingdom

Andrea Falini, MD, PhD
Full Professor
Department of Neuroradiology
Vita-Salute San Raffaele University
Milan, Italy

Juan C. Fernandez-Miranda, MD, FACS
Associate Professor
Director, Complex Brain Surgery Program
Associate Director, Center for Skull Base Surgery
Director, Surgical Neuroanatomy Lab
Director, Fiber Tractography (HDFT) Lab
University of Pittsburgh Medical Center
Pittsburgh, Pennsylvania, USA

Filippo Gagliardi, MD, PhD
Neurosurgeon
Department of Neurosurgery and
    Gamma Knife Radiosurgery
San Raffaele Scientific Institute
Vita-Salute University
Milano, Italy

Virginio Garcia-Lopez, PhD
Postdoc
Department of Human Anatomy and Embryology
University of Extremadura
BABYFARMA
FARMADIEX
Badajoz, Spain

Virginio Garcia-Martinez, MD, PhD
Professor
Department of Human Anatomy and Embryology
Institute of Molecular Pathology Biomarkers
University of Extremadura
Badajoz, Spain

Anand V. Germanwala, MD, FAANS
Associate Professor & Residency Program Director
Department of Neurological Surgery
Loyola University Stritch School of Medicine
Maywood, Illinois, USA

Chad A. Glenn, MD
Cerebrovascular and Skull Base Fellow
Department of Neurological Surgery
Case Western Reserve University
Cleveland, Ohio, USA

Pablo González-López, MD, PhD
Assistant Professor
Neurooncology and Skull Base Division
Department of Neurosurgery
Hospital General Universitario Alicante
Miguel Hernandez University
Alicante, Spain

Cristian Gragnaniello, MD, PhD, MSurg, MAdvSurg, FICS
Surgical Director
Harvey H. Ammerman Microsurgical Laboratory
Department of Neurosurgery
George Washington University
Washington, DC, USA

Ellina Hattar, MD
Resident
Department of Neurosurgery
Thomas Jefferson University Hospital
Philadelphia, Pennsylvania, USA

Katie Huynh, DO
Neurosurgeon
Inland Neurosurgery and Spine
Providence Sacred Heart
Spokane, Washington, USA

Jeremiah Johnson, MD
Assistant Professor
Department of Neurosurgery
Baylor College of Medicine
Houston, Texas, USA

Paulo A. S. Kadri, MD
Adjunct Professor
Department of Neurosurgery
Federal University of Mato Grosso do Sul
Campo Grande, Brazil

Brian Kang
Department of Neurosurgery
Saint Louis University School of Medicine
St. Louis, Missouri, USA

Joanna Kemp, MD
Assistant Professor
Division of Pediatric Neurosurgery
Department of Neurosurgery
Saint Louis University School of Medicine
St. Louis, Missouri, USA

Edward E. Kerr, MD
Baylor Neurosurgery Associates
Baylor University Medical Center
Dallas, Texas, USA

Sneha Koduru

S. Alexander König, MD
Consultant Neurosurgeon
Department of Neurosurgery
Klinikum Karlsruhe
Karlsruhe, Baden-Württemberg, Germany

John Y. K. Lee, MD, MSCE
Associate Professor
Department of Neurosurgery & Otolaryngology
University of Pennsylvania
Philadelphia, Pennsylvania, USA

Zachary Litvack, MD, MCR
Director, Skull Base & Minimally Invasive Neurosurgery
Department of Neurosurgery
Swedish Neuroscience Institute
Seattle, Washington, USA

James K. Liu, MD
Professor, Director of Skull Base and
   Cerebrovascular Surgery
Department of Neurological Surgery
Rutgers University, New Jersey Medical School
Rutgers Neurological Institute of New Jersey
Newark, New Jersey, USA

Carmen Lopez-Sanchez, PhD
Associate Professor
Department of Human Anatomy and Embryology
Institute of Molecular Pathology Biomarkers
University of Extremadura
Badajoz, Spain

Brandon P. Lucke-Wold, MD, PhD, MCTS
Department of Neurosurgery
University of Florida
Gainesville, Florida, USA

Sam Maghami, MD
Division of Cardiac Surgery
University of Maryland School of Medicine
Baltimore, Maryland, USA

Erin McCormack, MD
Preliminary Resident
Department of Surgery
Ochsner Clinic Foundation
Jefferson, Louisiana, USA

Gráinne S. McKenna, MA(Cantab) MB BChir FRCS (SN)
Neurosurgery Resident
Victor Horsley Department of Neurosurgery
The National Hospital for Neurology and Neurosurgery
Queen Square, London, United Kingdom

Marzia Medone, MD
Neurosurgeon
Department of Neurosurgery and Gamma Knife
   Radiosurgery
San Raffaele Scientific Institute
Vita-Salute University
Milano, Italy

Anthony Melot, MD
Doctor
Department of Neurosurgery
Hopital Nord, APHM-AMU
Marseille, France

Veronika Messelberger, MD, MSc
Intern
Department of Neurology
SRH Klinikum Karlsbad-Langensteinbach
Karlsbad, Baden-Württemberg, Germany

Ashkan Monfared, MD
Associate Professor
Department Neurosurgery
George Washington University
Washington, DC, USA

Michael Kerin Morgan, MD, MMedEd, FRACS
Professor
Department of Clinical Medicine
Macquarie University
Sydney, New South Wales, Australia

Pietro Mortini, MD
Professor and Chairman
Department of Neurosurgery and Gamma Knife
   Radiosurgery
San Raffaele Scientific Institute
Vita-Salute University
Milano, Italy

Remi Nader, MD, CM, FRCS(C), FACS, FAANS
President, Texas Center for Neurosciences
Houston, Texas, USA
Adjunct Clinical Professor of Neurosurgery
University of Texas Medical Branch
Galveston, Texas, USA

Peter Nakaji, MD
Professor of Neurological Surgery
Department of Neurological Surgery
Barrow Neurological Institute
Phoenix, Arizona, USA

Mateus Reghin Neto, MD
Neurosurgeon
Instituto de Ciências Neurológicas
Hospital BP – Beneficência Portuguesa de São Paulo
São Paulo, Brazil

Javier Abarca Olivas, MD
Adjunct Professor
Department of Neurosurgery
Hospital General Universitario de Alicante
Alicante, Comunidad Valenciana, España

Sacit Bulent Omay, MD
Assistant Professor
Department of Neurosurgery
Yale School of Medicine
New Haven, Connecticut, USA

Chirag R. Patel, MD
Assistant Professor
Department of Otolaryngology, Head and Neck Surgery
Loyola University Medical Center
Maywood, Illinois, USA

Francesco Pilolli, MD
Department of Otorhinolaryngology
San Raffaele Scientific Institute
Vita-Salute University
Milan, Italy

Martina Piloni, MD
Resident
Department of Neurosurgery and Gamma Knife
   Radiosurgery
San Raffaele Scientific Institute
Vita-Salute University
Milano, Italy

Luis Porras-Estrada, MD, PhD
Neurosurgeon
Department of Neurosurgery
Experimental Neurosurgical Unit. Neuroanatomy.
University Hospital Complex of Extremadura
Badajoz, Spain

Daniel M. Prevedello, MD
Professor
Department of Neurosurgery
The Ohio State University
Columbus, Ohio, USA

Marcio S. Rassi, MD
Assistant Professor of Neurosurgery
School of Medicine of Faculdade Evangélica do Paraná
Curitiba, Paraná, Brazil

Pierre-Hugues Roche, MD
Professor
Department of Neurosurgery
Hopital Nord, APHM-AMU
Marseille, France

Francesco Ruggieri, MD
Staff Anesthesiologist and Intensivist
Neuro-Anesthesia and Neuro-Intensive Care Unit
San Raffaele Scientific Institute
Milan, Italy

Parisa Sabetrasekh, MD
Post-doctoral Research Fellow
Department of Neurological Surgery
George Washington University School of Medicine and
Health Sciences
Washington, DC, USA

George Samandouras, MD, FRCS
Consultant Neurosurgeon
The National Hospital for Neurology and Neurosurgery
Queen Square, London, United Kingdom

Stephen Santoreneos, MBBS, FRACS
Director, Department of Neurosurgery
Royal Adelaide Hospital and Women's and Children's
    Hospital
Adelaide, South Australia, Australia

Sven-Martin Schlaffer, MD
Consultant Neurosurgeon
Department of Neurosurgery
University Erlangen-Nuremberg
Erlangen, Germany

Theodore H. Schwartz, MD, FACS
David and Ursel Barnes Professor of Minimally Invasive
    Neurosurgery
Director, Anterior Skull Base and Pituitary Surgery
Director, Epilepsy Research Laboratory
Departments of Neurological Surgery, Otolaryngology and
    Neuroscience
Weill Cornell Medicine
New York, New York, USA

Savannah Scott

Laligam N. Sekhar, MD, FACS, FAANS
Professor and Vice Chairman
Director of Cerebrovascular and Skull Base Surgery
Department of Neurological Surgery
University of Washington
Seattle, Washington, USA

Ameet Singh, MD, FARS
Associate Professor of Otolaryngology & Neurosurgery
Department of Surgery
George Washington University Medical Center
Washington, DC, USA

Harminder Singh, MD, FACS, FAANS
Clinical Associate Professor of Neurosurgery
Stanford University School of Medicine
Stanford, California, USA

Alan Siu, MD, MS
Department of Neurosurgery
George Washington University
Washington, DC, USA

Sananthan Sivakanthan, MD
Department of Neurosurgery and Brain Repair
University of South Florida
Tampa, Florida, USA

Claudio V. Sorrilha, MD
Head of Neurosurgery Service
Department of Neurosurgery
Regional Hospital of Mato Grosso do Sul
Campo Grande, Brazil

Uwe Spetzger, MD
Professor and Chairman
Department of Neurosurgery
Klinikum Karlsruhe
Karlsruhe, Germany

Alfio Spina, MD
Neurosurgeon
Department of Neurosurgery and Gamma Knife
    Radiosurgery
San Raffaele Scientific Institute
Vita-Salute University
Milano, Italy

Eleonora F. Spinazzi, MD
Resident
Department of Neurological Surgery
Columbia University Medical Center
New York, New York, USA

Gary K. Steinberg, MD, PhD
Bernard and Ronni Lacroute-William Randolph Hearst
    Professor of Neurosurgery and the Neurosciences
    Chairman Department of Neurosurgery
Stanford University School of Medicine
Stanford, California, USA

Michael E. Sughrue, MD
Associate Professor
Neurosurgery
Prince of Wales Hospital
Randwick, New South Wales, Australia

Kevin Swong, MD
Chief Neurosurgery Resident
Department of Neurosurgery
Loyola University Medical Center
Chicago, Illinois, USA

Mario Teo, MBChB(Hons), BMedSci(Hons), FRCS(SN)
Consultant Neurosurgeon
Department of Neurosurgery
Bristol Institute of Clinical Neuroscience
North Bristol University Hospital
Bristol, United Kingdom
Clinical Instructor
Department of Neurosurgery
Stanford University Medical Centre
Stanford, California, USA

Salvatore Toma, MD
Department of Otorhinolaryngology
San Raffaele Scientific Institute
Vita-Salute University
Milan, Italy

Matteo Trimarchi, MD
Professor
Department of Otorhinolaryngology
San Raffaele Scientific Institute
Vita-Salute University
Milan, Italy

Lucas Troude, MD
Department of Neurosurgery
Hopital Nord, APHM-AMU
Marseille, France

Asterios Tsimpas, MD, MSc, MBA, FACS, FAANS, FEBNS
Director of Cerebrovascular & Endovascular Neurosurgery
Section of Neurosurgery
Advocate Illinois Masonic Medical Center
Clinical Assistant Professor of Neurosurgery
University of Illinois at Chicago
Chicago, Illinois, USA

Kerry A. Vaughan, MD
Senior Resident
Department of Neurosurgery
University of Pennsylvania
Philadelphia, Pennsylvania, USA

Iván Verdú-Martínez, MD
Consultant Neurosurgeon
Department of Neurosurgery
Hospital General Universitario de Alicante
Alicante, Comunidad Valenciana, España

Wei-Hsin Wang, MD
Department of Neurosurgery
Taipei Veterans General Hospital
National Yang-Ming University
Taipei, Taiwan

Peter-John Wormald, MD, FRACS, FRCS, FCS (SA), MBChB
Professor and Chairman
Otolaryngology Head and Neck Surgery
Professor of Skull Base Surgery
University of Adelaide, Adelaide, Australia

Hasan A. Zaidi, MD
Assistant Professor
Department of Neurosurgery
Harvard Medical School
Brigham & Women's Hospital
Dana Farber Cancer Institute
Boston, Massachusetts, USA

Mehdi Zeinalizadeh, MD
Attending Neurosurgeon
Brain and Spinal Cord Injuries Repair and Research Center
Imam Khomeini Hospital Complex, Tehran University of
Medical Sciences
Tehran, Iran

Yi Chen Zhao, MBBS, FRACS, PhD
Consultant ENT Surgeon
Department of Otolaryngology and Head and Neck Surgery
University of Melbourne
Royal Melbourne Hospital
Melbourne, Victoria, Australia

Tommaso Zoerle, MD
Staff Physician
Department of Anaesthesia and Critical Care, Neuroscience
Intensive Care Unit
Fondazione IRCCS Ca' Granda – Ospedale Maggiore
    Policlinico
Milan, Italy

**Part I
Presurgical Training**

1 Training Models in Neurosurgery

Cristian Gragnaniello, Nicholas J. Erickson, Filippo Gagliardi, Pietro Mortini, and Anthony J. Caputy

1.1 Introduction

- Neurological surgery is one of the most technically demanding medical specialties, with a steep learning curve.
- Neurosurgery has benefited from several technical advancements in the last 3 decades that involved visualization, instrumentation, and approaches.
- In recent years there has been the development of an increasing number of training models and courses to augment the training of new generations of surgeons and in an attempt to lessen the steep learning curve mentioned earlier.
- Changes in regulations regarding working hours for neurosurgical trainees have challenged the neurosurgical community to develop methods to maintain high quality standards without compromising the neurosurgical training, which is a necessary component of each residency. This is extremely important when dealing with highly complex lesions that are not routinely encountered such as deep-seated tumors and vascular lesions.
- To augment the clinical exposure to the pathology, an alternative option of reliable training that simulates life-like conditions is needed.
- Laboratory training is usually advocated to master the intricate anatomy of the brain and micro-neurosurgical technique.
- Both physical and computer-simulated training models are becoming increasingly available. These include models based on synthetic materials, animals, and human cadaver.
- Human cadaveric models are still deemed the most beneficial as they resemble life-like anatomical and technical challenges however there is a lack of blood circulation.
- Excellent spinal and cranial models have been created, focusing on performing surgical approaches with normal surgical anatomy. Some expose the residents to anatomy altered by pathological processes.

1.2 Simulation Models in Neurosurgery

- There have been widespread advancements over recent years when it comes to simulation in neurosurgery.
- The majority of simulators are divided into either physical or virtual reality (VR) subtypes.

1.2.1 Physical Simulators

- The physical simulators include cadaver models, live animal models, and synthetic models. Despite many recent advancements, the cadaver model has remained the most effective and most commonly used method for neurosurgical training.
- Cadavers and mannequins are particularly useful for the practice of basic skills such as drilling techniques, neuroendoscopy, spinal decompression and instrumentation.
- Microsurgical training is among the most practiced type of simulation, and it can involve the use of synthetic models such as silicon tubes, dead tissue models such as the chicken wing artery (**Fig. 1.1**), human and bovine placental vessels, and more recently three-dimensional printing.
- Live models provide the most realistic method for many types of training with pulsatile blood flow, natural viscosity and coagulation. Utilizing these models, however, has become more difficult as institutional protocols and review boards continue to impose necessary but significant constraints regarding the use of live animals.

1.2.2 Virtual Reality

- Computer generated graphics along with CT and MRI data have allowed for the re-creation of human anatomy in a virtual space. This has become particularly useful for understanding the complex anatomy of the central nervous system and the spatial relationship between anatomical structures in three dimensions.
- Currently there are three main types of virtual simulators: they are simplified, augmented, and immersive.
  - Simplified VR systems are the most basic consisting of only a computer-user interface with no sensory interaction by the user.
  - Augmented VR systems allow for more interaction and manipulation by the user with the use of external props. The 'Robo-Sim-Endoscopic neurosurgical simulator' is an example.
  - Immersive VR systems are the most technologically advanced and involve creating a physical presence in a virtual world utilizing primary sensory input/output and haptic and kinesthetic modalities.
- Three-dimensional printing for neurosurgical training is a more recent advancement, which produces a multi-texture reconstruction and allows for the planning and training of specific and complex operative procedures (**Fig. 1.2**).

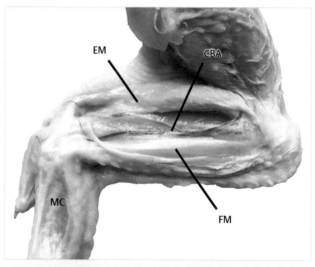

Fig. 1.1 Chicken wing dissection. The brachial artery is 5-6 cm long. Abbreviations: CBA = chicken brachial artery; EM = extensor muscle; FM = flexor muscle; MC = metacarpus.

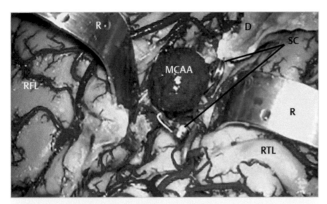

Fig. 1.2 Implantation of a 3D printed aneurysm in a right sided opercular artery. (Copyright © 2015 Arnau Benet et al. Reproduced from Benet A, Plata-Bello J, Abla AA, Acevedo-Bolton G, Saloner D, Lawton MT. Implantation of 3D-printed patient-specific aneurysm models into cadaveric specimens: a new training paradigm to allow for improvements in cerebrovascular surgery and research. BioMed Res Int 2015;2015:939387.)
Abbreviations: D = dura; MCAA = middle cerebral artery aneurysm; R = retractor; RFL = right frontal lobe; RTL = right temporal lobe; SC = surgical clips.

1.3 Training Models in Vascular Neurosurgery

1.3.1 Chicken Wing Artery

- The brachial artery is harvested from a chicken wing and can be used to practice end-to-end, end-to-side, or side-to-side anastomosis under a microscope (**Fig. 1.1**).
- Shapes of the arteriotomy, type of sutures as well as incident angle of the bypass graft may vary between surgeons; however, the basic yet crucial principles of microsuturing are exercised in this model.
- The distance the sutures are placed from the vessel edge is precise and the needle must penetrate the entire thickness of the vessel wall without touching the intima. It is important to keep the vessel and material moist throughout the anastomosis to prevent the structures from drying out.
- The integrity of the anastomosis can be evaluated by injecting water into the vessel and looking for leaks. In addition, the technique can be evaluated by cutting the artery, placing it under a microscope, and looking at the intimal appearance surrounding the anastomosis in search of kinks or strangulation.
- One of the drawbacks of this model is the variability in vessel diameter across different wings. Also, many of the wings suffer from freezing artifact after thawing which creates many difficulties when attempting to harvest the arteries.

1.3.2 Human and Bovine Placental Vessels

- Recently, the utility of both human and bovine placental vessels in microsurgical training has been explored and validated as an effective way to train neurosurgeons in low-flow and high-flow neurosurgical bypass techniques.

- Human placental arteries have wall thicknesses, amounts of connective tissue and diameters that closely resemble those in the human brain. Bovine placenta can be readily used if human specimens are not available as acquisition it does not require institutional review board or Institutional Animal Care and Use Committee approval, which makes it an easy replacement.
- The two umbilical arteries and the vein are cannulated and colored normal saline is incorporated into a flow circuit at around 100 to 180 mmHg. This allows for the trainee to encounter "bleeding" if a vessel is damaged and practice hemostatic techniques using bipolar coagulation or ligation.
- The placenta is placed into a skull with a previously created bone window to simulate depth and the restrictions of a craniotomy. Vessels with diameters of 0.8 to 1.5 mm and 1.0 to 2.0 mm are used to mimic the human middle cerebral artery (MCA) and superficial temporal artery (STA), respectively. Vessels with diameters of 8.0 mm to 9.0 mm and 2.0 to 3.0 mm are used to model the human ICA and radial artery (RA), respectively.
- End-to-side, end-to-end, and side-to-side bypasses with a long interposition graft are several of the microvascular techniques that can be practiced using this model.
- Some of the limitations of this model include the viability of placentas, the exposure to potential infectious agents using human placentas and the absence of adjacent soft-tissue that would need to be dissected in a real case.

1.3.3 Three-Dimensional Printing

- Recent advancements in endovascular surgery have changed the surgical indications for aneurysm clipping such that aneurysms not amenable to endovascular approaches are most often highly complex and challenging lesions. This decrease in the number of aneurysms considered amenable for surgery has led to an increase in the level of expertise required to handle those that need to be clipped. It is important that new methods are available for future neurosurgeons to practice and refine the techniques necessary to address these during their careers.
- In this model, 3D models of aneurysms are printed based on real patient data and implanted in human cadavers at the same anatomical region as the modeled patient (**Fig. 1.2**).
- The cadavers are connected to two liquid reservoirs inside pressure bags to simulate surgical bleeding during the simulation.
- Benet et al demonstrated this method by printing both patient specific middle cerebral artery and basilar apex aneurysms, placing them in human cadavers using standard surgical techniques and evaluating their utility in the operative training as well as case management and planning.
  - It was found that the flexibility of the neck and branches of the aneurysm were similar to those of the modeled patient.
  - The aneurysm domes were also sufficiently rigid to produce mass effect without compromising the aneurysm's integrity.
  - To simulate mass effect, a Foley catheter was introduced beforehand and progressively inflated to allow room for implantation of the modeled giant aneurysm.
- This 3D aneurysm implantation model may help supplement the declining number of aneurysms treated surgically by incorporating hands-on training for patient specific aneurysms considered for surgery.

- Currently 3D printers can only produce aneurysm models at least 1 mm in size. Patients with aneurysms smaller than this cannot be represented with this model. There is also a limit to how closely the 3D printed aneurysm will represent the source image in the patient, as MRI does not always pick up perforators, especially ones coming off the aneurysm dome.

1.4 Training Models In Neuro-Oncology

1.4.1 Injectable Tumor Model

- In 2010, Gragnaniello et al proposed an injectable skull based tumor model, using Stratathane resin ST-504 polymer (SRSP), that could be used to train future neurosurgeons for the delicate dissection of a tumor from surrounding neural and vascular structures (**Fig. 1.3**).
- Stratathane resin ST-504 polymer (SRSP) is used for its characteristics to emulate brain tumors different in consistency ranging from rubbery meningioma to suckable pituitary adenomas. The polymer, developed in cooperation with the scientists of the Nanotechnology Center, reflects most of the properties of real extra-axial central nervous system (CNS) tumors.

- It causes displacement of surrounding neural and vascular structure, and because of its non-adhesive nature, it affords us a dissection plane very similar to the one described in the aforementioned tumors. It also has a consistency similar to these tumors; it can be incised by micro-instruments, but it cannot be suctioned like a jelly, which helps in imitating the exact conditions of live surgery.
- The polymer has a distinct characteristic on T2-weighted MR images that enables its superb delineation and further assists the preoperative planning of the procedure.
- The pressurized heads consisted of cadavers in whom an artificial circulation was established in the existing vasculature using a red solution imitating real blood infused via a mechanical pumping device.

1.4.2 Intraventricular Tumor Model

- As endoscopic approaches to intraventricular tumors become more common, there is an increasing demand for appropriate laboratory training models.
- Ashour et al describe a model in which the polymer mentioned above is injected into the lateral ventricle of formalin-fixated, latex injected cadaveric heads under direct endoscopic and neuro-navigated guidance (**Fig. 1.4**).

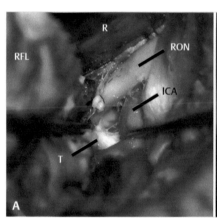
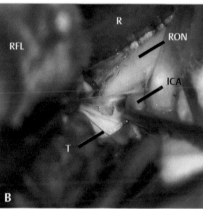

Fig. 1.3 Tumor dissection through the optic-carotid window (**A** and **B**). Abbreviations: ICA = internal carotid artery; R = retractor; RFL = right frontal lobe; RON = right optic nerve; T = tumor.

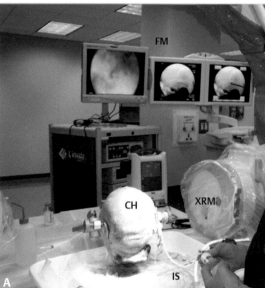
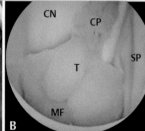
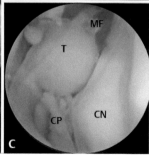

Fig. 1.4 Intraventricular tumor model. (**A**) Injection system of the intraventricular tumor model. (**B, C**) Endoscopic view of right lateral ventricle depicting tumor model injected into the ventricular atrium in two separate cases. Abbreviations: CH = cadaver head; CN = caudate nucleus; CP = choroid plexus; FM = fluoroscopy monitor; IS = injection system; MF = Monro foramen; SP = septum pellucidum; T = tumor; XRM = X-ray machine.

- This model allows the trainee to refine endoscopic techniques required for the resection of a solid intraventricular lesion in the presence of pathology-distorted anatomy. In addition, diluting the polymer at different ratios allows for the simulation of infiltrative and non-infiltrative tumor behavior toward the ependymal and surrounding critical structures.

1.5 Models To Simulate Blood Flow To The Brain

1.5.1 Garrett's Model

- In 2001 Garrett developed the first model to simulate circulation to the brain using a very neat and elegant design.
- Permico, a commercially available solvent, is used to create an arterial tree using two or three remote sites. An arterial-arterial circulation, which isolates the section of arterial tree under investigation, can be established, achieving inflow and outflow through catheters inserted at remote sites.
- Inflow is established through a large bore end hole catheter with balloon occlusion (Meditech OB, Boston Scientific, Natick, Mass) that is placed through a peripheral access site. Outflow is established through a variety of catheters placed distally to the area of interest.
- A variety of pumps and tubing may be used, including those used for cardiopulmonary bypass grafting. Pumps may produce pulsatile or non-pulsatile flow.
- Different solutions may be used to simulate blood, but a crystalloid solution colored with red dye is an inexpensive substitute.

1.5.2 Aboud's Model

- Without any doubt, the most powerful tool to simulate live conditions into cadaver heads is the one developed by Aboud et al at the University of Arkansas for Medical Sciences.

- Cadaver models injected with colored silicone, gelatin, or any other congealed material lack pulsation and vascular filling, which allow manipulation of vessels, hemostasis, clipping, and suturing. On the other hand, live anesthetized animals do not represent true human anatomy.
- In this model, in which vessels in a cadaveric head are filled with colored fluid under pulsating pressure for arteries and under static pressure for veins, the capability of bleeding, pulsation, vascular filling, and softness of the vascular tree makes it very close to live surgical condition.
- This model allows a trainee to perform many surgical procedures, among other, opening the Sylvian fissure, suturing vessels, practicing anastomosis, dissecting and clipping artificial aneurysms, and practicing surgical approaches.

References

1. Aboud E, Al-Mefty O, Yaşargil MG. New laboratory model for neurosurgical training that simulates live surgery. J Neurosurg 2002; 97(6):1367–1372
2. Ashour AM, Elbabaa SK, Caputy AJ, Gragnaniello C. Navigation-guided endoscopic intraventricular injectable tumor model: cadaveric tumor resection model for neurosurgical training. World Neurosurg 2016; 96:261–266
3. Belykh E, Lei T, Safavi-Abbasi S, et al. Low-flow and high-flow neurosurgical bypass and anastomosis training models using human and bovine placental vessels: a histological analysis and validation study. J Neurosurg 2016; 125(4):915–928
4. Benet A, Plata-Bello J, Abla AA, Acevedo-Bolton G, Saloner D, Lawton MT. Implantation of 3D-printed patient-specific aneurysm models into cadaveric specimens: a new training paradigm to allow for improvements in cerebrovascular surgery and research. BioMed Res Int 2015; 2015:939387
5. Nader R, van Doormaal T, et al. Skull base tumor model. J Neurosurg 2010; 113(5):1106–1111
6. Hino A. Training in microvascular surgery using a chicken wing artery. Neurosurgery 2003; 52(6):1495–1497, discussion 1497–1498

2 Assessment of Surgical Exposure

Alfio Spina, Filippo Gagliardi, Michele Bailo, Cristian Gragnaniello, Anthony J. Caputy, and Pietro Mortini

2.1 Introduction

Neurosurgery is one of the medical specialties that has experienced a rapid technological development. The advancements made in imaging technologies, surgical equipment, and the acquired knowledge in microanatomy and pathology have dramatically improved the safety and surgical outcomes of patients worldwide.

The careful evaluation of these features is essential in planning the most appropriate surgical approach, as well as in selecting the surgical tools that most afford a safe and extensive resection of the pathology.

In this chapter, we explain the operability score (OS), as an application of some simple geometrical concept to preoperatively evaluate not only the surgical target, but also the trajectory used to reach it, the maneuverability space around the target, and the surgical angle of attack.

2.2 Historical Perspectives

2.2.1 General Considerations

Lesions in the brain can be approached from many different angles and through different approaches, with the choice of the best approach for a specific lesion being still a matter of debate in Neurosurgery. The development of different approaches has been, and is still today, one of the main topics of the research in Neurosurgery.

The problem of safety and efficacy of surgeon's maneuvers have represented the leading subject of historical neurosurgical evolution, starting from the more extensive and invasive surgical approaches since the beginning of the 20th century, to the era of "Minimally Invasive Neurosurgery," passing through the development of the microscope, endoscope, and advanced imaging technologies.

In particular, skull base surgery, with the improvement of anatomic knowledge, the introduction and development of innovative instruments and diagnostic tools, the application of different display devices, such as microscope and endoscope, has evolved from more aggressive to less invasive tailored approaches based on a careful preoperative planning. The OS represents a further advance in this area.

2.2.2 Assessment of Operability and Surgical Exposure

Historically, several authors have analyzed the concept of operability under different perspectives.

- **Yasargil et al** first described the concept of operability related both to patient-linked variables (i.e., age, general and clinical conditions, previous therapies), as well as to pathology-linked patterns. In particular the latter did consider several factors: location and number of lesions (unilateral or bilateral), composition (size, vascularization), and characteristics of

the tumor (growth pattern, benign/malignant lesion, edema, presence of hydrocephalus). Considering these factors together with surgeons' personal skills, it was possible to qualitatively assess tumor operability. Again, Yasargil, by analyzing surgery of intraventricular tumors, demonstrated that, by drilling the sphenoid wing in a pterional approach, the surgical cone was significantly implemented, making it easier the opening of the Sylvian fissure and the maneuver around the sellar region.

In the last years, several authors have also comparatively analyzed different approaches and their variants in terms of operability on selected targets.

- In 2001, **Sindou et al** described the concept of working cone by approaching central skull base lesions. Authors quantitatively analyzed surgical trajectory, depth and width of the surgical field, as well as working space, to reach a selected target, by adding different osteotomies to a standard fronto-temporo-parietal craniotomy. The different working cones did provide a multiangle visualization of the selected target, depending on its anatomical location, morphology, neurovascular relationships, and pathological features. Authors concluded that additional orbital or zygomatic osteotomies were useful in implementing the working cone for tumor removal, avoiding brain retraction.
- **Gonzalez et al** in 2002 have further developed these concepts, defining the operability as the ability to execute surgical maneuvers on a target area. The application of the concept of defined surgical triangles in the pre-operative planning was found to be helpful in individualizing the approach, tailoring the surgical corridor according to tumor anatomic location.
- **Filipce et al** in 2009 qualitatively and quantitatively analyzed the extent of the working area, as obtained by microscope and endoscope, by treating anterior communicating artery aneurysms. They claimed as advantage of the endoscope the direct view and illumination, and the 3D visualization as main advantage of the microscope. By combining the advantages of each technique, they stated that endoscope-assisted microscopic approaches were the best way to look around corners and to guarantee an optimal 3D view. Interestingly, angled endoscopes allowed for a better visualization, which might not necessarily implicate a direct improvement of the working corridor.
- **Salma et al** in 2011 proposed a qualitative score system to compare the exposure obtained by pterional and supraorbital craniotomy. Even if supraorbital craniotomy did provide a less invasive way to reach the sellar region, the pterional approach presented a wider pyramidal-shaped surgical corridor as compared to the cylindrical-shaped one of the supraorbital approach, increasing the overall surgical operability.

2.3 Operability Score

As first described by **Gagliardi et al**, the OS summarizes all the analyzed variables mentioned above by applying some geometrical concepts in the surgical preoperative evaluation of the lesion, in order to evaluate the main criticisms that could be encountered.

These key points are easy to apply in most of the situations:

- **Depth of the surgical field (SF)**. The SF represents the length of the major axis of the surgical corridor. It is assessed, by measuring the distance between the maneuverability area and the target. The translational value of this measure is explained by the fact that dealing with deeply located lesions might represent a challenge in terms of surgical comfort and tumor control (**Fig. 2.1**).
- **Surgical angle of attack (SAA)**. The SAA corresponds to the angle of incidence of the surgical corridor toward an area of interest. The more the angle is wide, the more comfortable is the approach and this reflects the possibility to better control the target (**Fig. 2.2**).
- **Maneuverability arc (MAC)**. The MAC consists in the maximal degrees of maneuverability of surgical instruments around a target and is intrinsically influenced by the wideness of the surgical cone. As already stated for the SAA, the width of the arc directly determines the control of the target (**Fig. 2.1**).

Assigning a numerical score to each variable by comparing different surgical approaches or different targets within the same surgical approach enables to graduate surgical complexity, optimizing the pre-surgical planning.

The score system consists in assigning to each variable 0 or 1 according to **Table 2.1**.

Other geometrical concepts could be considered in selected cases, such as

- **Maneuverability area (MAR)**. The MAR is the cross-section area, as calculated at the narrowest point in the surgical corridor. From a geometrical perspective, it corresponds to an ellipsoid (**Fig. 2.3**).

Table 2.1 Score system of the variables of the OS.

Variables	Score 0	Score 1
Depth of the surgical field (SF)	> 5 cm	≤ 5 cm
Surgical angle of attack (SAA)	< 60°	≥ 60°
Maneuverability arc (MAC)	< 45°	≥ 45°

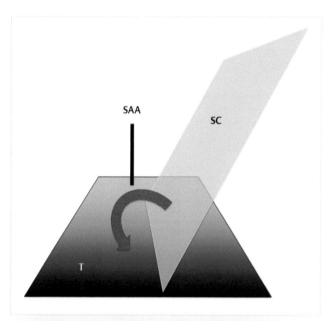

Fig. 2.2 Schematic drawing depicting the different variables analyzed by the operability score: surgical angle of attack. Abbreviations: SAA = surgical angle of attack; SC = surgical corridor; T = target.

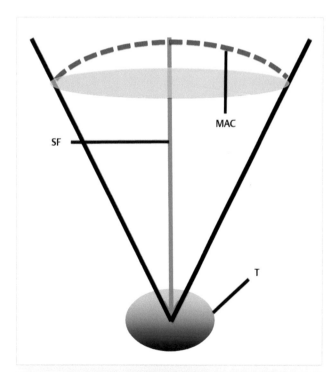

Fig. 2.1 Schematic drawing depicting the different variables analyzed by the operability score: depth of the surgical field and maneuverability arc.
Abbreviations: MAC = maneuverability arc; SF = depth of the surgical field; T = target.

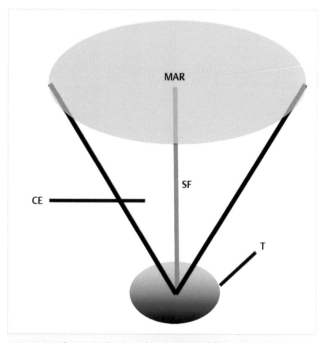

Fig. 2.3 Schematic drawing depicting the different variables analyzed by the operability score: maneuverability area. Abbreviations: CE = conizing effect; MAR = maneuverability area; SF = depth of the surgical field; T = target.

- **Conizing effect (CE).** The conizing effect corresponds to a co-efficient, calculated by dividing the MAR by the SF. It is directly correlated to the SF. The deeper is the field the narrower is the surgical cone, with a consequent decrease of the MAC.
- **Endoscopic index (EI).** The endoscopic index is the ratio obtained by dividing the area of the surgical field exposed by the endoscope and the whole area exposed by the approach itself. The higher is the score, the more technically demanding is the approach, being considered the endoscopic index as an indirect score of technical complexity.

2.4 Case Illustration

As case illustration, the comparative analysis on operability between the frontotemporal (FT) approach and the fronto-orbito-zygomatic (FOZ) approach is reported (**Fig. 2.4**). In particular, as illustrative example, the operability on the anterior clinoid process (AC) as obtained by a standard FT and by adding an additional orbital osteotomy (FOZ) were evaluated and compared.

2.4.1 Material and Methods

The study was performed at the Anatomical Laboratory of the Department of Neurosurgery at the George Washington University (Washington, DC, USA). Silicone-injected cadaveric heads were prepared using standard formaldehyde fixation techniques. Four cadaveric heads underwent a FT first and a FOZ thereafter on the same side. The surgical techniques are described in **Chapters 15 and 17**.

A Zeiss OPM 1 FC microscope was used for microsurgical techniques and morphometric measurements (Carl Zeiss, Oberkochen, Germany) and a Midas Rex drill was used for all bone drilling (Midas Rex, Fort Worth, TX, USA).

The morphometric measurements were accomplished with graded scales. The mean value of the measurements was recorded and served as the basis for the final tabulated data. The tip of the anterior clinoid process (AC) was selected as the anatomical target point. At this point the SF, SAA and MAC have been measured for each specimen.

2.4.2 Results

See **Table 2.2** for results.

By applying the OS, even if the FT showed the best score for SF, the FOZ, providing a better SAA and MAC, did show a higher OS on the ACP. **Table 2.3** summarizes the OS calculated for the two approaches.

These results must be analyzed, taking into consideration the extreme inter-individual variability of the pneumatization

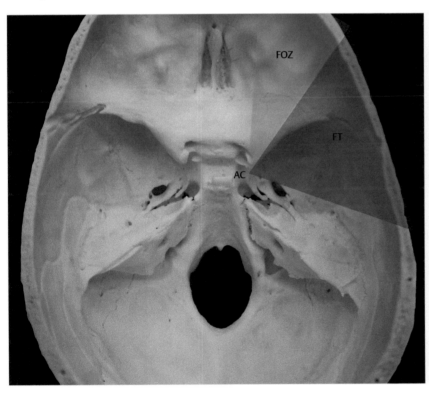

Fig. 2.4 Surgical exposure of fronto-temporal approach (red area) and fronto-orbito-zygomatic approach (blue area) of the anterior clinoid process.
Abbreviations: AC = anterior clinoid process; FOZ = fronto-orbito-zygomatic approach; FT = frontotemporal approach.

Table 2.2 Variables as calculated on the anterior clinoid process for each approach.

	SF (mm)			SAA (degrees)			MAC (degrees)		
	Mean	Range	SD	Mean	Range	SD	Mean	Range	SD
FT	39.5	37–43	2.51	57	53–61	3.65	57	53–61	3.65
FOZ	58.25	52–62	4.34	87.5	79–98	8.34	87.5	79–98	8.34

Abbreviations: FOZ = fronto-orbito-zygomatic approach; FT = fronto-temporal approach; MAC = maneuverability arc; SAA = surgical angle of attack; SD = standard deviation; SF = depth of the surgical field.

Table 2.3 Operability score for each approach to AC.

	SF	SAA	MAC	OS
FT	1	0	0	1
FOZ	0	1	1	2

Abbreviations: FOZ = fronto-orbito-zygomatic approach; FT = fronto-temporal approach; MAC = maneuverability arc; OS = operability score; SAA = surgical angle of attack; SF = depth of the surgical field.

of the sphenoid sinus and consequently of the development of the ACP.

References

1. Filipce V, Pillai P, Makiese O, Zarzour H, Pigott M, Ammirati M. Quantitative and qualitative analysis of the working area obtained by endoscope and microscope in various approaches to the anterior communicating artery complex using computed tomography-based frameless stereotaxy: a cadaver study. Neurosurgery 2009;65(6):1147–1152, discussion 1152–1153

2. Gagliardi F, Boari N, Roberti F, Caputy AJ, Mortini P. Operability score: an innovative tool for quantitative assessment of operability in comparative studies on surgical anatomy. J Craniomaxillofac Surg 2014;42(6):1000–1004

3. Gonzalez LF, Crawford NR, Horgan MA, Deshmukh P, Zabramski JM, Spetzler RF. Working area and angle of attack in three cranial base approaches: pterional, orbitozygomatic, and maxillary extension of the orbitozygomatic approach. Neurosurgery 2002;50(3):550–555, discussion 555–557

4. Salma A, Alkandari A, Sammet S, Ammirati M. Lateral supraorbital approach vs pterional approach: an anatomic qualitative and quantitative evaluation. Neurosurgery 2011;68 (2, Suppl Operative):364–372, discussion 371–372

5. Sindou M, Emery E, Acevedo G, Ben-David U. Respective indications for orbital rim, zygomatic arch and orbito-zygomatic osteotomies in the surgical approach to central skull base lesions. Critical, retrospective review in 146 cases. Acta Neurochir (Wien) 2001;143(10):967–975

6. Yaşargil MG, Abdulrauf SI. Surgery of intraventricular tumors. Neurosurgery 2008;62(6, Suppl 3):1029–1040, discussion 1040–1041

**Part II
Planning, Patient Positioning,
and Basic Techniques**

3 Anatomical Landmarks and Cranial Anthropometry

Victor Fernández Cornejo, Javier Abarca Olivas, Pablo González-López, and Iván Verdú-Martínez

3.1 Introduction

In this chapter, we describe surface landmarks of the skull and how they relate to underlying important cortical structures.

These correlations are particularly important and a great aid, when planning surgical approaches, as they assist in tailoring the approach, avoiding unnecessary exposure and minimizing risk of injuries to the brain parenchyma.

Even though there is an individual variability among skulls and underlying vascular and cortical anatomy, the knowledge of these markers is of paramount importance to "outline" the position of vital structures, which will be uncovered during the surgical approach.

3.2 Main Cranial Landmarks (Fig. 3.1)

Looking at the skull, these landmarks become readily available in the different aspects as seen in **Fig. 3.1**.
• **Frontal view**: Nasion, Bregma, and Frontozygomatic point (**Fig. 3.1A**).
• **Lateral view**: Coronal Suture, Stephanion, Pterion, Frontozygomatic Point, Squamous Suture, and Temporal Line (**Fig. 3.1B**).
• **Superior view**: Bregma, Lambda, Sagittal Suture, and Coronal Suture (**Fig. 3.1C**).
• **Posterior view**: Lambdoid suture, Opisthocranion, Inion, Asterion, and Superior Nuchal Line (**Fig. 3.1D**)

While some of these landmarks represent intersections of different bones of the neurocranium, some are marks left on the bone by the attachment of muscles or are simply relevant to the palpation of the skull (*i.e.,* opisthocranion).
• **Nasion (Na):** Point of intersection between the two nasal bones and the frontal bone.
• **Bregma (Br):** Point of intersection between the coronal and sagittal suture.
• **Frontozygomatic Point (FzP):** Suture in the lateral wall of the orbit, between the frontal and zygomatic bones.
• **Superior Temporal Line (STL):** Line of attachment of the temporal fascia to the skull, crossing the middle of the parietal bone in an arched direction.
• **Stephanion (St):** Point of intersection between the superior temporal line and coronal suture.
• **Pterion (Pt):** Area where frontal, parietal, temporal, and sphenoid bones join together.
• **Lambda (La):** Point of intersection between the sagittal and lambdoid sutures.
• **Opisthocranion (Op):** Most prominent point of the occipital bone.
• **Inion (In):** External occipital protuberance.
• **Asterion (As):** Posterior end of the parieto-mastoid suture.
• **Superior Nuchal Line (SNL):** Line of insertion of the semispinalis capitis muscle in the occipital bone.

3.3 Cranial Anthropometry (Fig. 3.2)

Once the work of memorizing these landmarks is done, they can be put to good use in calculating distances and relationships among these landmarks and the underlying brain.

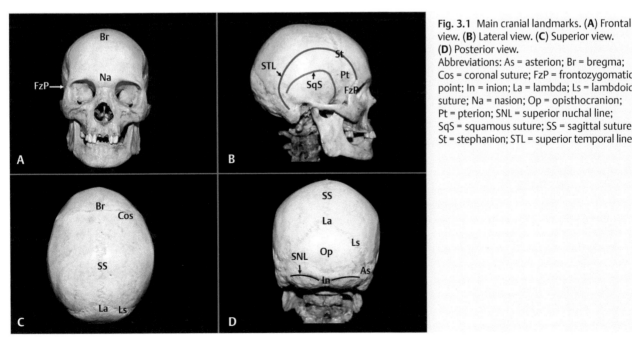

Fig. 3.1 Main cranial landmarks. (A) Frontal view. (B) Lateral view. (C) Superior view. (D) Posterior view.
Abbreviations: As = asterion; Br = bregma; Cos = coronal suture; FzP = frontozygomatic point; In = inion; La = lambda; Ls = lambdoid suture; Na = nasion; Op = opisthocranion; Pt = pterion; SNL = superior nuchal line; SqS = squamous suture; SS = sagittal suture; St = stephanion; STL = superior temporal line.

3.3.1 Main Measurements of The Skull

Approximate distance between important landmarks in adult skull:
- Nasion- Bregma: 13 cm
- Nasion-Lambda: 24-25 cm
- Bregma-Lambda: 12-13 cm
- Pterion-Frontozygomatic Suture: 3 cm
- Opisthocranion-Inion: 2 cm
- Lambda-Opisthocranion: 2-4 cm
- Inion-Lambda: 4-6 cm

3.3.2 Location of the Main Cerebral Sulci And Gyri

Some of the important cerebral landmarks can be located with good approximation with the help of artificial lines constructed on the previously described bony and surface markers, considering the variability among patients related to individual anatomy and concurrent pathologies.
- **The Sylvian Fissure (SF).** A line that is constructed along the sagittal convexity helps determine the distance from **Nasion** to **Inion**. It is important to locate the **Sylvian Fissure** as it courses parallel (a few mm above or below) a line that joins the **Frontozygomatic Point** to the three-quarter point of the **Nasion-Inion** mid-sagittal line on the lateral surface of the head (**Fig. 3.2A**).
- **The Central Sulcus (CS).** It runs parallel or along a line constructed connecting the **Superior Rolandic Point (SRP)** and the **Inferior Rolandic Point (IRP)**. SRP is 5 cm behind the **Bregma** and IRP is 2.5 cm behind the **Pterion** (**Fig. 3.2B**).
- **Precentral Gyrus (PreCG).** It is located 4.5 cm posterior to the **Bregma** (midline) and 2.5 cm posterior to the **Stephanion** (lateral surface) (**Fig. 3.2C**).
- **Postcentral Gyrus (PostCG).** Situated 6.5 cm posterior to the **Bregma** (midline) and 4 cm posterior to the **Stephanion** (lateral surface) (**Fig. 3.2C**).

- **Calcarine Sulcus.** It is located 3-4 cm inferior to the **Lambda** and 2 cm superior to the **Inion**, on the mesial aspect of the occipital lobe (**Fig. 3.2D**).

3.4 Sulcal Key Points. Correlation with Craniometric Points

3.4.1 Anterior Sylvian Point (ASP) (Fig. 3.3)

- **Description:** It is an enlargement of the **Sylvian Fissure**, just inferior to the triangular part and anterior to the opercular part of the **Inferior Frontal Gyrus (IFG)** (**Fig. 3.3A**).
- **Craniometric correlation:** On the cranial surface, it relates well to the **Anterior Squamous Point (ASqP)**. This is located on the most anterior segment of the **Squamous Suture (SqSut)** just posterior to the **Pterion** (**Fig. 3.3B, Fig. 3.3C**).
- **Clinical implications:** It represents the starting point to open the SF and localizes the insular apex. Middle cerebral artery bifurcation is deeper and 1-2 cm anterior to it.
- **Correlation:** The distance between the **Anterior Sylvian Point (ASP)** and the **Inferior Rolandic Point (IRP)** along the **Sylvian Fissure** is 2-3 cm (**Fig. 3.3D**).

3.4.2 Inferior Rolandic Point (IRP) (Fig. 3.4)

- **Description:** It represents the intersection of the lower extremity of the **Central Sulcus** and the **Sylvian Fissure** (**Fig. 3.4A**).
- **Craniometric correlation:** On the cranial surface the **Superior Squamous Point (SSqP)** is a good landmark. It represents the intersection between the **Squamous Suture** and a vertical line coming from the preauricular depression, just in front of the tragus. The average vertical height of this segment is 4 cm above the zygoma. (**Fig. 3.4B**). The **Inferior Rolandic Point** is located 2.5 cm posterior to the **Pterion** along the **Sylvian Fissure**.

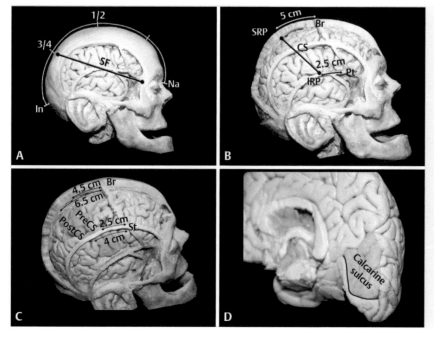

Fig. 3.2 Location of the main cerebral sulci and gyri. (**A**) Measure the distance along the sagittal convexity from nasion to inion. Mark the midpoint (1/2) and the three-quarter point (3/4). The line from the frontozygomatic point and the three-quarter point represent approximately the Sylvian fissure (SF). (**B**) The central sulcus (CS) is represented by the line connecting the superior rolandic point (SRP) and the inferior rolandic point (IRP). (**C**) Location of the precentral and postcentral gyri. (**D**) The calcarine sulcus.
Abbreviations: Br = bregma; CS = central sulcus; In = inion; IRP = inferior rolandic point; Na = nasion; PostCS = postcentral sulcus; PreCS = precentral sulcus; Pt = pterion; SF = Sylvian fissure; SRP = superior rolandic point; St = stephanion.

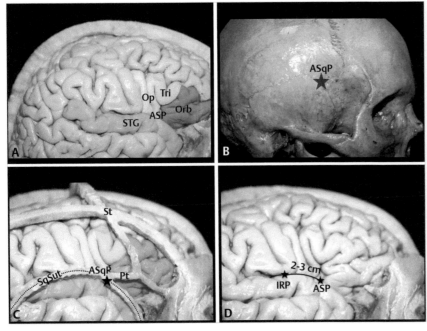

Fig. 3.3 The **Anterior Sylvian Point (ASP)**. (**A**) The ASP is surrounded by the pars orbitalis (red), pars triangularis (green) and pars opercularis (yellow) of the inferior frontal gyrus (IFG) superiorly and by the superior temporal gyrus (STG) (blue) inferiorly. (**B**) The anterior squamous point (ASqP) is the craniometric point for the ASP. (**C**) The anterior squamous point (ASqP) is located on the most anterior segment of the SqSut just in the pterion. (**D**) Correlation of the ASP with the inferior rolandic point (IRP). Abbreviations: ASP = anterior Sylvian point; ASqP = anterior squamous point; IRP = inferior rolandic point; Op = pars opercularis; Orb = pars orbitalis; Pt = pterion; SqSut = squamous suture; St = stephanion; STG = superior temporal gyrus; Tri = pars triangularis.

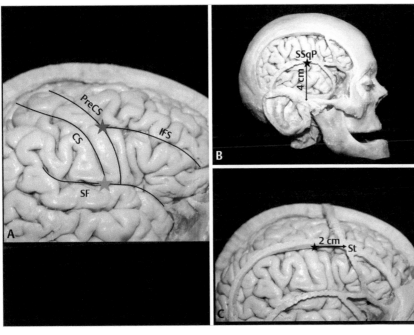

Fig. 3.4 The **Inferior Rolandic Point (IRP)** and the **Inferior Frontal Sulcus/Precentral Sulcus Intersection Point (IFS/PreCS)**. (**A**) The IRP is the intersection of the central sulcus (CS) (or its prolongation) with the Sylvian fissure (SF) (blue). IFS/PreCS intersection point is the point of intersection of the inferior frontal sulcus (IFS) and the precentral sulcus (PreCS) (red). (**B**) IRP is underneath the superior squamous point (SSqP). (**C**) IFS/PreCS intersection point lies 2 cm posterior to the Stephanion (St). Abbreviations: CS = central sulcus; IFS = inferior frontal sulcus; PreCS = precentral sulcus; SF = Sylvian fissure; SSqP = superior squamous point; St = stephanion.

- **Clinical correlation:** The **Inferior Rolandic Point** indicates the lower position of the **Central Sulcus** and with a good approximation the position of the Heschl's Gyrus. Removal of the superior and middle temporal gyri posterior to the **Inferior Rolandic Point** in the dominant hemisphere has a high risk of causing permanent dysphasia as it damages Wernicke's Area.

3.4.3 Point of Intersection Between Inferior Frontal Sulcus and Precentral Sulcus (IFS/PreCS) (Fig. 3.4)

- **Description**: It is the point of intersection between the **Inferior Frontal Sulcus** and the **Precentral Sulcus** (**Fig. 3.4A**).

- **Craniometric correlation**: On the cranial vault the **Stephanion (St)** corresponds to the intersection of the **Coronal Suture (Cos)** and the **Superior Temporal Line**. Normally the point of intersection between the **Inferior Frontal Sulcus** and **Precentral Sulcus (IFS/PreCS)** lies 2 cm posterior to the **Stephanion** (**Fig. 3.4C**).
- **Clinical implications**: It helps localizing the **Precentral Gyrus** in the inferior third level, which corresponds to the motor activation area of the face and indicates the posterior and superior limits of the opercular portion of the **Inferior Frontal Gyrus**.
- **Correlation**: The point of intersection between the **Inferior Frontal Sulcus** and the **Precentral Sulcus** corresponds to the superior limit of the **Inferior Frontal Gyrus** at its opercular part at a distance of 2.5-3 cm from the **Sylvian Fissure**.

3.4.4 Point of Intersection Between the Superior Frontal Sulcus and Precentral Sulcus (SFS/PreCS) (Fig. 3.5)

- **Description:** It represents the intersection of the **Superior Frontal Sulcus** and the **Precentral Sulcus** (**Fig. 3.5A**).
- **Craniometric correlation:** On the cranial surface, it relates well to the **Posterior Coronal Point (PCoP)**. It corresponds to the area located 3 cm lateral to the sagittal suture and 2 cm posterior to the coronal suture (**Fig. 3.5B, 3.5C**).
- **Clinical implications:** It is an important neurosurgical corridor for the frontal and anterior ventricular access. It represents the posterior limit for the **Superior Frontal Sulcus** opening.
- **Correlation:** It has an anatomical relationship with the underlying ventricular frontal horn. Just behind it, the

Precentral Gyrus lies at the level of the hand motor activation area.

3.4.5 Superior Rolandic Point (SRP) (Fig. 3.6)

- **Description:** It represents the intersection between the **Central Sulcus** and the **Interhemispheric Fissure (IHF)** (**Figs. 3.6A, 3.6B**).
- **Craniometric correlation:** On the cranial surface, it corresponds to the **Superior Sagittal Point (SSP)**, which is located 5 cm posterior to the **Bregma** (**Fig. 3.6C**). The **Superior Rolandic Point** is situated approximately 18 cm behind the **Nasion** and 5 cm posterior to the **Bregma.**
- **Clinical correlations:** Central craniotomies for the exposure of the **Precentral** and **Postcentral Gyri**, the **Cingulate Gyrus**, and the **Corpus Callosum**.

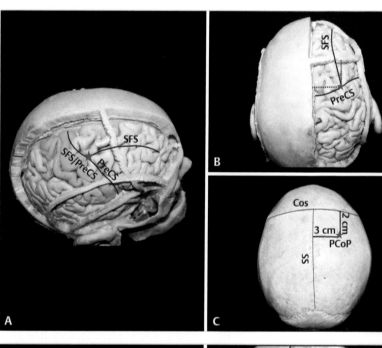

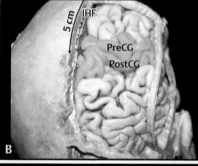

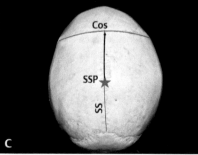

Fig. 3.5 **Superior Frontal Sulcus and Precentral Sulcus Intersection Point (SFS/PreCS).** (**A**) Intersection of the superior frontal sulcus (SFS) and precentral sulcus (PreCS). (**B**) SFS/PreCS location (red) (superior view). (**C**) Posterior coronal point (PCoP) is 3 cm lateral to the sagittal suture (SS) and 2 cm posterior to the coronal suture (Cos).
Abbreviations: Cos = coronal suture; PCoP = posterior coronal point; PreCS = precentral sulcus; SFS = superior frontal sulcus; SFS/PreCS = superior frontal sulcus and precentral sulcus intersection point; SS = sagittal suture.

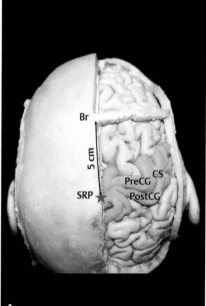

Fig. 3.6 **Superior Rolandic Point (SRP).** (**A**) The SRP corresponds to the intersection of the interhemispheric fissure (IHF) and the central sulcus (CS). It is the most medial point of the CS. (**B**) Posterolateral view of the SRP. (**C**) The craniometric point of the SRP is the superior sagittal point (SSP). It is the point 5 cm posterior to Bregma (Br) along the sagittal suture (SS).
Abbreviations: Br = bregma; Cos = coronal suture; CS = central sulcus; IHF = interhemispheric fissure; PostCG = postcentral gyrus; PreCG = precentral gyrus; SRP = superior rolandic point; SS = sagittal suture; SSP = superior sagittal point.

3.4.6 Point of Intersection Between the Intraparietal Sulcus and Postcentral Sulcus (IPS-PostCS) (Fig. 3.7)

- **Description:** It is the intersection point of the **Intraparietal Sulcus** and the **Postcentral Sulcus** (**Fig. 3.7A**). The **Intraparietal Sulcus** represents the posterior limit of the **Postcentral Gyrus**. It can be found as a continuous or interrupted sulcus; it is normally parallel to the **Interhemispheric Fissure** and separates the superior from the inferior parietal lobule.
- **Craniometric correlation:** On the cranial surface, it relates to the **Intraparietal Point (IPP)**. It is located 6 cm anterior to the **Lambdoid Suture** and 5 cm lateral to the **Sagittal Suture (SS)** (**Fig. 3.7C**).

- **Clinical correlation:** It represents a safe starting point for the microsurgical opening of the **Postcentral Sulcus**. It holds a deep relationship with the ventricular trigone. Posteriorly it is usually continuous with the **Transverse Occipital Sulcus**.

3.4.7 The External Occipital Fissure (EOF) Medial Point (Fig. 3.8)

- **Description:** The **External Occipital Fissure** corresponds to the extension of the medial **Parieto-Occipital Sulcus (POS)** into the brain convexity (**Fig. 3.8A**) The most medial point represents the intersection of the **External Occipital Fissure (EOF)** and **Parieto-Occipital Sulcus (POS)** (**Fig. 3.8B**).
- **Craniometric correlation:** On the cranial surface, it corresponds to the **Lambdoid/Sagittal Point** with its paramedian

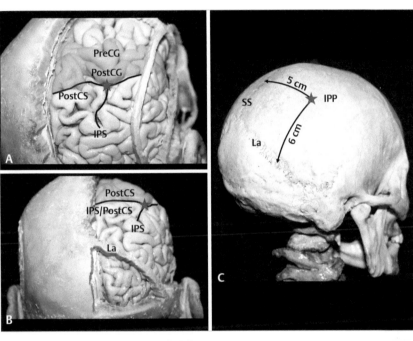

Fig. 3.7 **Intraparietal Sulcus and Postcentral Sulcus Intersection Point (IPS/PCS).** (**A**) Intersection of the intraparietal sulcus (IPS) and the postcentral sulcus (PCS). (**B**) IPS/PCS (posterior view). (**C**) The intraparietal point (IPP) is located underneath a point 6 cm anterior to the Lambda (La) and 5 cm lateral to the sagittal suture (SS). Abbreviations: IPP = intraparietal point; IPS = intraparietal sulcus; IPS/PostCS = intraparietal sulcus and postcentral sulcus intersection point; La = lambda; PostCS = postcentral sulcus; PostCG = postcentral gyrus; PreCG = precentral gyrus; SS= sagittal sulcus.

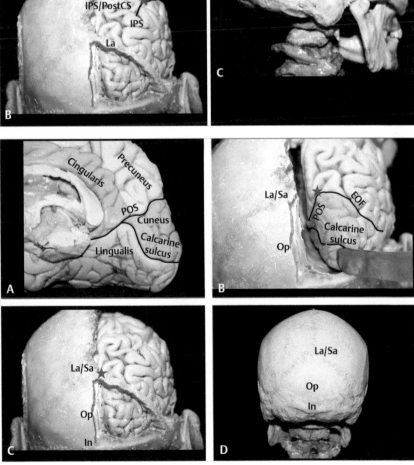

Fig. 3.8 The **External Occipital Fissure Medial Point** and the **Calcarine Sulcus.** (**A**) The external occipital sulcus (EOF) corresponds to the extension of the medial parieto-occipital sulcus (POS) into the brain convexity. The Calcarine Sulcus separates the cuneus and lingual gyrus. (**B**) EOF/POS (red). Calcarine sulcus (blue). (**C**) The craniometric point for EOF/POS is the lambdoid/sagittal point (La/Sa) and for the calcarine sulcus is the opisthocranion (Op). (**D**) La/Sa is 13 cm posterior to Bregma and 3 cm superior to Op. Op is 2 cm superior to inion (In). Abbreviations: EOF = external occipital fissure; EOF/POS = external occipital fissure and parieto-occipital sulcus intersection point; In = inion; La/Sa = lambdoid/sagittal point; POS = parieto-occipital sulcus; Op = opisthocranion.

area corresponding to the angle between the sagittal and lambdoid sutures (**Fig. 3.8C**).
- **Clinical correlation:** Its identification is important while performing occipital craniotomies for exposure of the **cuneus**. The **Lambdoid/Sagittal Point** defines the position of the **Parieto-Occipital Sulcus** and, thus, the posterior aspect of the precuneus along the **Interhemispheric Fissure.**
- **Notes: Lambda/Sagittal Point** is 13 cm posterior to the **Bregma** and 3 cm superior to the **Opisthocranion.** The distance between the point of intersection of **External Occipital Fissure/Parieto-Occipital Sulcus (POS)** and **Postcentral Sulcus** is 4 cm (equivalent to the longitudinal extension of the precuneus along the Interhemispheric Fissure (**Fig. 3.8D**).

3.4.8 Calcarine Sulcus (Fig. 3.8)

- **Description:** The **Calcarine Sulcus** corresponds to the sulcus between the cuneus and the lingual gyrus (**Fig. 3.8A**).
- **Craniometric correlation:** It corresponds to the **Opisthocranion (Op)**, the most prominent occipital cranial point (**Fig. 3.8C**).
- **Clinical correlations:** Its identification is important while performing occipital craniotomies for exposure of medial aspects of the occipital lobe and occipital craniotomies for transtentorial approaches to the retro-callosal area and pineal region.

- **Notes: Opisthocranion** is found 3 cm inferior to the **Lambda** and 2 cm superior to the occipital base **(Inion)** (**Fig. 3.8D**).

References

1. Campero A, Ajler P, Emmerich J, Goldschmidt E, Martins C, Rhoton A. Brain sulci and gyri: a practical anatomical review. J Clin Neurosci 2014; 21(12):2219–2225
2. Kendir S, Acar HI, Comert A, et al. Window anatomy for neurosurgical approaches. Laboratory investigation. J Neurosurg 2009; 111(2):365–370
3. Naidich TP, Valavanis AG, Kubik S. Anatomic relationships along the low-middle convexity: Part I—Normal specimens and magnetic resonance imaging. Neurosurgery 1995; 36(3):517–532
4. Ribas GC, Yasuda A, Ribas EC, Nishikuni K, Rodrigues AJ Jr. Surgical anatomy of microneurosurgical sulcal key points. Neurosurgery 2006; 59(4, Suppl 2):ONS177–ONS210, discussion ONS210–ONS211
5. Sampath R, Katira K, Vannemreddy P, Nanda A. Quantifying sulcal and gyral topography in relation to deep seated and ventricular lesions: cadaveric study for basing surgical approaches and review of literature. Br J Neurosurg 2014; 28(6):713–716

4 Presurgical Planning By Images

Antonella Castellano and Andrea Falini

4.1 Role of Imaging in Preoperative Planning

- This chapter provides an overview of common preoperative imaging protocol advices as they relate to different cranial neurosurgical approaches.
- **CT** (computed tomography) **scans** yield an excellent definition of bone anatomy and are useful to identify highly calcified lesions, but cannot distinguish subtle differences between tissues in the brain.
- **Conventional MRI** (magnetic resonance imaging) sequences (i.e., T2-weighted, FLAIR or fluid-attenuated inversion-recovery, T1-weighted images before and post-contrast administration) have an excellent contrast resolution and bring information about the location, signal intensities, and enhancement features of the lesions.
- Beside conventional morphologic evaluation, **advanced MRI** techniques can improve the specificity of preoperative imaging diagnosis and are useful tools for surgical planning. In this regard, the next sections will propose an integrated approach that includes magnetic resonance angiography (MRA), diffusion MR-based techniques (DWI/DTI: diffusion-weighted imaging/diffusion tensor imaging), functional MRI, perfusion MR imaging, and MR spectroscopy.

4.2 Anterior Cranial Fossa (Fig. 4.1.)

4.2.1 General Features

- Presurgical imaging of lesions in the anterior compartment of the skull base includes meningioma (common), dural metastasis, paranasal sinus tumor invasion, olfactory neuroblastoma or esthesioneuroblastoma (rare), aneurysms, intra-axial frontal tumors.

4.2.2 MR Imaging

- **Pre- and post-contrast MRI (Figs.4.1A–1F)** are the best imaging tool for the diagnosis and characterization of anterior cranial fossa lesions. Tissue signal and enhancement are variable in appearance across different lesions.
  - In *meningiomas, T2-w* images well delineate trapped hyperintense cerebrospinal fluid (CSF) clefts **(Figs. 4.1A, 4.1C)** and vascular flow-voids. The extent of perilesional edema is well demonstrated on *FLAIR* images **(Fig. 4.1F)**. Meningiomas usually enhance homogeneously and intensely **(Figs. 4.1D, 4.1E)** on *T1-w* post-contrast images and usually show a thickening of the adjacent dura *(dural tail)*.
  - *Metastasis* and other anterior cranial fossa lesions may differ according to their tissue of origin.
- **MRA (Fig. 4.1G)** demonstrates the mass effect of the lesion on arterial vessels, as well as their possible encasement and narrowing. MRV (magnetic resonance venography) may help to identify dural sinus invasion (superior sagittal sinus).

4.2.3 CT Imaging

- **Non-contrast CT** (**Figs. 4.1H, 4.11**) may show calcifications and intra-lesional hemorrhages. *Bone CT* scans of the maxillofacial region are useful to detect *hyperostosis* (**Fig. 4.11**) (typical for meningiomas abutting the dura of the skull base), *bone erosion* or *destruction* (**Fig. 4.1H**) (typical for higher grade or lytic lesions), and enlargement of the paranasal sinuses (*pneumosinus dilatans*).

4.2.4 DSA (Digital Subtraction Angiography)

- **Conventional and interventional DSA** may be used for detailed delineation of lesion vascular supplies and for preoperative embolization of anterior cranial fossa lesions, which may substantially reduce operative time and blood loss.

4.3 Sellar and Parasellar Region (Fig. 4.2)

4.3.1 General Features

- Located in the central compartment of the skull base (middle cranial fossa), it includes the sella turcica in the sphenoid bone, which houses the pituitary gland.
- Surrounding structures are the sphenoid sinus (inferiorly), the suprasellar cistern, the optic chiasm and the infundibular recess of the third ventricle (superiorly) and the cavernous sinuses (laterally).
- Presurgical imaging firstly aims at determining the anatomical sub-location of the lesion: intrasellar, suprasellar, or in the infundibular stalk (alone or in combination).
  - *Intrasellar lesions*: Pituitary adenomas, Rathke cleft cyst, craniopharyngioma, neurosarcoidosis (less common).
  - *Suprasellar lesions*: Pituitary macroadenoma, meningioma, aneurysm, craniopharyngioma, and astrocytoma; less common suprasellar masses are arachnoid cyst, dermoid cyst, and neurocysticercosis (usually multiple lesions).
  - *Infundibular stalk lesions*: Metastasis, lymphoma, pituicytoma, germinoma (more common in children), histiocytosis, hypophysitis, neurosarcoidosis (rare).

4.3.2 MR Imaging

- **Pre- and post-contrast MRI** (**Figs. 4.2A–4.2F**) signal and enhancement varies across different lesions and cyst contents.
  - In *craniopharyngiomas, T2-w* images show large hyperintense cystic components, heterogeneous solid components and vascular flow-voids of surrounding arteries (**Figs. 4.2A–4.2C**). *T1-w* post-contrast images usually show heterogeneous enhancement of the solid portions

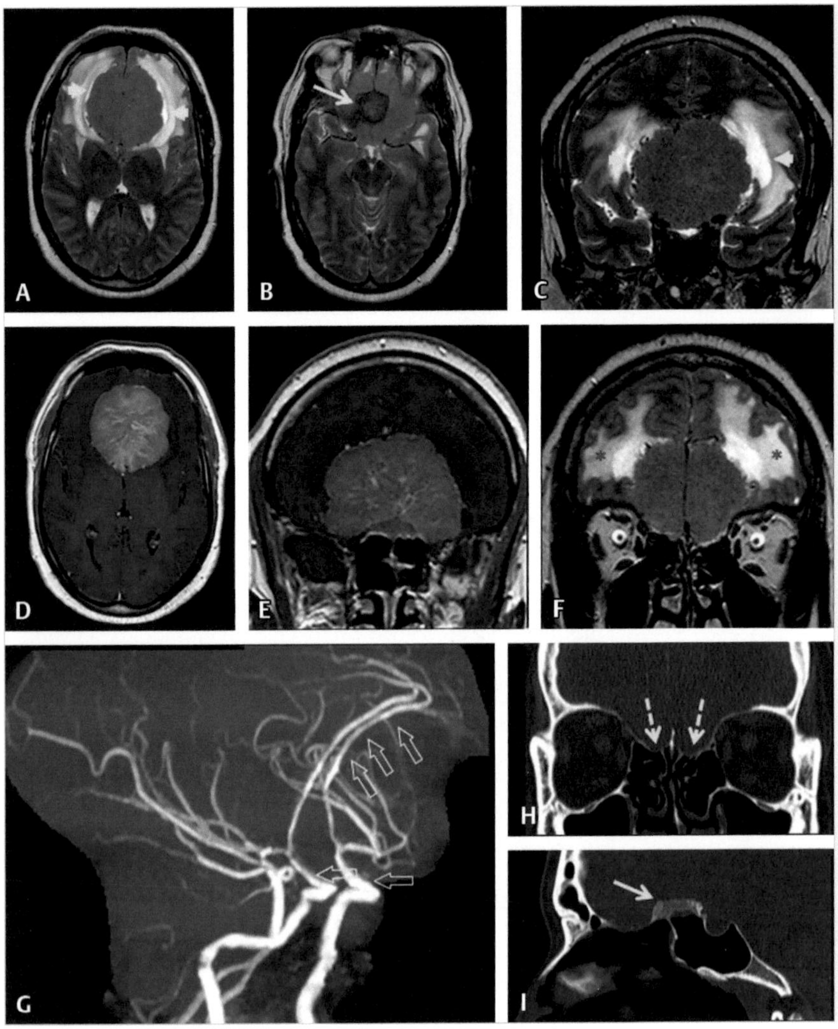

Fig. 4.1 Anterior cranial fossa meningioma. (**A, B, C**) Axial and coronal *T2-w* images show an extra-axial mass arising from the sphenoidal planum and extending into both anterior frontal lobes. The lesion is quite homogeneous, except for its calcified basal part, which is markedly hypointense (*yellow arrow*). Peripheral CSF clefts are seen as hyperintense rim between tumor and brain (*yellow arrowheads*). (**D, E**) *T1-w* post-contrast axial and coronal images demonstrates intense enhancement of the lesion, with even more hyperintense "sunburst" of the vessels. (**F**) Coronal *FLAIR* image shows markedly hyperintense peritumoral vasogenic edema (*asterisks*). (**G**) *MRA* shows posterior and cranial displacement of both the anterior cerebral arteries, and posterior displacement of both the intracranial carotid arteries (*open arrows*). (**H, I**) *Bone CT* shows enlargement of the olfactory groove bilaterally (*dashed arrows*) and hyperostosis of the sphenoidal planum and calcification at the basis of the lesion (*yellow arrow*).

of the lesions. Cyst walls of craniopharyngiomas enhance strongly (**Fig. 4.2D–4.2F**)

○ *Arachnoid cysts* behave like CSF, *dermoid cysts* appear like fat.

○ In *pituitary adenomas, dynamic T1-w* post-contrast images may help to detect slowly enhancing *microadenomas*.

• **DTI and MR Tractography** (**Figs. 4.2G–4.2I**) allow to depict the major white matter tracts in the brain. Preoperative DTI tractography may show the location and displacement of the main fiber bundles surrounding the lesions, including the anterior commissure, the fornix, the optic chiasm and tracts. This information may be particularly useful for the resection of large lesions growing toward the third ventricle.

• **MRA** (**Fig. 4.2L**) demonstrates the vascular displacement or encasement of the arterial vessels surrounding the lesions.

4.3.3 CT Imaging

• **Non-contrast CT** shows intra-lesional calcifications. The bone window of *CT* scans of the maxillofacial region are useful to evaluate the paranasal sinuses before surgery and to detect the *bone erosion* of sellar floor and sphenoid invasion.

4.4 Posterior Cranial Fossa, Lateral Approaches (Figs. 4.3, 4.4)

4.4.1 General Features

• Presurgical imaging of the lateral posterior compartment of the skull base includes cerebello-pontine angle (CPA) cisternal masses (usually involving the temporal bone or infratemporal fossa): most commonly demonstrate vestibular schwannoma (common), meningioma, epidermoid, arachnoid cyst, trigeminal or facial nerve schwannoma and metastasis.

4.4.2 MR Imaging

• **Pre- and post-contrast MRI** (**Figs. 4.3, 4.4**) help to characterize CPA cistern masses.

○ The MR signal of *schwannomas* is similar to that of lesions involving other nerves. *Vestibular schwannomas*, the most common CPA lesions, are intensely enhancing masses with an 'ice cream on a cone' appearance (**Figs. 4.3A–4.3F**). The mass effect on the adjacent cerebellar and brainstem structures is well demonstrated on MR images (**Figs. 4.3A–4.3F**). *DWI* MR

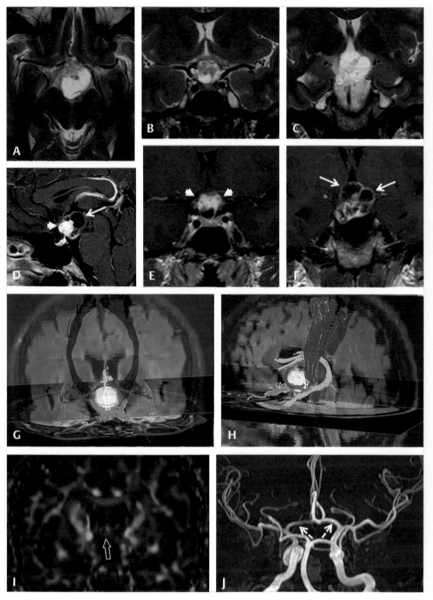

Fig. 4.2 Suprasellar intraventricular craniopharyngioma. (**A–C**) Axial and coronal *T2-w* images show a lobulated, partially cystic suprasellar mass; the posterior cystic portion is markedly hyperintense. (**D–F**) Sagittal and coronal post-contrast *T1-w* images show the enhancing rim (*white arrows*) and the solid components (*white arrowheads*) of the lesion. (**G–I**) Preoperative DTI tractography (**G**, anterior and **H**, lateral view) shows the anterior commissure (red), the fornix (green), the optic chiasm and tracts (orange), and the pyramidal tracts (purple): the anterior commissure is displaced cranially and anteriorly by the lesion (*open arrows*), confirmed on DTI color map (**I**, coronal section). (**J**) *MRA* shows divarication of the A1 segments of both the anterior cerebral arteries (*dashed arrows*).

sequence shows elevated ADC (apparent diffusion coefficient) values with respect to normal brain tissue, reflecting the increased amount of extracellular water in tumor matrix.

- ○ *Meningiomas* usually enhance strongly on *T1-w* post-contrast images, usually 'cap' the internal auditory canal (IAC) without extending into it and may show a thickening of the adjacent dura *(dural tail)*.
- ○ *Epidermoid* shows no enhancement on *T1-w* post-contrast images (**Fig. 4.4**) and restricted diffusion on *DWI* images (**Figs. 4.4D–4.4E**), which is typical of these lesions.
- ○ *Metastases* are usually multiple, and other lesions may be present.
- **MRV** may identify the involvement of adjacent dural sinuses (transverse and sigmoid sinuses) and jugular veins.

4.4.3 CT Imaging

- **Non-contrast bone CT window** (**Figs. 4.3G, 4.3H**) in schwannomas is useful to detect the possible enlargement

of bony foramina (IAC, facial nerve canal, hypoglossal canal and jugular foramen).

4.4.4 DSA

- **Conventional DSA** (**Figs. 4.3I–4.3L**) may be used for detailed delineation of displaced arterial vessels and vascular supplies, especially in large lesions.

4.5 Posterior Cranial Fossa, Medial Approaches (Fig. 4.5)

4.5.1 General Features

- Presurgical imaging of the medial posterior compartment of the skull base includes brainstem lesions, such as cerebral cavernous malformations, metastasis, primary brain gliomas, ependymomas, and imaging of neurovascular compression syndromes.

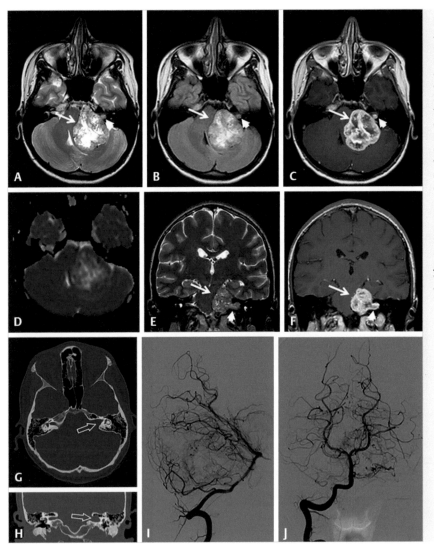

Fig. 4.3 Acoustic (vestibular) schwannoma. Axial and coronal *T2-w* (**A, E**) and FLAIR (**B**) images show a large lesion at the level of left CPA, with both a cisternal (*white arrows*) and an intracanalicular (*white arrowheads*) component. The tumor tissue inside the internal auditory canal represents the cone, the CPA cisternal component forms the "ice cream" on the cone. The lesion exerts an important mass effect on the adjacent cerebellum and brainstem and on the fourth ventricle. (**C, F**) *T1-w* post-contrast images demonstrate intense inhomogeneous, ring enhancement of the lesion with a central necrotic portion. (**D**) *DWI* shows increased intralesional ADC values with respect to normal brain tissue. (**G, H**) *Bone CT window* shows enlargement of the left IAC and porus acusticus (*open arrows*). (**I, J**) *DSA* (**I**, oblique; **J**, frontal view) shows an hypovascular mass with a diffuse blush and stretched adjacent vessels.

4.5.2 MR Imaging

- **Pre- and post-contrast MRI** (**Figs. 4.5A–4.5E**) are used to depict midline lesions in the posterior cranial fossa.
  - *Cerebral cavernous malformations* are intra-axial brainstem lesions with a reticulated 'popcorn-like' appearance on *T2-w* images (**Figs. 4.5A–4.5C**): the mixed signal core is surrounded by a complete, hypointense hemosiderin rim that 'blooms' on *T2-w* sequences. Enhancement is minimal (**Fig. 5.5D**) or absent. *Steady-state and dynamic post-contrast T1-w* sequences for venous flow depiction may help to identify associated venous malformations (**Figs. 4.5E**).
- **DTI and MR Tractography** (**Figs. 4.5F–4.5H**) allow to depict the brainstem white matter tracts and their relationships with intra-axial lesions in the posterior fossa. Preoperative DTI tractography of the motor and sensitive fibers as well as the cerebellar peduncles show the location and displacement of these bundles surrounding the lesions.
- The combination of 3D time-of-flight **MRA** with high-resolution *3D* heavily *T2-w* imaging and high-resolution *3D T1-w* post-contrast sequences with *steady-state* acquisition is considered the standard of reference for the detection of *neurovascular compression* and to guide neurosurgical treatment.

4.5.3 CT Imaging

- **Non-contrast bone CT window** is recommended to evaluate bone structures of the cranio-spinal junction.

4.6 Pineal Region (Figs. 4.6, 4.7

4.6.1 General Features

- This region is located under the falx cerebri, in close proximity to its confluence with the tentorium cerebelli, and includes the pineal gland and the adjacent CSF spaces (third ventricle and subarachnoid cisterns).
- Surrounding structures are the splenium of the corpus callosum, the quadrigeminal plate, the upper vermis, the medial and lateral posterior choroidal arteries, the internal cerebral veins and vein of Galen and the dural sinuses (inferior sagittal sinus, straight sinus).
- Preoperative imaging includes pineal region lesions and their relationships with the above-mentioned structures: pineal parenchymal tumors, germinoma (more frequent in young patients), meningioma, glioma, metastasis, neurocytoma and lymphoma (rare).

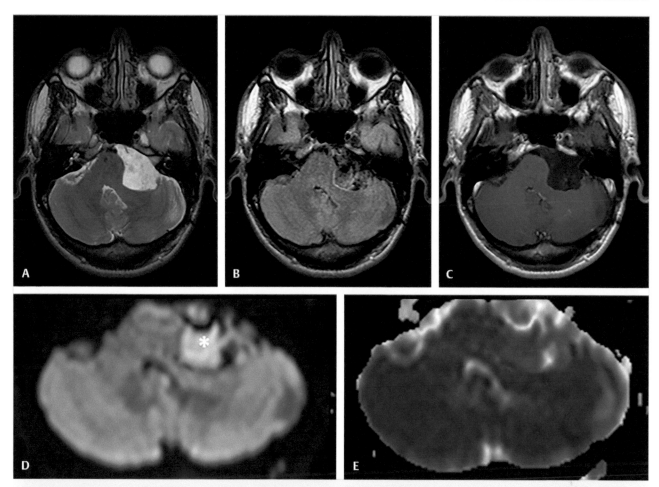

Fig. 4.4 Epidermoid cyst. **(A)** Axial *T2-w* image shows a CPA mass with signal intensity similar to CSF. **(B)** On the axial *FLAIR* image, the signal of the lesion is incompletely suppressed. **(C)** No enhancement is seen on the *T1-w* post-contrast image. **(D, E)** The *DWI* scan shows restricted water diffusion within the mass (*white asterisk*) and therefore very high signal intensity on DWI images **(D**, differently from the CSF in the fourth ventricle) and low ADC on the corresponding map **(E).**

4.6.2 MR Imaging

- **Pre- and post-contrast MRI** (**Figs. 4.6, 4.7**) are recommended for the diagnosis and characterization of pineal region lesions.
  - *Pineal parenchymal tumors* show heterogeneous signal on *T2-w* and *FLAIR* images, areas of cystic degeneration and flow-void images due to the encasement of deep cerebral veins (**Figs. 4.6A–4.6B**); *T1-w* post-contrast images show intense and heterogeneous enhancement (**Figs. 4.6C**). Extension into adjacent structures is typical of higher grade lesions (*pineal parenchymal tumor of intermediate differentiation* and *pineoblastoma*).
  - *Germinomas* typically show intratumoral cysts, often restrict on *DWI* images due to their high cellularity and enhance strongly on *T1-w* post-contrast images. CSF spread is common, thus the entire neuroaxis should be imaged in young patients with suspected germinoma, with particular attention to the pituitary stalk where synchronous lesions can be detected.
  - MR signal of *metastasis* may differ according to their tissue of origin (**Fig. 4.7**): multiple lesions are usually detected.
- **MRS (magnetic resonance spectroscopy)** may help in differential diagnosis of pineal region masses: *pineal parenchymal tumors* show elevated Choline (Cho) and decreased N-Acetil-Aspartate (NAA) (**Fig. 4.6G**), whereas *metastases* usually show a lipid peak and absence of all the typical cerebral metabolites (**Fig. 4.7D**).

4.6.3 CT Imaging

- **Non-contrast CT** may show intralesional calcifications (**Fig. 4.6D**).
- **Angio-CT scans** (venous phase) may demonstrate the relationships of the lesion with surrounding deep cerebral veins (internal cerebral veins and vein of Galen) (**Fig. 4.6E, 4.6F**).

4.7 Brain Convexity and Supratentorial Lesions (Figs. 4.8 and 4.9)

4.7.1 General Features

- Presurgical imaging of brain convexity and supratentorial lesions comprises all the intra-axial and extra-axial masses in the cerebral hemispheres.

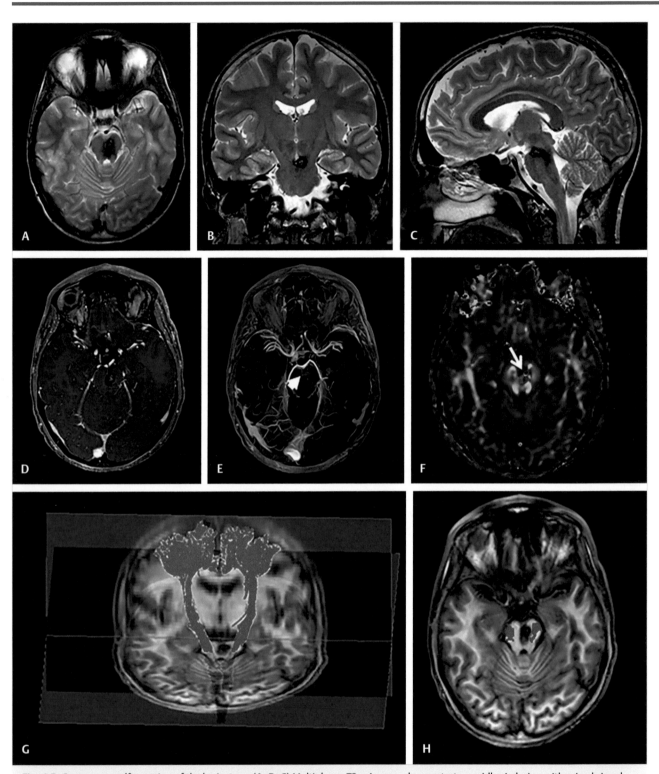

Fig. 4.5 Cavernous malformation of the brainstem. (**A, B, C**) Multiplanar *T2-w* images demonstrate a midbrain lesion with mixed signal in the core and a marked peripheral hypointensity due to hemosiderin. (**D**) Steady-state post-contrast *T1-w* sequence shows minimal enhancement in the core. (**E**) *Dynamic post-contrast T1-w* sequences for venous flow depiction help to identify a tiny, associated venous malformation (*white arrowhead*). (**F**) *DTI color map* show an area of signal loss (*white arrow*) between the decussation of superior cerebellar peduncles (red central spot) and the left corticospinal tract (blue area at the level of the cerebral peduncle). (**G, H**) Three-dimensional rendering of preoperative DTI tractography (**G**, frontal view and **H**, axial section) shows the left corticospinal tract lining laterally the cavernous malformation in the midbrain.

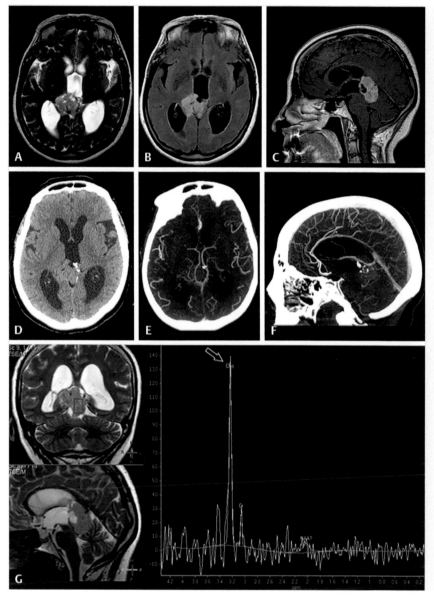

Fig. 4.6 Pineocytoma. (**A, B**) Axial *T2-w* and *FLAIR* images show a multilobulate, heterogeneously hyperintense pineal region lesion with small cystic components. (**C**) Intense enhancement is seen on the *T1-w* post-contrast image. (**D**) *Non-contrast CT* image demonstrates peripheral intralesional calcifications. (**E, F**) *Angio-CT scans* in the venous phase (**E**, axial, **F**, midsagittal) indicate encasement, divarication and cranial displacement of both the internal cerebral veins. (**G**) *Single voxel MRS* (TE = 144) shows elevated Choline (Cho) and decreased N-Acetil-Aspartate (NAA) in the sampled area of the lesion (*red box*).

4.7.2 MR Imaging

- **Pre- and post-contrast MRI** (**Figs. 4.8, 4.9**) are the exams of choice to characterize brain convexity and supratentorial lesions.
  - *Primary brain tumors* such as cerebral gliomas show heterogeneous signal on *T2-w* and *FLAIR* images and variable enhancement on *T1-w* post-contrast images.
- **MRS** may help in differential diagnosis and detection of glioma infiltration (**Fig. 4.9E**).
- **PWI** (perfusion-weighted imaging) MR enables to quantify tumor microvessel proliferation and permeability, and thus to measure changes associated to neoangiogenesis, which correlate with tumor malignancy.
- **DTI and MR Tractography** (**Figs. 4.8D, 4.8E; Figs. 4.9F–4.9H**) have become an integral part of the presurgical and intraoperative workup of supratentorial brain lesions and enable to depict a map of the main eloquent fiber bundles, like motor, visual, and language fascicles or subcortical connections involved in specific circuits, near or inside a lesion.

- **fMRI (functional magnetic resonance imaging)** (**Fig. 4.8D**) complements the anatomical tractography information by depicting the eloquent functional activations at a cortical level.
- **MRA** demonstrates the displacement of the major arterial vessels by the lesion.
- **MRV** may evaluate the venous anatomy of the interhemispheric fissure.

4.7.3 CT Imaging

- **Non-contrast CT** may show intralesional calcifications (**Figs. 4.6D–4.6F**) and hemorrhages.

4.8 Pearls

- MRI is the best imaging tool for presurgical characterization of brain lesions; CT is essential to depict bony anatomy.
- Advanced MRI techniques should be used in the clinical routine to provide relevant structural, hemodynamic,

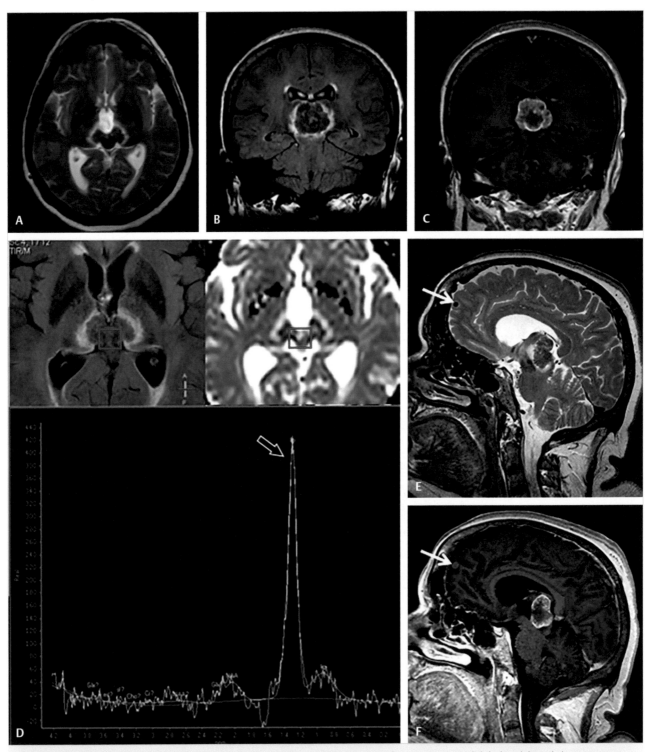

Fig. 4.7 Metastasis of adenocarcinoma. (**A, B**) Axial *T2-w* and coronal *FLAIR* images demonstrate a multilobulated, heavily hypointense pineal region lesion. Supratentorial hydrocephalus is seen. (**C**) *T1-w* post-contrast image shows peripheral enhancement of the lesion. (**D**) *Single voxel MRS* (TE = 144) shows a lipid peak at 1.3 ppm and absence of all the typical cerebral metabolites in the sampled area of the lesion (*red box*), which is characteristic of metastases. (**E, F**) A small, nodular lesion in the fronto-polar region is demonstrated on sagittal *T2-w* and *T1-w* post-contrast images (*white arrows*), with the same signal characteristics of the pineal region lesion, suggesting multiple metastatic localizations in the brain.

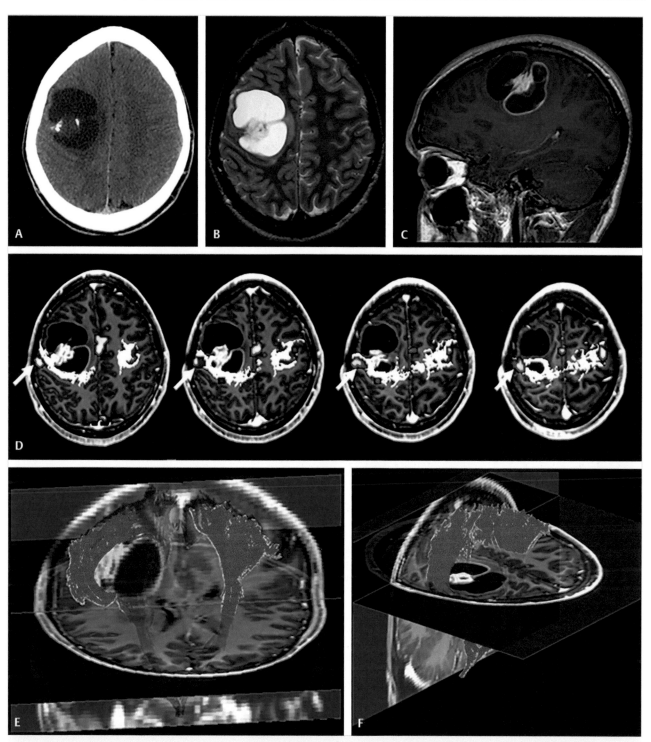

Fig. 4.8 Supratentorial pilocytic astrocytoma. (**A**) Axial *CT scan* shows a bilobed cystic lesion with an internal sepimentation and a partially calcific nodule. (**B**) Axial *T2-w* image demonstrates the mass effect of the lesion on the adjacent brain tissue. (**C**) Sagittal *T1-w* post-contrast image shows the intense and homogeneous enhancement of the solid nodule and the enhancing rim of the posterior cyst. (**D**) Four consecutive axial sections demonstrate preoperative *fMRI* cortical activations during bimanual finger tapping (red-yellow areas) and DTI tractography reconstructions of the corticospinal tracts (white) superimposed on *T1-w* images. Note the posterior displacement of the primary motor area of left hand by the lesion. (**E, F**) Three-dimensional rendering of preoperative DTI tractography shows posterior displacement of the subcortical fibers of the right corticospinal tract, wrapping the posterior cyst and lining the solid nodule.

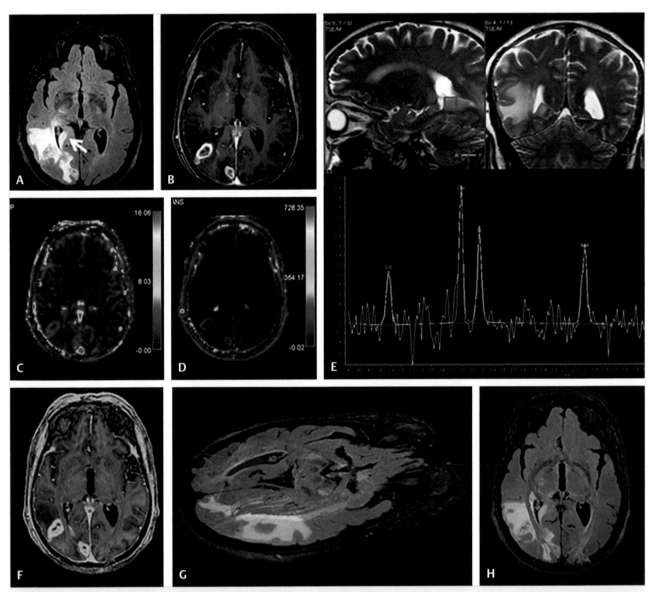

Fig. 4.9 Multifocal glioblastoma. (**A, B**) Axial *FLAIR* and *T1-w* post-contrast images demonstrate two solid nodules in the right occipital lobe with strong but irregular ring enhancement surrounding a central non-enhancing necrotic core, surrounded by heterogeneous *FLAIR* hyperintensity (*white arrow*). (**C, D**) *Dynamic-contrast enhanced PWI* plasma volume (v_p, **C**) and vascular permeability (K^{trans}, **D**) maps demonstrate increased perfusion and leakiness along the enhancing margins of the nodules. (**E**) *T2/FLAIR* heterogeneous hyperintensity surrounding the nodules is partly due to vasogenic edema; indeed, it extends along the medial wall of the occipital horn of the left lateral ventricle and the adjacent parahyppocampal gyrus. In this location (red box), *single voxel MRS* (TE = 144) shows mild elevation of Choline (Cho) and reduction of N-Acetil-Aspartate (NAA), corresponding to tumor spreading along white matter. (**F, G, H**) HARDI (high angular resolution diffusion imaging) Q-ball tractography reconstructions superimposed on post-contrast *T1-w* and *FLAIR* images enhance a high-resolution depiction of the optic pathways (orange) and of their relationships with the tumor tissue: the right optic radiation passes through the *FLAIR* hyperintensity between the two nodules, thus being infiltrated and slightly displaced medially with respect to the contralateral left optic radiation.

physiological, and metabolic information for the characterization of lesion biology and for supporting differential diagnosis.

References

1. Castellano A, Falini A. Progress in neuro-imaging of brain tumors. Curr Opin Oncol 2016;28(6):484–493
2. Haller S, Etienne L, Kövari E, Varoquaux AD, Urbach H, Becker M. Imaging of neurovascular compression syndromes: trigeminal neuralgia, hemifacial spasm, vestibular paroxysmia, and glossopharyngeal neuralgia. AJNR Am J Neuroradiol 2016;37(8):1384–1392
3. Mortini P, Gagliardi F, Bailo M, et al. Resection of tumors of the third ventricle involving the hypothalamus: effects on body mass index using a dedicated surgical approach. Endocrine 2017;57(1):138–147
4. Parizel PM, Carpentier K, Van Marck V, et al. Pneumosinus dilatans in anterior skull base meningiomas. Neuroradiology 2013;55(3):307–311

5 Patient Positioning

Francesco Ruggieri, Tommaso Zoerle, Filippo Gagliardi, Pietro Mortini, and Luigi Beretta

5.1 Introduction

Patient positioning for intracranial neurosurgical procedures represents a critical point for both the surgeon and the anesthesiologist. Some positions of the body for an extended period of time portend many intracranial, cardiovascular, or respiratory consequences that are often not well tolerated in some categories of patients. Hence a preoperative evaluation is mandatory to define any possible patient's limitation to postural and positional changes that may be required to obtain a satisfactory surgical access.

Adverse events are mainly related to peripheral nerve injury and pressure sources that must be prevented by using padding of critical areas. Positioning the head to avoid excessive rotation and flexion/extension helps to prevent neuro-vascular complications due to reduced arterial flow to the brain or reduced venous return that causes further increase in intracranial pressure due to venous engorgement at the neck level. Injuries of the eyes include corneal lesions and ischemic optic neuropathy, which is mostly seen in the prone position.

Here we describe how to perform patient positioning for intracranial surgery minimizing adverse events.

5.2 General Principles

- Any possible limitation to postural and positional changes should be assessed preoperatively.
- Principal positions for intracranial surgery include
  - Supine
  - Lateral
  - Prone
  - Sitting

- The last two may cause major physiological cardiovascular and respiratory changes.
- Positioning is performed after induction of general anesthesia and placement of monitoring systems. Endotracheal tube and vascular access must be secured carefully because they can be displaced during positioning maneuvers (**Fig. 5.1**).
- Head may be positioned on a horseshoe head holder or pins fixation to the skull (Mayfield frame). Pins application is a high pain stimulus, so an adequate anesthesia plan must be provided in order to blunt a cardiovascular response and accidental patient movements causing skin laceration and even spinal injuries.
- Padding is pivotal for prevention of pressure sores and peripheral nerve injury. Eyes protection is mandatory to prevent corneal lesions (**Fig. 5.1**).
- Intermittent pneumatic sequential compression devices are necessary both to help reduce blood pooling in the legs and to prevent deep venous thrombosis (**Fig. 5.2**).
- Serum creatine phosphokinase elevation is often observed after prolonged surgery.

5.3 Supine Decubitus

Supine decubitus is the most frequently used position in Neurosurgery. It is advised in case of pathology of the anterior skull base and frontal/parietal/temporal convexity, as well as endoscopic endonasal and intraventricular procedures. According to the disease, the head can be placed either in neutral position or slightly rotated toward the controlateral side. The neck might be either extended or flexed based on the selected approach.
- The supine position is easy and safe with minimal cardiovascular effect.

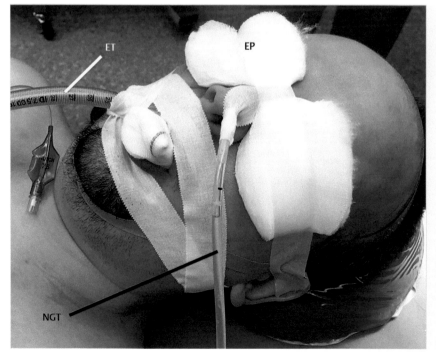

Fig. 5.1 Supine decubitus: head. Abbreviations: EP = eye protection; ET = endotracheal tube; NGT = nasogastric tube.

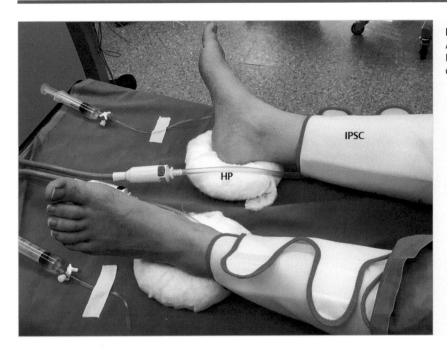

Fig. 5.2 Supine decubitus: legs. Abbreviations: HP = heel pad; IPSC = intermittent pneumatic sequential compression devices.

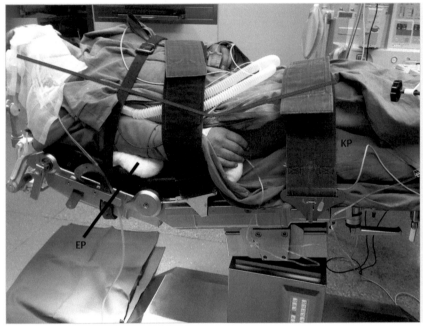

Fig. 5.3 Supine position. Abbreviations: EP = elbow pad; KP = knee pad.

- Slight head elevation improves cerebral venous outflow from the brain.
- A more physiological positioning of the lumbar spine, hips, and knees is achieved with the "lawn chair" position. It is a modification of the classical supine position with 15° angulation at the trunk and knees flexion. A roll is placed under the knees to keep them flexed and improve venous return (**Fig. 5.3**).
- Excessive neck flexion might result in tongue and pharyngeal edema. Thyromental distance must be kept greater than 3-4 cm (**Fig. 5.4**).
- Head rotation more than 45° and excessive neck extension/flexion could decrease flow into carotid and vertebral

arteries and might give subsequent spinal or cerebral ischemia. If head rotation more than 45° is required, a roll should be placed under the contralateral shoulder (**Fig. 5.5**).
- Arms should be kept alternatively adducted or abducted less than 90°, to minimize brachial plexus injury. Excessive downward traction of the shoulders must be avoided (**Fig. 5.6**).
- The hands and forearms should be kept supinated or in neutral position, to reduce external pressure on the spinal groove of the humerus and ulnar nerve. Elbows and heels must be protected with pads (**Fig. 5.6**).

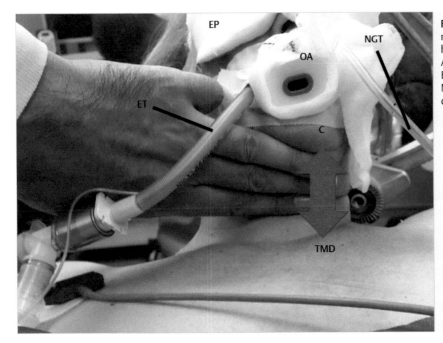

Fig. 5.4 Supine decubitus: to avoid excessive neck flexion keep thyro-mental distance higher than 3-4 cm (*arrow*).
Abbreviations: C = chin; OA = oral airway; EP = eye protection; ET = endotracheal tube; NGT = nasogastric tube; TMD = thyromental distance.

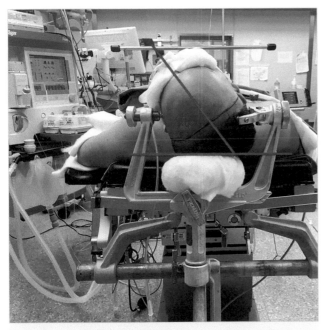

Fig. 5.5 Head should not be rotated more than 45°. A roller is positioned under the contralateral shoulder.

5.4 Lateral Decubitus

Lateral position is indicated in case of pathology involving the middle skull base as well as parieto-temporal convexity and lateral aspect of the posterior cranial fossa. The body lies with the face up, resting on the opposite side as compared to the pathology. The ipsilateral shoulder is usually elevated and the head is turned toward the contralateral side. Neck might be alternatively extended or flexed based upon the approach.

- Ventilation-perfusion mismatch in upper lung might deteriorate gas exchange in patients with functional impairment of the dependent lung.
- The high risk of brachial plexus injury and axillary artery compression of the dependent arm must be taken into consideration. Both arms on boards are positioned putting a roll under the upper chest away from the axilla.
- The arterial line must be placed on the non-dependent arm and a pulse oxymeter on the dependent arm, to verify its perfusion.
- A pillow is put between knees and ankles to prevent peroneal and saphenous nerve injuries (**Fig. 5.7**).

5.5 Park-Bench

The park-bench position is a modification of the standard lateral position; it is indicated in cases of pathology involving lateral aspect of the posterior cranial fossa and cranio-cervical junction. The body rests on the opposite side as compared to the pathology, lying on a plane which is inclined about 45° in relation to the floor. The head is flexed 30° and rotated 40-45° toward the contralateral side.

- The dependent arm is positioned in ventral position and placed on a low padded board, inserted between the table and head fixator (**Fig. 5.8**).
- The non-dependent arm is positioned on a pillow over the body (**Fig. 5.8**).
- The upper shoulder is taped toward the table.

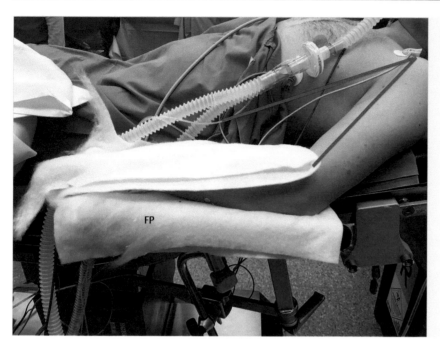

Fig. 5.6 Supine position: hand and forearm. Abbreviations: FP = forearm pad.

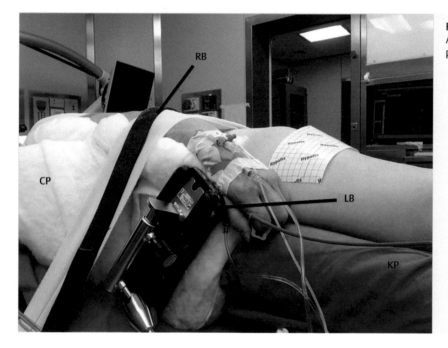

Fig. 5.7 Lateral decubitus. Abbreviations: CP = chest pad; KP = knee pad; LB = lateral buffer; RB = restraint belt.

5.6 Prone Decubitus

The prone position is used in case of pathology arising from the posterior cranial fossa and the occipital convexity and for approaches to the posterior aspect of the inter-hemispheric fissure and ventricular system. The body lies facing downward. According to the anatomy of the pathology, the head can be placed either in neutral position or slightly rotated toward the ipsilateral side. Neck might be alternatively extended or flexed based on the approach to be performed.

- The patient is anesthetized in the supine position and then is turned prone. If possible it is advisable to keep arterial line connected and pulsossimetry in place during patient positioning (**Fig. 5.9**).

- The most critical aspects, which must be taken into consideration are increased intra-abdominal pressure, decreased venous return, and increased systemic and pulmonary vascular resistance.

- A decrease in cerebral vein outflow can result in intracranial pressure elevation, increased surgical bleeding and risk of cerebral hemorrhage. Furthermore, it is associated with the development of ischemic optic neuropathy. Jugular veins and vertebral venous plexus compression can be prevented, by avoiding head down positioning and eyes compression.

- Thyromental distance must be kept as more than 3-4 cm to prevent excessive neck flexion, which can result in tongue and pharyngeal edema.

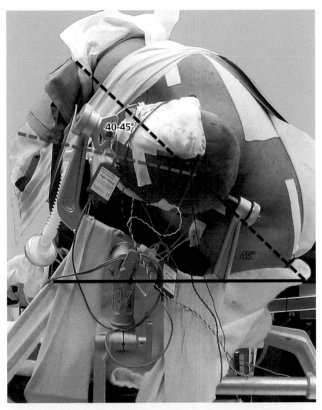

Fig. 5.8 Park-bench decubitus. The dependent arm is positioned on a board between the table and the Mayfield frame. The abundant paddings protect critical areas and the nondependent arm on which are positioned the vascular accesses and monitoring systems.

- Inferior vena cava compression should be avoided. Supporting frames for chest and pelvis, leaving the abdomen free, are advised.
- Knees are positioned on cotton doughnuts.
- Pressure sores are the most frequent complications of the prone position.
- Postoperative visual loss is a rare but devastating complication mainly due to ischemic optic neuropathy.

5.7 Sitting Decubitus

The sitting position is indicated for approaches to the pineal region as well as both the median and lateral compartments of the posterior cranial fossa. Patient lies on a sitting position with the head either in neutral or slightly flexed and rotated position, according to the approach, which must be performed. Beyond the advantage in surgical exposure in terms of parenchymal relaxation and gravity drainage of blood from the surgical field, potential position related morbidity must be taken into consideration.

- Blood pooling in the legs and decreased venous return could lead to hemodynamic instability. Semirecumbent position must be taken into consideration instead of classical sitting position. The table must be moved to the final position slowly.
- By positioning the patient in the sitting/semi-sitting position, the head is above the level of the heart, with consequent risk of air possibly being trapped in the venous system.
- A large venous air embolism may produce severe hypoxemia and hemodynamic instability by decreasing cardiac output.
- A preoperative echocardiographic evaluation is mandatory to exclude a patent foramen ovale. Intraoperative monitoring

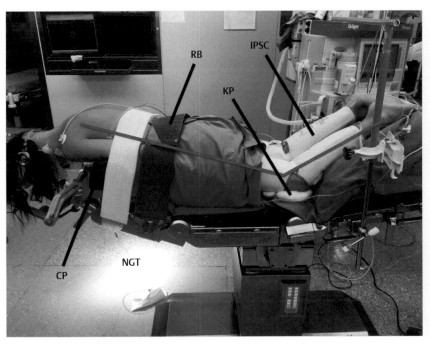

Fig. 5.9 Prone decubitus. Abbreviations: CP = chest pad; IPSC = intermittent pneumatic sequential compression; KP = knee pad; NGT = nasogastric tube; RB = restraint belt.

with transthoracic (or transesophageal) doppler and placement of an atrial catheter are recommended to detect and aspirate air embolisms.

- Thyromental distance must be kept more than 3-4 cm, to prevent excessive neck flexion, which can result in tongue and pharyngeal edema.
- Knees should be flexed to prevent peroneal nerve damage.
- The use of a pad minimizes risk of sciatic nerve compression.

References

1. American Society of Anesthesiologists Task Force on Prevention of Perioperative Peripheral Neuropathies. Practice advisory for the prevention of perioperative peripheral neuropathies: an updated report by the American Society of Anesthesiologists Task Force on prevention of perioperative peripheral neuropathies. Anesthesiology 2011; 114(4):741–754
2. Poli D, Gemma M, Cozzi S, et al. Muscle enzyme elevation after elective neurosurgery. Neurological complications of surgery and anesthesia. Br J Anaesth 2015;114:194–203
3. Zlotnik AI, Vavilala MS, Rozet I. Positioning the patient for neurosurgical operations. In: Brambrink AM, Kirsch JR, eds. Essentials of Neurosurgical Anesthesia & Critical Care. New York, NY: Springer; 2012; 151–157

6 Fundamentals of Cranial Neurosurgery

Filippo Gagliardi, Elena V. Colombo, Carmine Antonio Donofrio, Cristian Gragnaniello, Anthony J. Caputy, and Pietro Mortini

6.1 Principles of Mayfield Head Holder Positioning (Fig. 6.1)

- Variable holding pressure is used to fix the head holder and is defined by four tension rings on the outer aspect of each single pin, which should correspond to 20 Lbs/in^2 for each ring.
- Suggested holding pressure: adults 60 Lbs/in^2, children 30/40 Lbs/in^2.
- Pediatric holding pins have a smaller pinpoint compared to adults' one and they should be used for children aging up to 5 years.
- Mayfield head holder should not be used for children younger than 3 years.
- Maximum holding pressure allowed by the system: 80 Lbs/in^2.
- Mayfield head holder should not be used in case of skull fracture after head trauma.

6.1.1 Pins Positioning

- Pins should be placed away from
  - The course of the skin incision.
  - Pneumatized sinuses (*e.g.*, frontal sinus, mastoid).
  - Pterion and cranial sutures (considered as points of least resistance).
  - Dural venous sinuses and temporal artery because of risk of vascular damage.
- The line connecting the single pin and the center of the double pin clamp should bisect the intersection between the main sagittal and coronal diameters of the skull (**Fig. 6.2**).

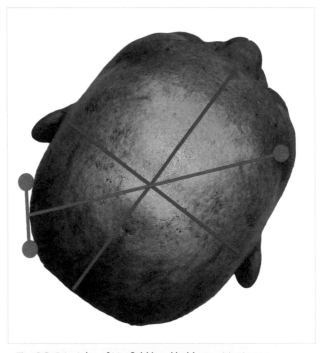

Fig. 6.2 Principles of Mayfield head holder positioning. Blue lines show the sagittal and coronal planes. Red lines with dots represent the Mayfield holder with its pins.

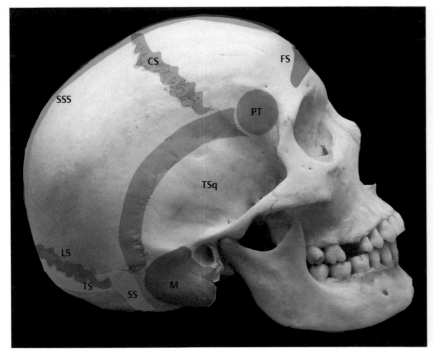

Fig. 6.1 Principles of Mayfield head holder positioning.
Abbreviations: CS = coronal suture; FS = frontal sinus; LS = lambdoid suture; M = mastoid; PT = pterion; TS = transverse sinus; TSq = temporal squama; SS = sigmoid sinus; SSS = superior sagittal sinus. *Colors:* Blue area = dural sinuses; Purple area = areas of least resistance.

6.2 Types of Skin Incisions (Fig. 6.3)

- **Linear incisions.** Incision should run parallel to the direction of the principal subcutaneous arteries (*i.e.*, temporal and occipital arteries) to preserve the regional vascular supply.

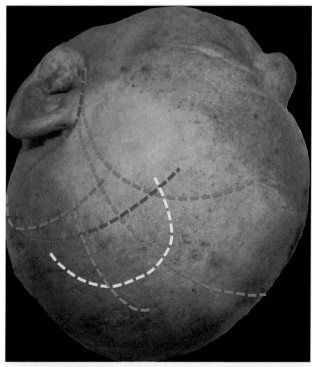

Fig. 6.3 Skin incisions.
Lines: Blue dotted lines (linear incisions); Green dotted line (C-shaped incision); Red dotted line (question mark incision); Yellow dotted line (horseshoe incision).

- **Horseshoe incision.** AKA U-shaped incision. The concavity of the incision trajectory must be directed downward to preserve the regional vascular supply. It reduces the mechanical tension on the skin as compared to linear incision.
- **Question mark incision.** It is usually performed for surgical approaches to the fronto-temporal region and skull base. It starts <1 cm in front of the tragus at the level of the zygoma, runs posteriorly around the superior margin of the ear and turns anteriorly after reaching the posterior aspect of the pinna. Incision ends on the midline just behind the hairline.
- **C-shaped incision.** It is usually performed for lateral approaches to the posterior cranial fossa and cerebellopontine angle. The incision starts 1 cm above the ear, at the lower temporal region, runs around the pinna toward the mastoid tip and turns down- and forward until it reaches the anterior margin of the sternocleidomastoid muscle. The concavity of incision trajectory is tailored according to the approach, which has to be performed.

6.3 Extracranial Soft Tissues Dissection (Fig. 6.4)

6.3.1 Extracranial Soft Tissues Encountered During Superficial Dissection:

- Skin
- Subcutaneous fat tissue
- Galea capitis (*aka* galea aponeurotica)
- Loose connective tissue
- Pericranium

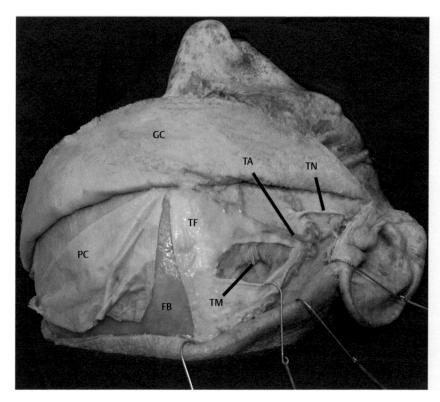

Fig. 6.4 Cranial soft tissues dissection. Abbreviations: FB = frontal bone; GC = galea capitis; PC = pericranium; TA = temporal artery; TF = temporal fascia; TM = temporal muscle; TN = temporal nerve.

6.3.2 Specific Anatomical Considerations

- The **superficial temporal artery** runs anteriorly to the tragus, in the subcutaneous tissue, lying on the superficial temporal fascia and bifurcates into its frontal and parietal branches at the temporal region, just 2 cm above the zygomatic arch.
  - The corresponding vein and the fronto-temporal branch of the facial nerve run anteriorly to the artery.
  - To preserve these structures, the skin incision is generally performed 0.5 to 1 cm anteriorly to the tragus.
- In the temporal region, the galea capitis divides into
  - The **deep temporal fascia** is located beneath the temporal muscle (TM) on the bone surface. It carries the blood supply to the temporal muscle.
  - The **superficial temporal fascia**, which covers the entire TM, goes from the zygomatic arch to the superior temporal line. The anterior third of the fascia is composed of two layers separated by the **interfascial fat pad** (a sickle-shaped layer of fat); here the frontal branch of the facial nerve and the deep temporal vessels run. The two layers can be recognized at the temporal attachment on the orbital rim.

6.4 Fundamental Techniques of Temporal Muscle Dissection (Figs. 6.5–6.7)

- Three different methods of temporal muscle dissection are described: interfascial, submuscular, and sub-fascial. We remind the reader to the dedicated chapter to see the nuances of the different techniques and their advantages **(see Chapter 8)**.

6.4.1 Main Principles

- Allows to preserve the frontal branch of the facial nerve and to optimize temporal bone and zygomatic arch exposure.
- The interfascial fat pad marks the separation of the superficial temporal fascia into its superior and inferior layers.
- The two layers are smoothly separated with a dissector starting from the pterion.
- They are then cut along their junction until their insertion at the superior margin of the zygomatic arch. The fat pad is exposed and the Yasargil vein is recognized.
- The deep temporal fascia together with the muscle are incised starting at the pterion and following the course of the superior temporal line until the zygomatic process of the temporal bone.
- The temporal muscle is subperiostally dissected from the bone, together with the superficial and the deep fascia, starting from the pterion.

6.5 Technique of Supraorbital Nerve Preservation (Figs. 6.8, 6.9)

- The supraorbital nerve may exit the skull through either a notch or a true foramen, which may be located at the junction between the medial and the lateral two thirds of the upper orbital rim. The supraorbital artery runs medial to it.
- If a supraorbital foramen is present, the nerve has to be freed to avoid damage during orbital osteotomies.
- To open the supraorbital foramen a chisel is used, while protecting the nerve and the artery.
- Once freed, the nerve is then gently mobilized and reflected anteriorly with the skin flap.

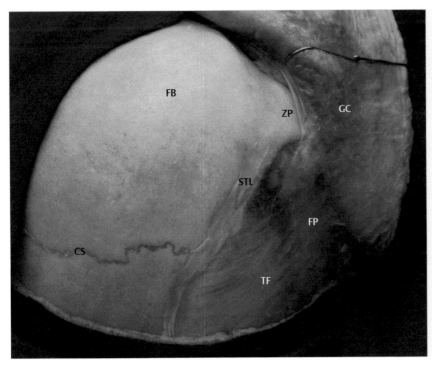

Fig. 6.5 Basic technique of temporal muscle interfascial dissection. **Step 1.** Abbreviations: CS = coronal suture; FB = frontal bone; FP = fat pad; GC = galea capitis; STL = superior temporal line; TF = temporal fascia; ZP = zygomatic process of the frontal bone.

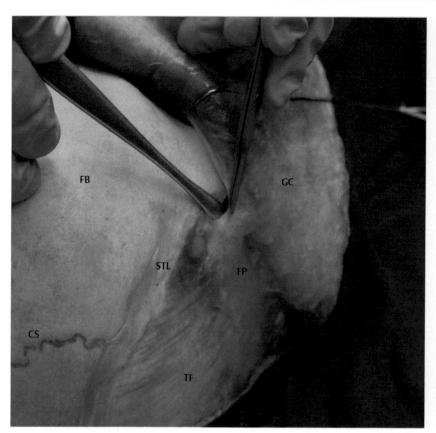

Fig. 6.6 Basic technique of temporal muscle interfascial dissection. **Step 2.**
Abbreviations: CS = coronal suture; FB = frontal bone; FP = fat pad; GC = galea capitis; STL = superior temporal line; TF = temporal fascia.

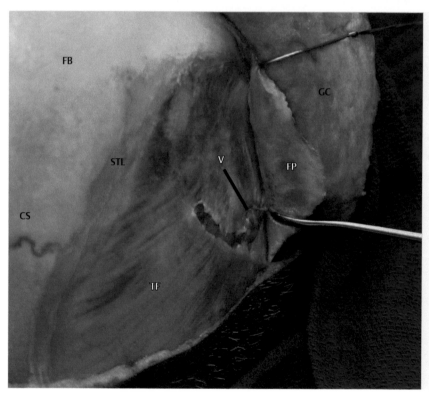

Fig. 6.7 Basic technique of temporal muscle interfascial dissection. **Step 3.**
Abbreviations: CS = coronal suture; FB = frontal bone; FP = fat pad; GC = galea capitis; STL = superior temporal line; TF = temporal fascia; V = vein.

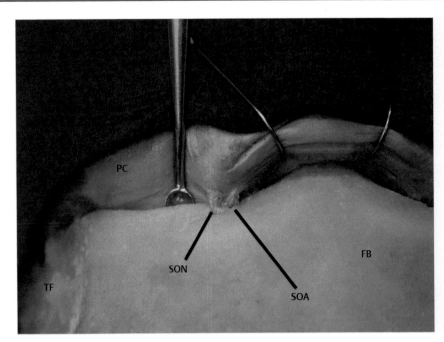

Fig. 6.8 Supraorbital nerve identification. Abbreviations: FB = frontal bone; PC = pericranium; SOA =supraorbital artery; SON = supraorbital nerve; TF = temporal muscle fascia.

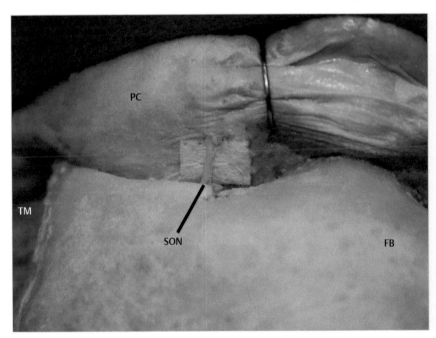

Fig. 6.9 Dissection of the supraorbital nerve and final view.The nerve has been mobilized from its notch in the frontal bone with the use of a dissector and under no tension. Abbreviations: FB = frontal bone; PC = pericranium; SON = supraorbital nerve; TM = temporal muscle.

6.6 Fundamentals of Harvesting A Pericranial Pedicled Flap (Figs. 6.10, 6.11)

- The length and width of the pericranial flap that one can harvest mostly depend on the skin incision used for the specific approach being utilized. Preservation and preparation of this layer is of utmost importance as it represents vascularized tissue that can be used to repair skull base defects. Following the principle that whatever has been opened will have to be closed in the end and that you truly never have enough pericranium, the incision of the pericranium can be extended way beyond the skin incision by elevating the skin

and sliding below it as far as it can be done without any skin disruption.
- Pericranium is cut 2 cm posteriorly to the margin of the skin incision and along the superior temporal lines bilaterally. It is dissected from the bone, taking care to preserve its anatomical integrity.
- It is very important to use a wide periosteal elevator and a lot of irrigation to safely elevate this flap, with special attention paid to the areas covering sutures that will be inevitably strongly adherent to the bone.
- It is then reflected anteriorly to maintain its blood supply, which arises from frontal vascular pedicles such as the anterior branches of the superficial temporal, supraorbital and supratrochlear arteries.

39

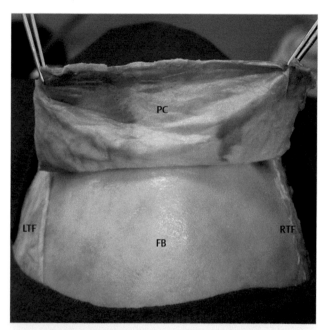

Fig. 6.10 Dissection and elevation of the pedicled pericranial flap. **Step 1.**
Abbreviations: FB = frontal bone; LTF = left temporal muscle fascia; PC = pericranium; RTF = right temporal muscle fascia.

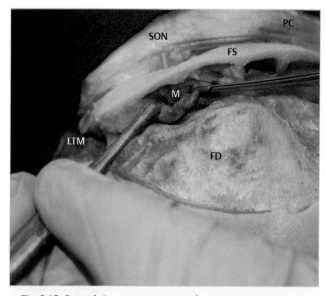

Fig. 6.12 Frontal sinus mucosa removal.
Abbreviations: FD = frontal dura; FS = frontal sinus; LTM = left temporal muscle; M = mucosa; PC = pericranium, SON = supraorbital nerve.

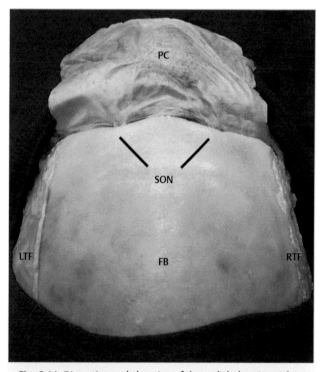

Fig. 6.11 Dissection and elevation of the pedicled pericranial flap. **Step 2.**
Abbreviations: FB = frontal bone; LTF = left temporal muscle fascia; PC = pericranium; RTF = right temporal muscle fascia; SON = supraorbital nerves.

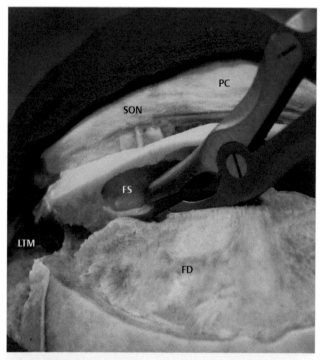

Fig. 6.13 Removal of the posterior wall of the frontal sinus with large rongeurs.
Abbreviations: FD = frontal dura; FS = frontal sinus; LTM = left temporal muscle; PC = pericranium, SON = supraorbital nerve.

6.7 Fundamentals of Skull Base Reconstruction with Pedicled Flap (Figs. 6.12, 6.13)

• Skull base reconstruction with pedicled pericranial flap is indicated in cases of opening of pneumatized sinuses and skull base reconstruction after skull base surgery, in order to reduce the rate of infection, cerebrospinal fluid leak, pneumocephalus and late mucocele formation.

- If the paranasal sinuses are violated during a craniotomy, the mucosa is exenterated before dural opening and the posterior wall of the frontal sinus is removed (frontal sinus cranialization).
- The ostium of the sinus is plugged with the pedicled pericranial flap, which is held in place with fibrin glue.

- All instruments used during the procedure are kept aside and discarded for the remainder of the operation to lower the risk of infections.

6.8 Burr Holes Placement: Technical Principles (Figs. 6.14–6.16)

- **Burr holes should be placed**
  - ○ Behind the hairline (aesthetic reason).

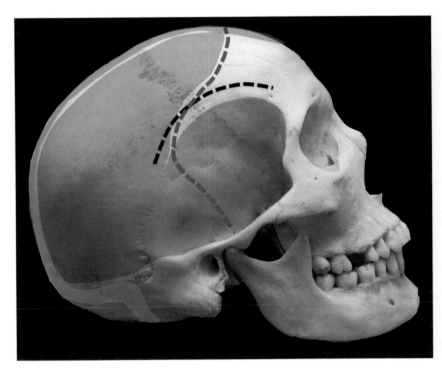

Fig. 6.14 Burr holes placement.
Colors and lines: Black dotted line = superior temporal line; Blue area = dural sinuses; Pink area = suggested area for burr holes placement; Red dotted line = hair line.

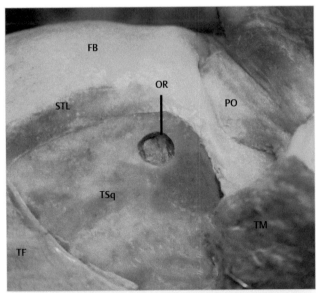

Fig. 6.15 McCarty hole.
Abbreviations: FB = frontal bone; OR = orbital roof; PO = periorbit; STL = superior temporal line; TF = temporal fascia; TM = temporal muscle; TSq = temporal squama.

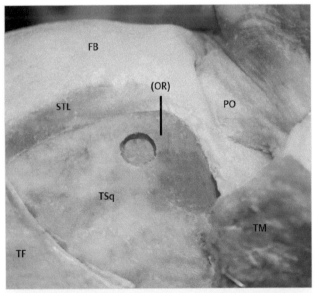

Fig. 6.16 Dandy hole.
Abbreviations: FB = frontal bone; (OR) = projection of orbital roof; PO = periorbit; STL = superior temporal line; TF = temporal fascia; TM = temporal muscle; TSq = temporal squama.

- Below the superior temporal line (aesthetic reason).
- Away from pneumatized areas (*i.e.,* frontal sinus, mastoid) and dural venous sinuses to avoid opening of paranasal sinuses or vascular damage, respectively.
- **Types of pterional holes**
  - **McCarty burr hole** is used to expose at the same time the anterior cranial fossa and the orbit. It is located 1 cm behind the fronto-zygomatic suture and along the fronto-sphenoidal suture.
  - **Dandy burr hole** is generally used for standard pterional craniotomy. It is placed just above the fronto-sphenoidal suture, below the superior temporal line and posteriorly to the fronto-zygomatic suture.

6.9 Craniotomy: Technical Principles (Figs. 6.17, 6.18)

- **General principles**
  - The pneumatized paranasal cavities, dural venous sinuses and the temporal squama are usually considered areas of concern when performing a craniotomy because of the potential risk of damaging vital structures such as the dural sinuses, of the increase of chances of infections or cerebrospinal (CSF) leaks, or of plunging into the temporal lobe, respectively.
  - Before using the craniotome, the dura has to be carefully detached from the inner table of the skull to reduce the risk of dural tearing.
  - The craniotome is directed perpendicularly to the skull surface.
  - The tip of the instrument is placed between the dura mater and the bone and it is slightly tilted backward 5-10°.
- **Principles of craniotomies over dural sinuses**

- Craniotomies over dural sinuses should be performed with a clear sequence of burr holes and bone cuts, in order to avoid injuries to the underlying dura.
- Even this needs to follow the principle of doing all the work away from the sinus first, so that if this would be

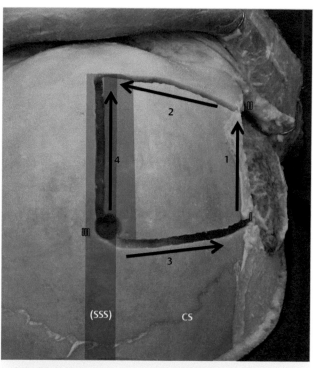

Fig. 6.18 Craniotomy over dural sinus. Case example. Abbreviations: I = first burr hole; II = second burr hole; III = third burr hole; 1 = first cut; 2 = second cut; 3 = third cut; 4 = fourth cut; CS = coronal suture; SSS = superior sagittal sinus. *Colors:* Blue area = sinus projection; Orange area = area at risk for draining veins

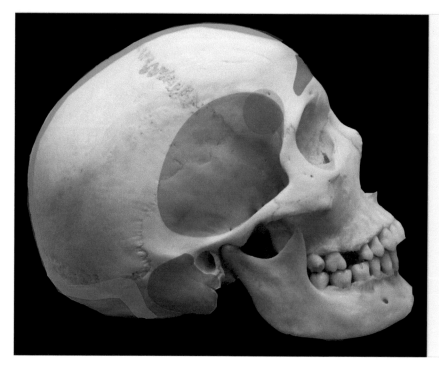

Fig. 6.17 Areas of concern for craniotomy. Colors: Blue area = dural sinuses; Green area = area of high risk of dural tearing; Pink area = area of minimum thickness of the bone and high risk of plunging; Red area: pneumatized areas.

injured the bone flap could be turned immediately and the bleeding dealt with promptly.

❖ **Burr holes**
  • **I:** Away from the sinus.
  • **II:** Over the sinus.
❖ **Craniotomy cuts**
  • **I:** Far from the sinus.
  • **II:** Starting from the sinus and going away.
  • **III:** Over the sinus.

6.10 Dural Tenting Technique (Figs. 6.19, 6.20)

• Dural tenting reduces the risk of progressive detachment of the dura from the bone and the consequent collection of blood in the epidural space. It also prevents the retraction of the dura, which can make the dural closure more challenging.
• Several holes are made on the margins of the craniotomy (about 2 mm in thickness) at a distance of approximately 1 cm from each other, away from venous sinuses and air pneumatized cavities.
• A free blade of smaller diameter to the one used for raising the bone flap is utilized for placing the holes.
• Holes must be placed close to the bone margin and directed obliquely, from the outer cortical table to the spongious bone, protecting the dura with a retractor to avoid damage to the underlying structures.
• Stiches (3/0, non-absorbable) are anchored to the dura, as close as possible to the bony margin, and then passed through the holes.

6.11 Dural Opening (Fig. 6.21)

• The dura is usually opened in a C-shaped fashion, keeping the pedicle toward the cranial base or the dural sinuses.

In areas such as the posterior fossa an X-shaped incision is preferred.
• The dura should be opened away from the bone (at least 2-4 mm) to facilitate dural closure.
• The dura is first incised with a small knife in a "safe point" (away from venous sinuses or underlying vessels, as well as neoplastic masses) and then it is gently cut with scissors, using cottonoid strips to protect the underlying neurovascular structures.

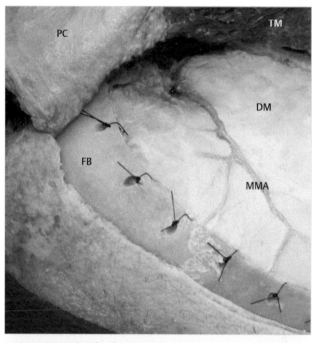

Fig. 6.20 Stiches for dural tenting.
Abbreviations: DM = dura mater; FB = frontal bone; MMA = middle meningeal artery; PC = pericranium; TM = temporal muscle.

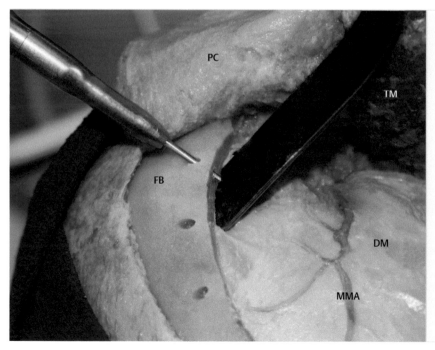

Fig. 6.19 Hole placement for dural tenting. Abbreviations: DM = dura mater; FB = frontal bone; MMA = middle meningeal artery; PC = pericranium; TM = temporal muscle.

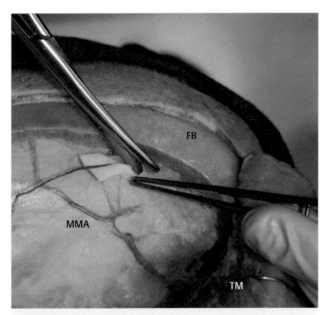

Fig. 6.21 Dural opening.
Abbreviations: FB = frontal bone; MMA = middle meningeal artery; TM = temporal muscle.

• The dura is then reflected and gently tented, paying attention not to compress underlying dural sinuses or to stretch draining veins.

References

1. Fossett D, Caputy AJ. Operative neurosurgical anatomy. New York, NY: Thieme Medical Publisher; 2002
2. Sekhar LN, Fessler RG. Atlas of Neurosurgical Techniques. Brain. Volume 1. New York, NY: Thieme Medical Publishers; 2016
3. Snyderman CH, Janecka IP, Sekhar LN, Sen CN, Eibling DE. Anterior cranial base reconstruction: role of galeal and pericranial flaps. Laryngoscope 1990;100(6):607–614
4. Yaşargil MG, Reichman MV, Kubik S. Preservation of the frontotemporal branch of the facial nerve using the interfascial temporalis flap for pterional craniotomy. Technical article. J Neurosurg 1987;67(3):463–466

7 Skin Incisions, Head and Neck Soft-Tissue Dissection

Virginio Garcia-Martinez, Luis Porras-Estrada, Carmen Lopez-Sanchez, and Virginio Garcia-Lopez

7.1 Introduction

An adequate planning of skin incision and selected flaps are essential in Neurosurgery. In order to do that, it is important to keep in mind the vascular pedicles of the scalp from the cervical region to the orbit. We also must consider the distribution of nerves, as well as muscle fascias and muscle insertions.

Ideally, all incisions should be hidden behind the hairline for cosmetic reasons.

Since specific cutaneous flaps could be performed through different myofascial and muscle incisions, the overall standard should consider flaps with a wide support, respecting a vascular-nervous axis in order to guarantee its functional preservation. This peculiarity optimizes flap viability, thus avoiding possible functional and/or aesthetic sequelae.

In this chapter, we will analyze head and neck soft-tissue structures, including vascular-nervous patterns, establishing the precise location for incisions and flaps used in Neurosurgery.

7.2 Soft-Tissue Structures

Head and neck soft-tissue structures consist of the following layers
- Skin (epidermis and dermis).
- Subcutaneous fibro-adipose tissue or superficial muscle-aponeurotic system (and facial muscles).
- Epicranial aponeurosis or galea.
- Temporal or deep fascia (including superficial and deep layers).
- Muscles.
- Periosteum.

7.3 Cutaneous Cranial Incisions

- **Longitudinal incisions (Fig. 7.1)**
  - Midline-suboccipital incision (**Fig. 7.1A**).
  - Retromastoid (retrosigmoid) incision (**Fig. 7.1B**).
  - Temporal incision (**Fig. 7.1C**).
- **L and/or S-shaped incisions (Fig. 7.1)**

Applied for:
- ***Inter-hemispheric approaches:*** A sagittal incision is followed by a limb orientated towards the lesion side (**Fig. 7.1D**).
- ***Unilateral posterior fossa approaches:*** A midline suboccipital incision is followed by a limb starting from the *Inion*, and running along the superior nuchal line to the mastoid process (**Fig. 7.1E**), also known as "hockey stick incision."

When **L-shaped** incisions are not sufficient for surgical exposure, **S-shaped** incisions might be considered; they are performed by extending the incision with an additional opposed limb to allow a wider exposure (**Fig. 7.1D**). Some surgeons also prefer a **lazy S-shaped** incision to those with very sharp turns, especially on the convexity for superior healing and reduced risk of infections.

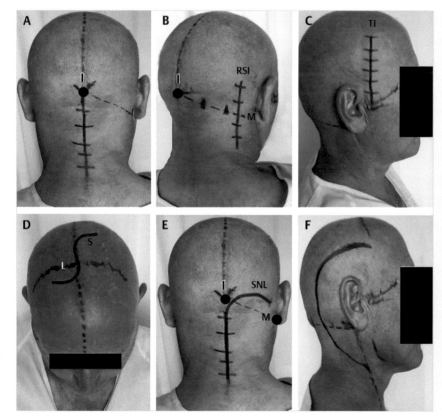

Fig. 7.1 Longitudinal incisions. (**A**) Midline-suboccipital incision: caudal to the inion. (**B**) Retromastoid (retrosigmoid) incision: longitudinal vertical incision at the level of the lateral third of the line joining the inion and the mastoid tip. (**C**) Temporal incision: vertical incision from the zygomatic arch (1 cm anterior to the tragus) and extended as needed. (**D**) Longitudinal incision with a lateral limb and/or S-shaped incision (longitudinal incision with two opposite limbs). (**E**) Midline suboccipital incision followed by a limb from the inion along the superior nuchal line to the mastoid process also known as "hockey stick incision." (**F**) Combined post-auricular C-shaped incision oriented to skull base approaches, from the margin of the sternocleidomastoid muscle to the superior temporal line in most cases. This incision can be combined with others to extend the approach to the anterior and middle cranial fossa, so it is important to preserve the vascularity of both anterior and posterior flaps. Abbreviations: I = inion; L = longitudinal incision; M = mastoid; RSI = retrosigmoid incision; S = S-shaped incision; SNL = superior nuchal line; TI = temporal incision.

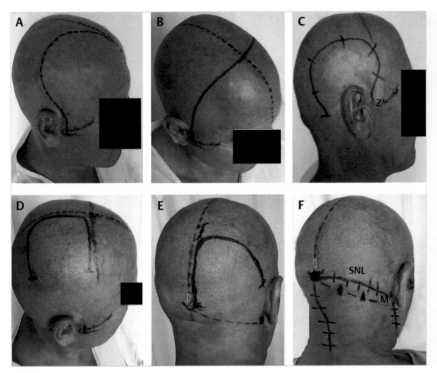

Fig. 7.2 C-shaped incisions. **(A)** Fronto-temporal: tragus - temporal line - midline. **(B)** Bicoronal. **(C)** Temporal: tragus - temporal line - mastoid process. **(D)** Parietal. **(E)** Occipital. **(F)** Horse-shoe incision. Abbreviations: I = inion; M = mastoid; SNL = superior nuchal line; Z = zygoma.

- **C-shaped incisions or cutaneous flaps (Fig. 7.2)**
  - Fronto-temporal (**Fig. 7.2A**)
  - Bicoronal (**Fig. 7.2B**)
  - Temporal (**Fig. 7.2C**)
  - Parietal (**Fig. 7.2D**)
  - Occipital (**Fig. 7.2E**)
  - Horseshoe incision (**Fig. 7.2F**)

In surgical anatomy, the dissection techniques and approaches have to be planned thoroughly, in order to obtain a successful reconstruction and prevent possible complications. The general planning should include

- Sufficiently wide incisions and cutaneous flaps.
- Avoidance of excessive edge tractions.
- Care to preserve myofascial and pericranial structures integrity.

The subgaleal layer is very important for several reasons. This virtual space is almost avascular, easily detachable, resistant to self-retaining retractors, and protects the related vascular-nervous pedicles. By means of subgaleal detachments we can obtain extensive layers of pericranium **(see Chapter 6)**. This is of great relevance as the replacement of the dura mater, since this may have to be removed in several instances. Furthermore, it is very useful both for sinuses occlusion in frontal exposures before dural opening and skull base approaches.

7.4 Cranial Vascular-Nervous Axes

Several vascular pedicles, originating from the external carotid artery, reach the scalp. They establish anastomosis among each other and with the opposite side.

7.4.1 Classification

- **Anterior group**
  - Supraorbital pedicle (supraorbital artery and lateral branch of supraorbital nerve).
  - Medial-frontal pedicle (supratrochlear artery branches and medial branch of supraorbital nerve).
- **Lateral group**
  - Temporal pedicle (superficial temporal artery and auriculo-temporal nerve).
  - Mastoid pedicle (posterior auricular artery and lesser occipital nerve).
- **Posterior group**
  - Occipital pedicle (occipital artery, greater occipital nerve and medial branch of the third cervical dorsal nerve).

7.5 Vascular-Nervous Structures of the Neck

- Cervical plexus (in particular, the great auricular nerve).
- Facial nerve (VII cranial nerve): mandibular branch.
- Spinal accessory nerve.
- Carotid sheath.
- Vertebral artery and glossopharyngeal (IX), vagus (X) and hypoglossal (XII) cranial nerves.

7.6 Flaps and Vascular-Nervous Axes

- At the **frontal level**, in case of orbital exposure, the periosteum must be detached reaching the supraorbital notch (**Fig. 7.3**) (**see Chapter 6**).

- At the **temporal level**, just above the zygomatic arch, the superficial temporal artery appears subcutaneously. The temporal and frontal branches of the facial nerve run superficial to the zygomatic arch, at about 2 cm from the tragus, and run parallel and anterior to the superficial temporal artery (**Fig. 7.4**).

Therefore, the incision must preserve the frontal branch of the facial nerve, by sectioning the superficial layer of deep temporal fascia, avoiding undesirable eyebrow asymmetry.

Immediately after this step, the temporal muscle is detached leaving a cuff of muscle for further reconstruction (**Fig. 7.5**).

- At occipital level (**Figs. 7.6, 7.7**) attention should be paid to the occipital artery and greater occipital nerve. Its injury may lead to a sensitive alteration or neuralgic pain at the ipsilateral occipital region. Artery and nerve are located about 3 cm lateral to the inion, between trapezius muscle fibers.

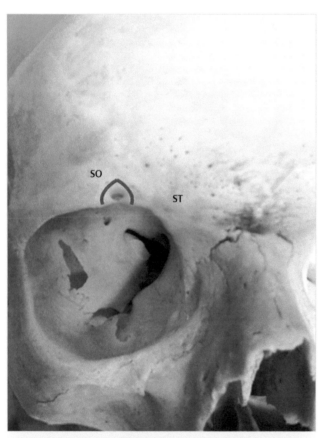

Fig. 7.3 Frontal view of the orbital fossa. Note the "V" cut must be performed when the supraorbital foramen is present. Abbreviations: SO = supraorbital area; ST = supratrochlear area.

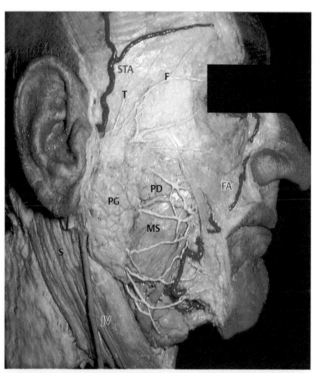

Fig. 7.4 Lateral sub-fascial dissection in a cadaveric specimen. Abbreviations: F = frontal branches of facial nerve; FA = facial artery; JV = jugular vein; MS = masseter muscle; PD = parotid duct; PG = parotid gland; S = sternocleidomastoid muscle; STA = superficial temporal artery; T = temporal branches of facial nerve.

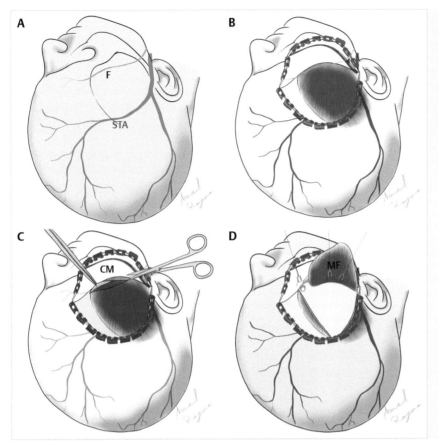

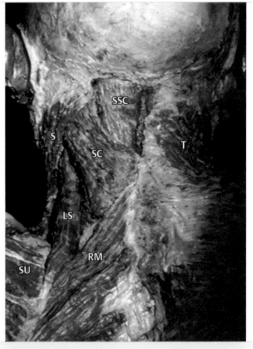

Fig. 7.5 **(A–D)** Schematic surgical view of the temporal approach showing the incision to preserve the superficial temporal artery and the frontal branch of the facial nerve. The superficial layer of deep temporal fascia is sectioned leaving a cuff of muscle for further re-approximation of the muscle flap. Abbreviations: CM = cuff of muscle; F = frontal branch of the facial nerve; MF = muscle flap; STA = superficial temporal artery. (Figure provided courtesy of Dr. Manuel Royano Sanchez.)

This region contains three muscle layers:
- **Superficial layer:** Sternocleidomastoid muscle and splenius capitis (**Figs. 7.6, 7.7A**).
- **Middle layer:** Longissimus capitis and semispinalis capitis (**Fig. 7.7B**).
- **Deep layer:** Rectus capitis posterior major, obliquus capitis superior and obliquus capitis inferior (**Figs. 7.7C, 7.7D**).

The muscles of the deep layer define the suboccipital triangle, where the V3 horizontal segment of the vertebral artery and the first cervical nerve dorsal ramus can be exposed. The greater occipital nerve appears below, in ascending direction.

7.7 Latero-Cervical Flaps

Cranial incisions reaching the latero-cervical region should avoid any injury to the carotid sheath and cranial nerves.

The basic procedure involves a post-auricular C-shaped incision, which runs from the fronto-temporal region to the anterior edge of the sternocleidomastoid muscle (**Fig. 7.1F**); it is performed for approaches directed toward the cavernous sinus and middle cranial fossa, temporal region, posterior cranial fossa, mastoid process, occipito-cervical region, carotid sheath and descending cranial nerves. Through this flap, extended middle fossa approach, mastoidectomy, exposure of posterior fossa and upper cervical region, as well as cervical vascular-nervous control can be performed.

As key references during the dissection, the surgeon must pay attention to the posterior edge of the sternocleidomastoid muscle (**Fig. 7.8**), identifying the greater auricular nerve, 2-3 cm below the mastoid tip. The transverse process of the atlas (C1)

Fig. 7.6 Dorsal superficial dissection in a cadaveric specimen showing trapezius muscle fibers orientation as well as sternocleidomastoid, splenius capitis, semispinalis capitis, levator scapulae, rhomboid minor and supraspinatus muscles in the left side. Abbreviations: LS = levator scapulae; RM = rhomboid minor; S = sternocleidomastoid muscle; SSC = semispinalis capitis; SU = supraspinatus muscle; T = trapezius muscle; SC = splenius capitis.

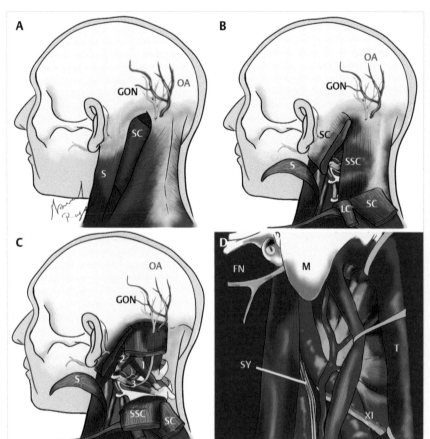

Fig. 7.7 Schematic drawing showing the lateral aspect of the head and neck to indicate the muscular layers. **(A)** Sternoclei-domastoid muscle and splenius capitis. **(B)** Longissimus capitis and semispinalis capitis. Please note that longissimus capitis attaches superiorly to the posterior aspect of the mastoid process. **(C)** Rectus capitis posterior major, obliquus capitis superior and obliquus capitis inferior. Greater occipital nerve and occipital artery. **(D)** Lateral view to indicate the mastoid process, facial nerve, trapezius muscle as well as cranial nerves X, XI and XII and sympathetic cervical component.

Abbreviations: 1 = rectus capitis posterior major; 2 = obliquus capitis superior; 3 = obliquus capitis inferior; FN = facial nerve; GON = greater occipital nerve; LC = longissimus capitis; M = mastoid; OA = occipital artery; S = sternocleidomastoid muscle; SC = splenius capitis; SSC = semispinalis capitis; SY = sympathetic cervical component; T = trapezius muscle; XI = accessory nerve. (Figure provided courtesy of Dr. Manuel Royano Sanchez.)

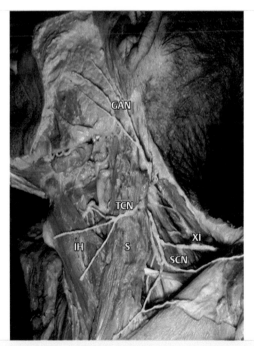

Fig. 7.8 Preparation of a dissection in a cadaveric specimen to observe the superficial branches of the cervical plexus in relation with the sternocleidomastoid and infra-hyoid muscles. XI cranial nerve runs to the trapezius muscle.
Abbreviations: GAN = greater auricular nerve; IH = infra-hyoid muscles; S = sternocleidomastoid muscle; SCN = supraclavicular nerve; TCN = transverse cutaneous nerve; XI = eleventh cranial nerve.

must be recognized (the tip can be palpated) to identify, about 1 cm infero-lateral to it, the XI cranial nerve running between the jugular vein and digastric muscle (posterior belly) and reaching sternocleidomastoid muscle medially.

The anatomic landmarks to identify the VII cranial nerve include the following:
- 1 cm ventral-caudal to "the pointer" (the tip of the external canal cartilage).
- 1 cm medial to the ventral edge of the posterior belly of digastric muscle.
- 7 mm distal to the end point of tympano-mastoid fissure (**Fig. 7.7D**).

Any cranial surgery must be carefully planned by choosing the most appropriate incisions and flaps and by performing a thorough dissection by layers. A wide anatomical knowledge of the anatomy is absolutely necessary to achieve a successful result. Muscular, vascular and nervous complications should be avoided by all means in order to prevent ischemia and/or nerve lesions.

References

1. Fukushima T, Bloch JI. Manual of skull base dissection. AF1996. Neurovideo Inc
2. Gray H, Standring S, Ellis H, et al. Gray's Anatomy: the anatomical basis of clinical practice. Edinburgh: Elsevier Churchill Livingstone;2005
3. Mitz V, Peyronie M. The superficial musculo-aponeurotic system (SMAS) in the parotid and cheek area. Plast Reconstr Surg 1976;58(1):80–88

8 Techniques of Temporal Muscle Dissection

Marcio S. Rassi, Paulo A. S. Kadri, Claudio V. Sorrilha, and Luis A. B. Borba

8.1 Introduction

Temporal muscle preservation is a key point in planning surgical approaches to the fronto-temporal convexity as well as to the anterior and middle cranial fossa.

Adopting adequate dissection techniques aims to improve surgical exposure, preserve anatomical and functional integrity of superficial temporal neurovascular structures, optimizing further reconstruction and cosmetic results.

8.2 Objectives of Temporal Muscle Preservation

- Optimize the surgical exposure.
- Preserve functionality.
- Avoid injuries to the superficial temporal artery.
- Avoid injuries to the frontotemporal branch of the facial nerve.
- Prevent cerebrospinal fluid (CSF) leak.
- Preserve craniofacial symmetry.

8.3 Temporal Muscle Anatomy

To better understand the general principles underlining surgical techniques of muscle dissection the temporal muscle anatomy must be analyzed.

- **Temporal muscle is formed by four structures** (Fig. 8.1)
  - Main portion.
  - Anterior medial bundle.
  - Anterior lateral bundle.
  - Middle lateral bundle.

- **Blood supply to muscle fibers** (Fig. 8.2)
  - Middle temporal artery: branch of the superficial temporal artery.

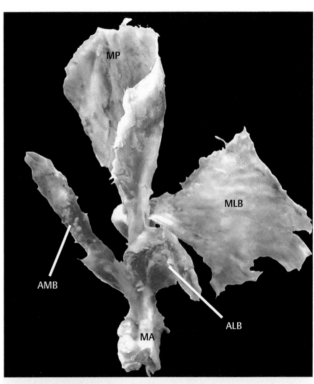

Fig. 8.1 The four portions of the temporal muscle. Abbreviations: ALB = anterior lateral bundle; AMB = anterior medial bundle; MA = mandible; MLB = middle lateral bundle; MP = main portion.

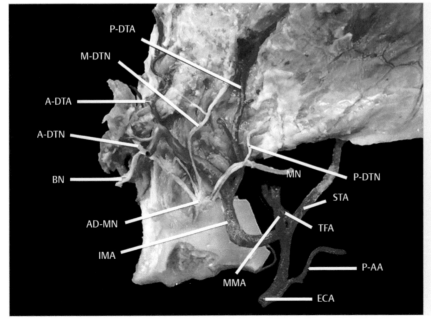

Fig. 8.2 Blood supply and innervation of the temporal muscle. (Reproduced with permission from Kadri PAS, Al-Mefty O. The anatomical basis for surgical preservation of temporal muscle. J Neurosurg 2004; 100 (3): 517–522.)
Abbreviations: A-DTA = anterior deep temporal artery; A-DTN = anterior deep temporal nerve; AD-MN = anterior division of mandibular nerve; BN = buccal nerve; ECA = external carotid artery; IMA = internal maxillary artery; M-DTN = middle deep temporal nerve; MMA = middle meningeal artery; MN = mandibular nerve; P-AA = posterior auricular artery; P-DTA = posterior deep temporal artery; P-DTN = posterior deep temporal nerve; STA = superficial temporal artery; TFA = transverse facial artery.

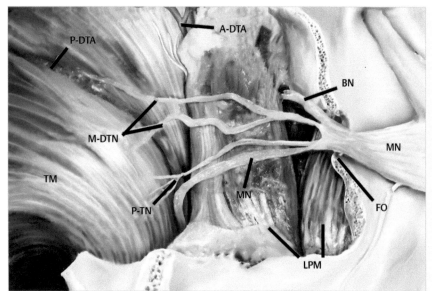

Fig. 8.3 Innervation of the temporal muscle (Reproduced with permission from Kadri PAS, Al-Mefty O. The anatomical basis for surgical preservation of temporal muscle. J Neurosurg 2004; 100 (3): 517–522.) Abbreviations: A-DTA = anterior deep temporal artery; BN = buccal nerve; FO = foramen ovale; LPM = lateral pterygoid muscle; M-DTN = middle deep temporal nerve; MN = mandibular nerve; P-DTA = posterior deep temporal artery; P-TN = posterior temporal nerve; TM =temporal muscle.

○ Anterior and posterior deep temporal arteries: branches of the internal maxillary artery.

- **Innervation** (**Fig. 8.3**)

The innervation to the temporal muscle is provided by the anterior division of the mandibular nerve (V3), through 3 branches:

○ Masseteric nerve (most posterior).
○ Middle deep temporal nerve.
○ Buccal nerve (most anterior).

8.4 Muscle Preservation in Temporal Approaches

- **Superficial temporal artery preservation, surgical steps:**
  ○ Superficial temporal artery identification.
  ○ The artery is dissected from the subcutaneous tissue, downward, preserving its attachment to the muscle.
  ○ The skin incision has to be continued upward until the desired ending point.
  ○ It is advisable not to reflect the artery together with the skin flap.
  ○ The anterior branch of the artery can be cut and elevated with the skin flap.
- **Frontotemporal branch of the facial nerve preservation.** (**Fig. 8.4**)
- **Sub-facial dissection, surgical steps:**
  ○ Straight incision 1 cm posteriorly and parallel to the frontotemporal branch of the facial nerve, along the zygomatic arch.
  ○ The incision has to run through the superficial fascia, fat pad and deep fascia, until muscle fibers are identified.

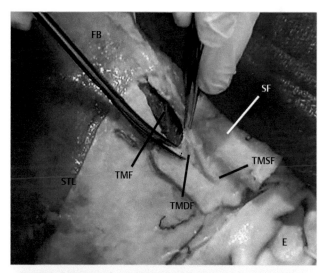

Fig. 8.4 Preserving frontal branch of the facial nerve through a subfascial dissection.
Abbreviations: E = ear; FB = frontal bone; SF = skin flap; STL = superior temporal line; TMF = temporal muscle fibers; TMDF = temporal muscle deep fascia; TMSF = temporal muscle superficial fascia.

○ The deep fascia, fat pad and the superficial fascia (containing the nerve fibers) are then reflected with the skin flap.

- **Muscle releasing, surgical steps** (**Fig. 8.5**):

Subperiosteal retrograde dissection is mandatory to preserve the neurovascular structures.

○ Section of the muscle, if needed, should be performed at its posterior aspect.

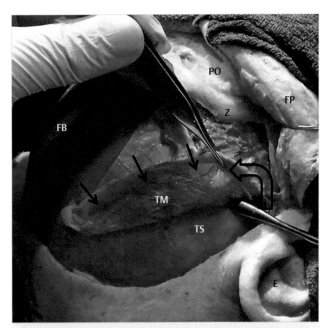

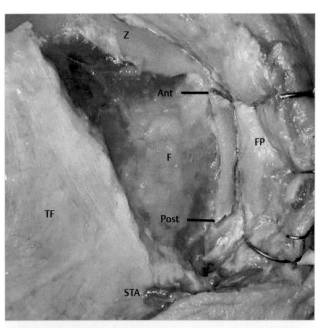

Fig. 8.5 Releasing the muscle through a subperiosteal dissection. Abbreviations: E = ear; FB = frontal bone; FP = fat pad; PO = periorbit; TM = temporal muscle; TS = temporal squama; Z = zygoma. Black arrows = periosteum; Curved arrow = proper movement of the periosteum elevator against the calvaria.

Fig. 8.6 Zygomatic osteotomy. Abbreviations: Ant = anterior cut; F = fat; FP = fat pad; Post = posterior cut; STA = superficial temporal artery; TF = temporal fascia; Z = zygoma.

- Periosteal elevator has to be driven from inferior to superior and from posterior to anterior, beginning at the posterior root of the zygoma.
- Muscle insertion detachment is made at the superior temporal line.
- The muscle is then deflected inferiorly.
- **Improving the exposure through a zygomatic osteotomy, surgical steps** (**Fig. 8.6, 8.7**):
  The zygomatic osteotomy provides a better access to the temporal fossa, avoiding excessive muscle retraction.
  - **Anterior cut** is made oblique, through the malar eminence.
  - **Posterior cut** is made oblique, through the root of the zygoma.
  - The arch is displaced downward, kept attached to the masseter muscle.
  - The muscle is displaced downward through the zygomatic osteotomy.
- **Reattaching the muscle, surgical steps** (**Fig. 8.8**):
  The muscle must be repositioned in anatomical position, to preserve fibers function and craniofacial symmetry.
  - At the beginning the superior aspect of the muscle is fixed to multiple holes made along the superior temporal line with simple suture.
  - The anterior portion, dissected to protect the frontal branch of the facial nerve (FFN), is then reattached to the main portion.
  - The posterior aspect, if incised, is sutured with the same technique.

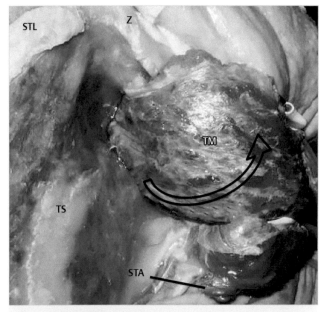

Fig. 8.7 Temporal muscle displacement. Abbreviations: STA = superficial temporal artery; STL = superior temporal line; TM = temporal muscle; TS = temporal squama; Z = zygoma. Curved arrow = proper displacement of the temporal muscle to allow maximum exposure to the temporal fossa.

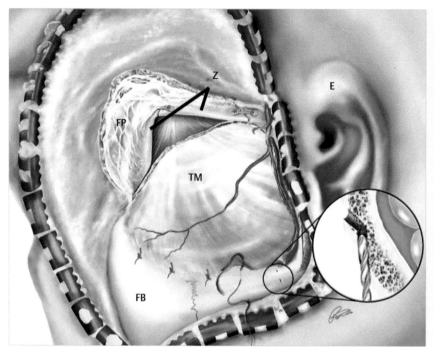

Fig. 8.8 Reconstruction of the temporal muscle. (Reproduced with permission from Kadri PAS, Al-Mefty O. The anatomical basis for surgical preservation of temporal muscle. J Neurosurg 2004; 100 (3): 517–522.) Abbreviations: E = ear; FB = frontal bone; FP = fat pad; TM = temporal muscle; Z = zygoma.

- **Use of temporal muscle to avoid CSF leak, surgical steps:**
Temporal muscle is mostly used for surgical reconstruction following opening of the frontal sinus, sphenoid sinus and infratemporal fossa.
  - The temporal muscle is sectioned according to current needs.
  - The selected portion is laid in the middle fossa to cover the flaw.
  - The bone flap is fixed above that portion and the remaining part of the muscle.

8.5 Frontal Approaches

- **Unilateral or bilateral approaches**
  - The pericranium should be detached from the calvaria just above the superior temporal line.
  - The muscle is then released according to the need, in a subperiosteal fashion as previously described.
  - The pericranium is then mobilized and reflected anteriorly.
- **Use of temporal muscle to avoid CSF leak**
The use of temporal muscle in surgical reconstruction is particularly indicated following resection of lesions involving the anterior fossa floor and craniofacial sinuses.
  - The pericranium is kept pedicled to the temporal muscles and used for packing air sinuses and the anterior fossa floor (**see Chapter 6**).
  - In large exposures, the muscle can be directly plugged to those areas in order to promote proper sealing.

8.6 Posterior Approaches (Figs. 8.9–8.11)

- **Posterolateral approaches**
  - The superficial fascia of the posterior portion of the temporal muscle is dissected, preserving its attachment to the sternocleidomastoid muscle.
  - The sternocleidomastoid muscle is detached from the mastoid process and displaced inferiorly and posteriorly.
  - The posterior aspect of the temporal muscle is dissected from the calvaria in a subperiosteal fashion and reflected anteriorly.
- **Use of temporal muscle to avoid CSF leak**
Temporal muscle is used for surgical reconstruction following approaches to the petrous portion of the temporal bone and the craniocervical junction.
  - The part of muscle fascia attached to the sternocleidomastoid muscle is placed over the dural flaw together with the temporal muscle, which lays above it.
  - The bone flap is fixed over the muscle.

8.7 Complications

- Muscular atrophy.
- Ischemia and necrosis.
- Infection.
- Pain.
- Functional impairment.

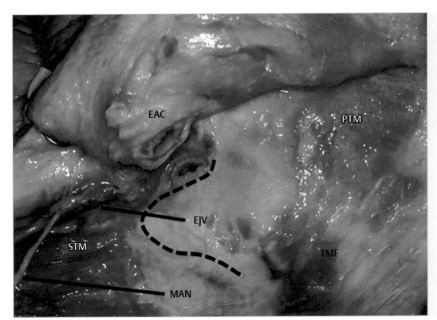

Fig. 8.9 Temporal muscle dissection in a posterior lateral approach. Abbreviations: EAC = external auditory canal (divided); EJV = external jugular vein; MAN = major auricular nerve; PTM = posterior aspect of the temporal muscle; STM = sternocleidomastoid muscle; TMF = temporal muscle fascia. Dotted line = approximate location of the mastoid process.

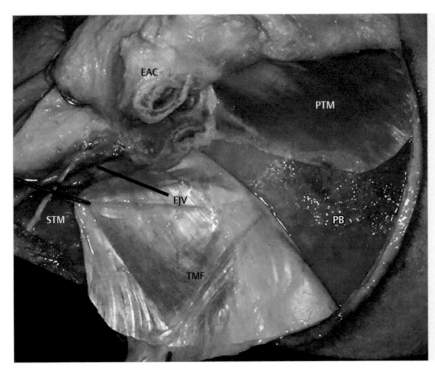

Fig. 8.10 Temporal muscle fascia dissection (posterior lateral approach). Abbreviations: EAC = external auditory canal (divided); EJV = external jugular vein; PB = parietal bone; PTM = posterior aspect of the temporal muscle; STM = sternocleidomastoid muscle; TMF = temporal muscle fascia.

- Craniofacial asymmetry.
- Palsy of the frontotemporal branch of the facial nerve.

8.8 Pearls

- The muscle should be protected from retractors and other fixed rigid instruments to avoid ischemia (a gauze or sponge can be used to protect the muscle).

- Keeping the muscle and fascia moisturized during surgical procedure helps maintaining their elasticity.
- Bleeding from the muscle should be controlled by simple compression when possible; the electrocautery, as bipolar and bovie, should be used with caution to avoid burning damage.
- If miniplates are used for cranioplasty at the level of the superior temporal line, the temporal muscle can be fixed by suturing it to them.

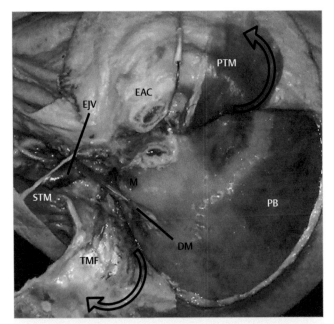

Fig. 8.11 Temporal and sternocleidomastoid muscles displacement (posterior lateral approach).
Abbreviations: DM = digastric muscle; EAC = external auditory canal (divided); EJV = external jugular vein; M = mastoid; PB = parietal bone; PTM = posterior aspect of the temporal muscle; STM = sternocleidomastoid muscle; TMF = temporal muscle fascia. Curved arrow = proper direction of muscle fibers displacement.

References

1. Al-Mefty O, Ayoubi S, Gaber E. Trigeminal schwannomas: removal of dumbbell-shaped tumors through the expanded Meckel cave and outcomes of cranial nerve function. J Neurosurg 2002;96(3):453–463
2. Borba LAB, Ale-Bark S, London C. Surgical treatment of glomus jugulare tumors without rerouting of the facial nerve: an infralabyrinthine approach. Neurosurg Focus 2004; 17(2):E8
3. Kadri PAS, Al-Mefty O. The anatomical basis for surgical preservation of temporal muscle. J Neurosurg 2004; 100(3):517–522
4. Obeid F, Al-Mefty O. Recurrence of olfactory groove meningiomas. Neurosurgery 2003;53(3):534–542, discussion 542–543

9 Intraoperative Imaging

George Samandouras and Gráinne S. McKenna

9.1 Optical Neuronavigation

9.1.1 Indications

- Frameless stereotactic biopsy.
- Hemispheric gliomas.
- Pituitary and skull base tumors.
- Intraventricular tumors.
- Ventricular catheter/shunt placement.

9.1.2 System Components

- Most optical neuronavigation systems are composed of a compact-footprint, free-standing computer workstation on wheels, a camera array that emits (illuminator) and detects (sensor) the infrared light from light-emitting diodes (LEDs) sources and reflecting spheres attached to the instruments and reference frame (**Fig. 9.1**).
- The most commonly used localizer is the Polaris localization system, which transmits a flash of infrared light from outer rings on each side of the hardware. The flash is reflected by the retroflective spheres in the reference frame and surgical probe, and is detected by the sensors on the transmission unit.

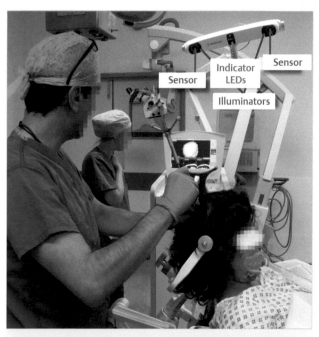

Fig. 9.1 Example of the Polaris type localizer (NDI, Northern Digital Inc., Bakersfield, CA, USA) with the Medtronic StealthStation S7®Navigation System (Medtronic, Minneapolis, MN, USA). Note that patient's head is fixed rigidly in the Mayfield clamp, and to this is attached the blue reference frame (*aka* "star") with retroflective spheres.

9.1.3 Setup

- Images are transferred to the computer workstation, via ethernet cable, memory stick or CD, where surgical planning is taking place.
- In optical navigation systems, the patient's head should be fixed in a head clamp (**Fig. 9.1**). Any subsequent head movement will invalidate the registration accuracy.
- A direct line of sight is required between the LEDs and the camera array (**Fig. 9.1**).
- Efforts should be made to ensure that the star housing the reflective spheres is not too far from the patient (usually a fist's width away) and will not be blocked by subsequent patient's draping and surgeon's or assistant's positions.
- Patient's registration and referencing to the pre-operative MRI (Magnetic Resonance Imaging) or CT (Computed Tomography) images, depending on the system, can be obtained by touching the pointer to fiducials (**Fig. 9.1**), performing surface matching without fiducials, or contact-free, laser registration based on surface matching (**Fig. 9.2**).
- For surgeon's convenience, for right-side lesions the camera and monitors should be placed to the left of the patient and vice versa (**Fig. 9.1**).

9.1.4 Tips And Tricks

- Interruptions in tracking are often due to reflective spheres; cleaning them with a wet swab or replacing them with new ones can restore navigation.
- Although brain shift can reduce navigational accuracy, skull base landmarks remain accurate reference points.
- System generated registration accuracy depends on the size of the lesion. A 2.0 mm registration error might be too large for a biopsy of a 10 mm deep-seated lesion but is acceptable in resecting a 6 cm convexity meningioma.
- The surgeon should not be relying on navigation only and should be prepared to perform the operation based on surgical anatomy and pathology in case of equipment malfunction or hardware failure.

9.2 Electromagnetic Neuronavigation

9.2.1 Indications

- Ventricular catheter placement in small or compressed ventricles (secondary to trauma or idiopathic intracranial hypertension).
- Awake craniotomies avoiding a fixed head position.
- Endoscopic ventricular navigation.

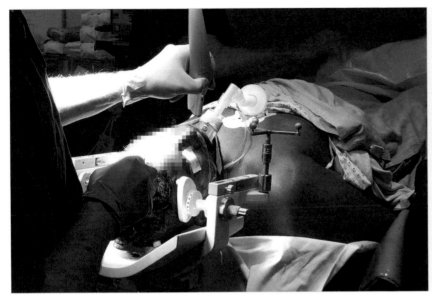

Fig. 9.2 Contact-free, laser, surface-match registration using Z-touch® with the Brain-Lab Cranial navigation system (BrainLab, Feldkirchen, Germany) in the intraoperative MRI for subsequent awake resection of a dominant frontal low-grade glioma. The Z-touch® allows the surgeon to sweep laser beams over the patient's head and acquire a dataset of surface points for registration. Note the projected red laser beam near patient's right eye.

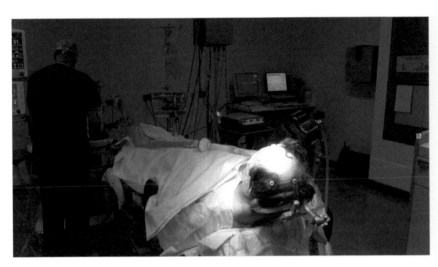

Fig. 9.3 Set up of the StealthStation S7® AxiEM Electromagnetic Tracking System (Medtronic, Louisville, CO, USA). Note that the patient's head is resting on a horseshoe; the black emitter is attached to the articulated vertek arm on the right side of the patient and the distance to the patient's head is not more than a fist's width. The brown adhesive tape fixing the patient's tracker is seen on the right side of the patient's forehead.

9.2.2 System Components

- StealthStation® AxiEM™ Electromagnetic Tracking System (Medtronic, Louisville, CO, USA).
- The portable computer workstation is identical to the optical navigation systems.
- Patient tracker attached to the patient's head.
- Registration probe.
- Emitter of electromagnetic signal (**Fig. 9.3**).
- The AxiEM™ Portable system box where patient tracker, registration probe and emitter are connected.

9.2.3 Setup

- Similar to optical navigation systems images are transferred to the computer workstation, via ethernet cable, memory stick or CD, where surgical planning is taking place.
- Patient tracker is attached to the patient's head with a strong adhesive tape (**Fig. 9.3**).
- The emitter is attached to the articulated vertek arm and placed close to the patient's head (**Fig. 9.3**).

- Registration is performed with fiducials or surface match similar to optical navigation systems (**Fig. 9.3**).

9.2.4 Tips And Tricks

- The main advantage of the electromagnetic navigation system is that it
  - ○ Allows patient's head movement.
  - ○ Can incorporate a stylet that can be introduced to ventricular catheters for targeting small or slit ventricles, or to guide an endoscope into the ventricle.
- Keeping the patient's tracker fixed is paramount. Movement of the tracker is equivalent to movement of reference frame in optical navigation systems and will result in impaired or completely invalid registration.
- The top of the forehead is a good position to place the patient's tracker. The practice of the senior author is to place strong adhesive tape over the tracker and further secure with four staples.
- All other components including the emitter and the patient's head can be moved without affecting the registration.

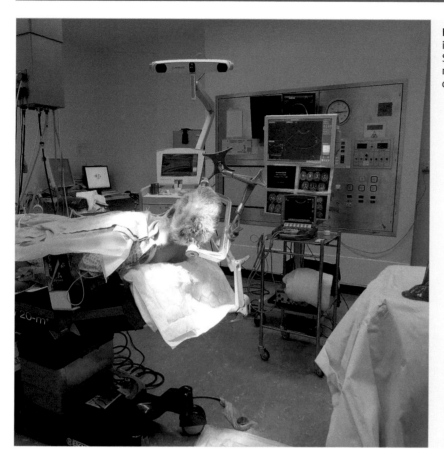

Fig. 9.4 A portable ultrasound machine integrated with the Medronic StealthSation S7® using the SonoNav™ ultrasound navigation interface to aid orientation of the ultrasound probe.

- All metals close to the operative field can affect neuronavigation. Although can be used with a Mayfield clamp, (Integra, Plainsboro, NJ, USA) navigation may be impaired or lost due to magnetic interference.
- During catheter placements removing self-retaining retractors from the operative field can restore impaired neuronavigation.

9.3 Intraoperative Ultrasound

9.3.1 Indications

- Real time neuronavigation to determine extent of resection during tumor surgery (glioma or metastasis).
- Localization of cystic lesions/ventricles in the brain.
- Localization of intradural spinal lesions before opening the dura.

9.3.2 System Components

- There are two main types of ultrasound based neuronavigation
  - Ultrasound systems that can be integrated with optical neuronavigation systems, including Medtronic (Medtronic, Louisville, CO, USA) and BrainLab (BrainLab, Feldkirchen, Germany) (**Figs. 9.4–9.6**).
  - All-in-one systems combining preoperative CT/MRI with intraoperative 3D (three dimensional) ultrasound images, 3D Power Doppler and classic neuronavigation, as for example in SonoWand™ (Sonowand AS, Trondheim, Norway) (**Fig. 9.7**).

9.3.3 Setup

- Portable ultrasound systems are less expensive and can be integrated to optical neuronavigation systems. The ultrasound probe and cable are inserted into a sterile plastic sleeve (**Fig. 9.5**). The probe houses reflective spheres allowing real-time navigation. The software allows to swap the image between ultrasound and optical navigation (**Fig. 9.6**).
- Sonowand™ (Sonowand AS, Trondheim, Norway) is a single-rack system with an ultrasound scanner and a built in navigational computer and an optical tracking system (**Fig. 9.7**).

9.3.4 Tips And Tricks

- Knowledge of normal ultrasound anatomy is essential to differentiate normal anatomy from pathology.
- Rotating the head of the ultrasound probe produces images in different planes. Knowledge of 3D-anatomy in all planes is required to avoid confusion.
- Ultrasound systems that integrate neuronavigation can be more useful, especially when surgeons have limited experience with normal ultrasound anatomy.
- As the learning curve is steep, gaining experience with ventricular surgery or cysts are good starting points before moving to gliomas and particularly to diffuse low grade gliomas that can be more challenging to differentiate from normal structures.

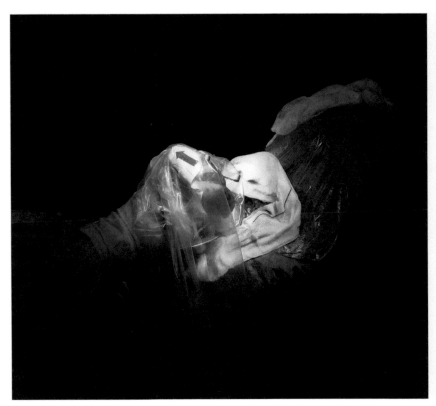

Fig. 9.5 The handheld ultrasound probe, with an attached reflective blue star, provides ultrasound-based neuronavigation when integrated with the Medronic Stealth-Sation S7® during intracranial navigation in an awake craniotomy for glioma.

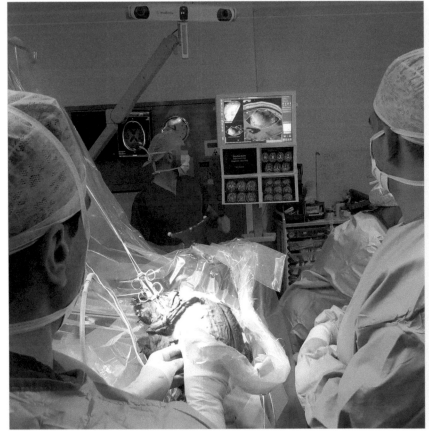

Fig 9.6 Awake craniotomy for dominant parieto-occipital glioma. Note the green ultrasound window within the optical neuronavigation image that can be adjusted from pure MRI image to pure ultrasound image facilitating surgical orientation.

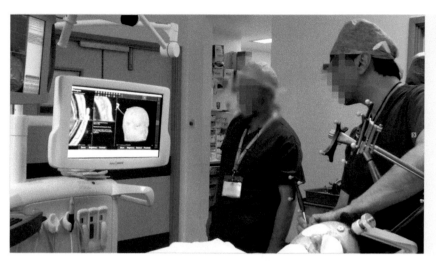

Fig. 9.7 Preoperative registration using the SonoWand™ system (Sonowand, Trondheim, Norway).

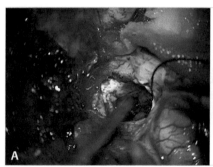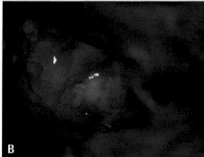

Fig. 9.8 **(A)** Intraoperative appearance of a glioblastoma under the normal, white light of the operating microscope with no appreciable visual difference between neoplastic and normal cells; **(B)** after switching to the blue UV filter of the operating microscope, the neoplastic cells fluoresce with a bright pink color.

9.4 Immunofluorescence-Guided Surgery

9.4.1 Indications

- Anaplastic gliomas
- Glioblastomas

9.4.2 System Components

- 5-aminolevulinic acid (5-ALA) is a photosensitive drug, which is converted to Protoporphyrin IX (PpIX) in malignant gliomas via an oral-intake of exogenous 5-ALA.
- Illumination of PpIX at an appropriate ultraviolet (UV) wave length (440 nm, nanometer) induces a visible (635 nm) red fluorescence.

9.4.3 Set Up

- 5-ALA dose 20 mg/kg (Medac GmbH, Wedel, Germany) is administered orally, 5 to 6 hours prior to the estimated time of dural opening.
- Patients should avoid direct sunlight/bright external light exposure after taking 5-ALA and immediately postoperatively to avoid the rare complication of superficial burns.
- The operating microscope should have been manufactured or adapted to emit ultraviolet light of wavelength 440 nm.
- During surgery, and under the UV light the tumor appears bright pink/red while the adjacent normal brain does not fluoresce (**Figs. 9.8A, 9.8B**).

9.4.4 Tips and Tricks

- The presence of even a thin layer of blood can obscure the fluorescence. A completely dry surgical field is required for optimal visualization.
- 5-ALA is more useful at the edges of malignant gliomas rather than in the necrotic center.
- Only parts of the tumor cavity with direct exposure to UV light will fluoresce. Extra care should be taken to inspect and illuminate all corners of the tumor cavity.
- The fact that a part of the tumor is fluorescent does not mean it cannot be functional. Knowledge of surgical and functional anatomy or cortical/subcortical mapping during awake procedures may be required in gliomas affecting eloquent areas.
- With experience, time spent under the UV will gradually increase as surgeons will be more comfortable operating in darker surgical field.
- Vessels will not fluoresce under the blue light. When operating in this less well illuminated environment, extra care should be taken to avoid vascular injury.

9.5 Intraoperative MRI (iMRI)

9.5.1 Indications

- Glioma surgery (High-grade or low-grade gliomas).
- Pituitary surgery.
- Skull base surgery.
- Brain biopsies.
- Deep brain stimulation.
- Cyst drainage/ventricular surgery.

9.5.2 System Components

- Low field magnets [<0.3T (Tesla)] are housed below the table and are raised during scanning, with minimal interruption to the surgical workflow. *Surgical instruments and materials must be MRI compatible.*
- High field magnets (1.5T - 3.0T) lie within dedicated operating room (OR) suites. Surgery is performed using normal surgical instruments and anesthetic equipment in an area outside a 5G (Gauss) line (usually 4.2-4.5 m from the magnet) to avoid radiofrequency interference with the MRI.
- Neuronavigation is integrated in the iMRI software allowing integration of functional data (fMRI and DTI), if required.

9.5.3 Set Up Low-Field IMRI

- In low-field iMRI the magnet is stored under the OR table and raised for imaging only, resulting in a fast, minor remodeling of the OR. Example is the PoleStar™ N-20 (Medtronic Navigation, Louisville, CO, USA) with a vertical gap of 27 cm.
- Major advantages of the low-field iMRI systems is they do not require patient movement in and out of the MRI; there is no need for undraping and re-draping of patients; offers closer to real time imaging and freedom of surgical access to the patient. In addition, the magnetic field's fall-off is rapid.
- In low-field (<0.3T) iMRI systems, MRI compatible instruments and materials must be used.

9.5.4 Set Up High-Field IMRI

- High-field iMRI systems (**Fig. 9.9**) are practically fully diagnostic MRI scanners providing diagnostic image quality and allowing acquisition of all MRI sequences with decreased susceptibility to radiofrequency interference (RFI).
- When not used during surgery, high-field scanners can be used for diagnostic imaging of inpatients or outpatients.
- High-field iMRI systems have demanding space requirements, requiring major remodeling of the OR with significant cost implications.

- High field iMRI systems are, at present, either 1.5T or 3.0T and have a design featuring either a fixed MRI scanner with a moving operating room table (**Fig. 9.9**) or a fixed operating room table with a ceiling-mounted, mobile magnet that moves on tracts from one room used for diagnostic imaging to the operating room used for intraoperative imaging. Systems of the former design include the BrainLab intraoperative MRI (BrainLab AG, Feldkirchen, Germany) incorporating image-guided surgery with high-field diagnostic MR imaging from different manufacturers and the Philips Gyroscan (Philips Medical Systems, Best, The Netherlands) while systems of the later design include the mobile VISIUS Surgical Theatre (IMRIS, Deerfield, New York, USA).
- In high field (1.5–3.0T) iMRI systems ferrous materials and instruments can be used provided that they remain outside the 5 Gauss (G) line (**Fig. 9.10**). The 5G line specifies a perimeter line the flux density of the static magnetic field is strong enough, so that ferrous materials are at risk of developing kinetic properties and becoming a ballistic hazard. On high-field MRIs, and according to the magnetic field, the 5G-line is typically 4.2 to 4.5 meters from the gantry aperture.
- High-field iMRI systems allow combination of neuronavigation systems with integration of functional data including fMRI, DTI, and trans-cranial magnetic stimulation data (TMS) (**Fig. 9.11**).

9.5.5 Tips And Tricks

- iMRI cases are lengthy due to intraoperative preparation and scanning time. Patient selection is crucial to maximize benefits without underutilizing operative time.
- On average 1-2 intraoperative MRIs are required for tumor surgery with an approximate preparation and scanning time of 40 minutes per scan.
- Certain iMRI models have head fixation devices with minimal freedom of movement. Parietal and occipital pathologies cannot always be reached.
- Recent models allow more degree of freedom in head positioning. Certain models allow MR-compatible head-clamp.

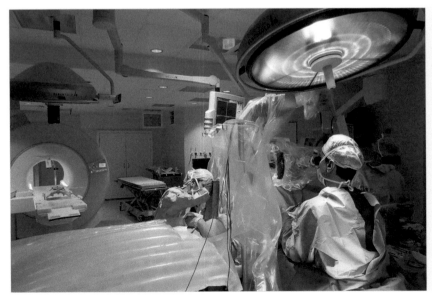

Fig. 9.9 Setup of the iMRI suite at the National Hospital for Neurology and Neurosurgery, Queen Square, London, United Kingdom during an awake craniotomy for dominant temporal low grade glioma. The system features a wide-bore, high-field, 1.5T MRI and the Vector Vision version of BrainLab.

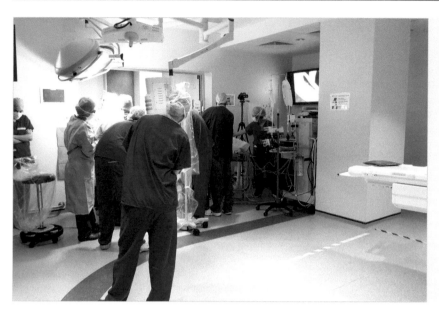

Fig. 9.10 The operating table and the surgical team are outside the 5G line allowing use of routine surgical instruments and anesthetic equipment.

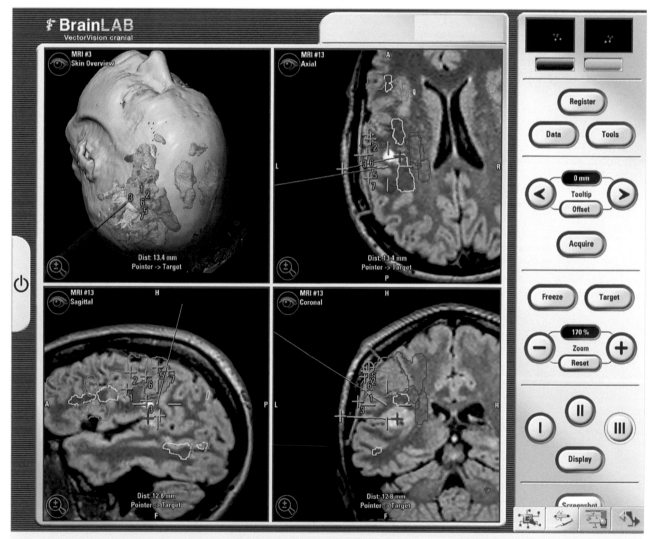

Fig. 9.11 Real-time intraoperative navigation with overlay of functional data; transcranial magnetic stimulation (TMS), blue pegs; arcuate fasciculus, yellow; corticospinal tract, red; verbal fluency, orange. The numbers correspond to areas of direct cortical stimulation (DCS) marked with sterile tickets intraoperatively.

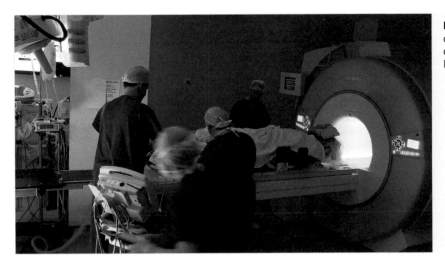

Fig. 9.12 The patient is transferred from the operating table to the MRI table with the coil placed over his head and connected to MRI-compatible anesthetic equipment.

- Extra care should be taken during un-draping/re-draping cycles to minimize the risk of infection.
- Awake craniotomies on iMRI are possible (**Figs. 9.9, 9.12**) but require strict patient selection as in addition to being placed within the scanner, the awake patients have a coil placed close to their faces (**Fig. 9.12**).
- Expert anesthetic involvement is mandatory in awake resections on iMRI (**Fig. 9.12**).
- Care should be taken not to cross the 5G-line (**Fig. 9.10**). where surgical instruments and anesthetic equipment can acquire ballistic properties, and become hazard to patients, personnel, and the MRI magnet itself.
- iMRI is not a replacement for surgical skills, knowledge of anatomy, and operative technique. This statement applies for all technologies of intraoperative imaging.

References

1. Barone DG, Lawrie TA, Hart MG. Image guided surgery for the resection of brain tumours. Cochrane Database Syst Rev 2014;1(1):CD009685
2. D'Amico RS, Kennedy BC, Bruce JN. Neurosurgical oncology: advances in operative technologies and adjuncts. J Neurooncol 2014;119(3):451–463
3. Hall WA, Truwit CL. Intraoperative MR-guided neurosurgery. J Magn Reson Imaging 2008;27(2):368–375
4. Wu JS, Gong X, Song YY, et al. 3.0-T intraoperative magnetic resonance imaging-guided resection in cerebral glioma surgery: interim analysis of a prospective, randomized, triple-blind, parallel-controlled trial. Neurosurgery 2014; 61(Suppl 1):145–154

10 Precaruncular Approach to the Medial Orbit and Central Skull Base

Jeremy N. Ciporen and Brandon P. Lucke-Wold

10.1 Introduction

In order to decrease scarring and improve healing times, the medial precaruncular approach was developed to address pathology of the anterior cranial fossa and orbit.

The approach follows the preseptal plane to the medial orbit, which provides minimal vascular disruption. The initial fifteen cases showed no complications with quick recovery times.

When the precaruncular port of entry is combined with a neuroendoscopic transorbital approach, it can be used to access the entire cranial fossa. The technique is especially useful for addressing intraorbital pathology of the anterior skull base.

To enhance working space for instrumentation, the precaruncular approach can be combined with the transnasal approach. This dual port approach allows the surgeon to adequately treat and manage complex pathology in the central portion of the anterior cranial fossa. The fourhanded technique increases visualization, which is important for treating pathology affecting the pituitary gland, cavernous carotid arteries, and optic chiasm.

The approach allows appreciation of important anatomical landmarks including the clivus, planum sphenoidale, tuberculum sella, and suprasellar region. In addition to treating pathology of the anterior cranial fossa, the precaruncular approach has been used for minimal dissection repairs of blowout fractures to the medial orbit. The approach provides adequate reduction of soft tissue to allow for the correct placement of implants.

This chapter focuses on the important considerations regarding patient positioning, location of incision, endoscopic portal site, and variations on the technique. Additionally, the primary indications are highlighted with supported evidence from both case series and cadaveric models.

10.2 Indications

- Intra-orbital pathology.
- Pathology affecting the clival, sella, suprasellar, parasellar, cavernous sinus and brainstem regions.
- Decompression of the orbit/optic nerve.
- Fracture repair of the medial orbital wall.
- Cerebrospinal fluid leak repair.

10.3 Patient Positioning

- **Position:** The patient is positioned supine, the head can either be secured to a Mayfield head holder or placed on a foam or gel donut.

- **Body:** The body is placed in neutral position.
- **Head:** The head is kept neutral, avoiding extension or flexion, it may be slightly turned toward the surgeon 10-15°. A sense of midline should be maintained at all times.
- **Endotracheal tube**: The tube is placed on the midline and directed inferiorly over the chin.
- **Eye protection**: Bilateral corneal shields with lubricant are used. Betadine is preferred for the preparation, avoiding alcohol.

10.4 Skin Incision (Figs. 10.1–10.3)

- **Precaruncular**
  - Self-retaining superior and inferior eyelid retractor is placed.
  - The caruncle is identified and lateralized with a pick up.
  - The superior and inferior lacrimal ducts are identified.
  - Incision is made medial to the caruncle with a Colorado tip bovie along the avascular plane.

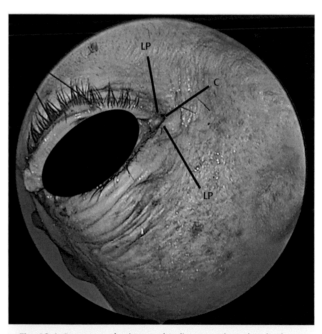

Fig. 10.1 Precaruncular (transorbital) approach to the clival, sellar, suprasellar, and parasellar regions. Anatomy. Abbreviations: C = caruncle; LP = lacrimal punctum.

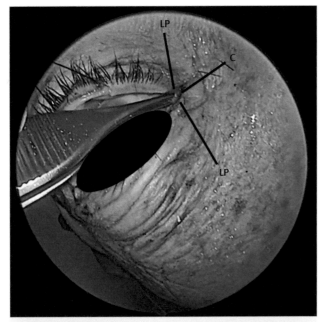

Fig. 10.2 Precaruncular (transorbital) approach. Caruncular lateralization.
Abbreviations: C = caruncle; LP = lacrimal punctum.

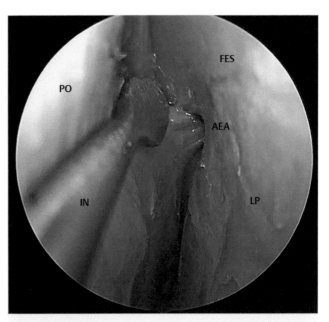

Fig. 10.4 Appreciation of intraoperative anatomy. Anterior ethmoidal artery and lamina papyracea.
Abbreviations: AEA = anterior ethmoidal artery; FES = fronto-ethmoidal suture; IN = instrument; LP = lamina papyracea; PO = periorbit.

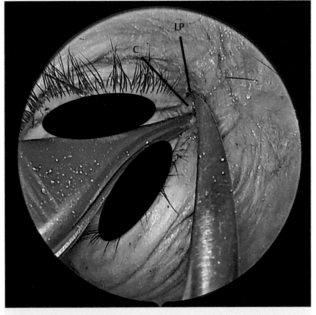
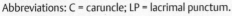

Fig. 10.3 Precaruncular (transorbital) approach. Dissection.
Abbreviations: C = caruncle; LP = lacrimal punctum.

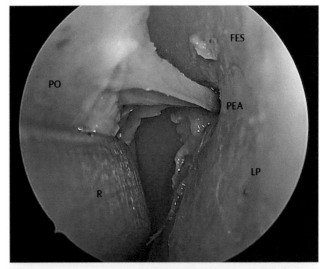

Fig. 10.5 Appreciation of intraoperative anatomy. Posterior ethmoidal artery and fronto-ethmoidal suture.
Abbreviations: FES = fronto-ethmoidal suture; LP = lamina papyricea; PEA = posterior ethmoidal artery; PO = periorbit; R = retractor.

10.5 Soft Tissue Dissection (Figs. 10.4–10.6)

- Scissors are used to dissect the avascular plane.
- Avoid the lacrimal sac by remaining posterior to the lacrimal impression.
- The trajectory of dissection is medial toward the medial orbital wall (lamina papyracea).

- The periosteum is incised to optimize the dissection plane.
- The periorbit has to be maintained throughout the dissection.
- **Bone Exposure**
  - The fronto-ethmoidal suture is identified.
  - The dissection is continued posteriorly along the suture.

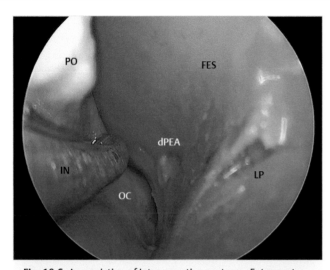

Fig. 10.6 Appreciation of intraoperative anatomy. Entrance to optic canal.
Abbreviations: dPEA = divided posterior ethmoidal artery; FES = fronto-ethmoidal suture; IN = instrument; LP = lamina papyracea; OC = optic canal; PO = periorbit.

○ The anterior ethmoidal artery is identified, coagulated and divided as well as the posterior ethmoidal artery if more posterior exposure is needed.
○ Further dissection posteriorly along the plane of the fronto-ethmoidal suture will lead to the optic canal and nerve.

10.6 Removal of Bone (Figs. 10.7, 10.8)

- Removal of bone **inferior** to the fronto-ethmoidal suture leads to the middle turbinate anteriorly and the ethmoidal air cells more posteriorly.
- Removal of the face of the sphenoid via an endonasal approach affords access through the transorbital precaruncular approach to the sphenoid sinus for visualization and instrumentation access to the clival region and posterior circulation, brainstem, sella, tuberculum, optic-carotid recesses, bilateral cavernous sinuses and the cavernous carotid arteries.
- Removal of bone **superior** to the fronto-ethmoidal suture leads to sub-frontal region intra-cranially.

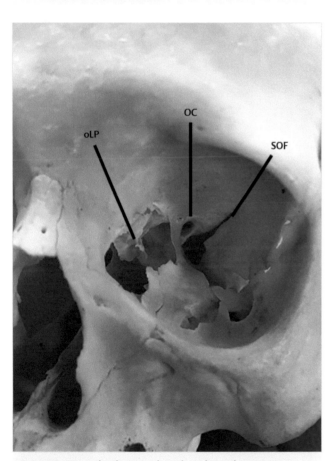

Fig. 10.7 Transorbital approach to the sphenoid sinus is obtained by removing the medial orbital wall, by performing an ethmoidectomy, and middle turbinectomy. Anatomical view: orbital anatomy.
Abbreviations: OC = optic canal; oLP = opened lamina papyracea; SOF = superior orbital fissure.

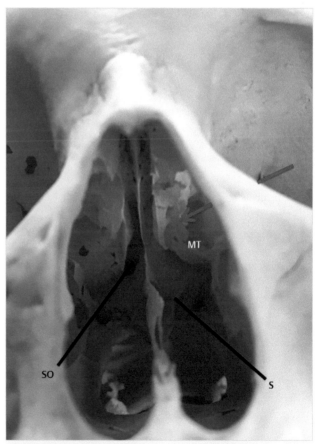

Fig. 10.8 Transorbital approach to the sphenoid sinus is obtained by removing the medial orbital wall, by performing an ethmoidectomy, and middle turbinectomy. Anatomical view: nasal anatomy.
Abbreviations: MT = middle turbinate; S = sphenoid; SO = sphenoid ostia.

10.7 Dual Port: Endoscopic Transorbital and Transnasal Access (Figs. 10.9, 10.10)

- Combined endoscopic precaruncular transorbital and endonasal transphenoidal approach to the clival, sella, suprasellar, parasellar, cavernous sinus and brainstem regions.

10.8 Critical Anatomy (Figs. 10.11–10.13)

- Optic nerve/Chiasm
- Pituitary gland/Infundibulum
- Cavernous sinuses and carotid arteries
- Anterior communicating and cerebral arteries
- Brainstem

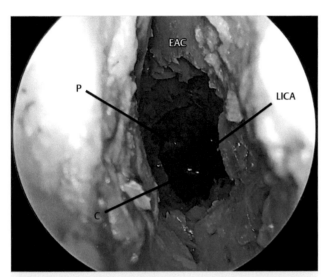

Fig. 10.9 Right transorbital view through the defect in the medial orbital wall. An ethmoidectomy, middle turbinectomy has been performed, in addition to the removal of the face of the sphenoid and the bone over the sella and tuberculum. Abbreviations: C = clivus; EAC = ethmoidal air cells; LICA = left internal carotid artery; P = pituitary.

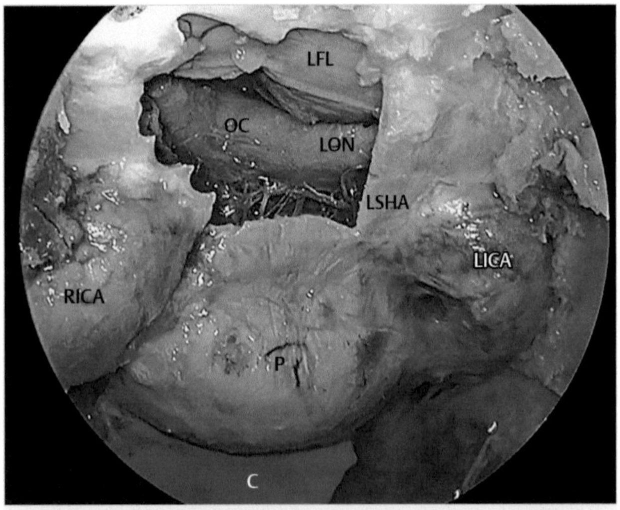

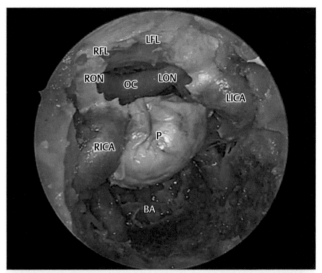

Fig. 10.11 Right transorbital view (0-degree endoscope) of the clival, sellar, suprasellar and parasellar regions. The tuberculum and the clivus have been removed and the dura opened. Abbreviations: BA = basilar artery; LFL = left frontal lobe; LICA = left internal carotid artery; LON = left optic nerve; OC = optic chiasm; P = pituitary; RFL = right frontal lobe; RICA = right internal carotid artery; RON = right optic nerve.

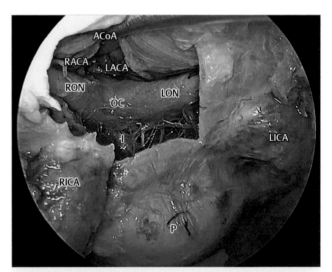

Fig. 10.10 Right transorbital view (0-degree endoscope) of the clival, sellar, suprasellar and parasellar regions. The tuberculum has been removed and the dura opened. Abbreviations: C = clivus; LFL = left frontal lobe; LICA = left internal carotid artery; LON = left optic nerve; LSHA = left superior hypophiseal artery; OC = optic chiasm; P = pituitary; RICA = right internal carotid artery.

Fig. 10.12 Right transorbital view (0-degree endoscope) of the sella, suprasellar and parasellar regions. The tuberculum has been removed and the dura opened. An endonasal transsphenoidal port is used for the instrument. Dual Port access. Abbreviations: ACoA = anterior communicating artery; LACA = left anterior cerebral artery; LICA = left internal carotid artery; LON = left optic nerve; OC = optic chiasm; P = pituitary; RACA = right anterior cerebral artery; RICA = right internal carotid artery; RON = right optic nerve.

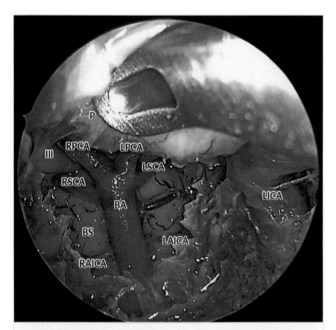

Fig. 10.13 Right transorbital view (0-degree endoscope) of brainstem and posterior circulation. The clival dura has been opened. An endonasal trans-sphenoidal port is used for the instrument. Dual Port access.
Abbreviations: BA = basilar artery; BS = brainstem; III = third cranial nerve; LAICA = left anterior inferior cerebellar artery; LICA = left internal carotid artery; LPCA = left posterior cerebral artery; LSCA = left superior cerebellar artery; P = pituitary; RAICA = right anterior inferior cerebellar artery; RPCA = right posterior cerebral artery; RSCA = right superior cerebellar artery.

References

1. Ciporen JN, Moe KS, Ramanathan D, et al. Multiportal endoscopic approaches to the central skull base: a cadaveric study. World Neurosurg 2010;73(6):705–712
2. Moe KS, Kim LJ, Bergeron CM. Transorbital endoscopic repair of cerebrospinal fluid leaks. Laryngoscope 2011; 121(1):13–30
3. Moe KS. The precaruncular approach to the medial orbit. Arch Facial Plast Surg 2003;5(6):483–487
4. You HJ, Kim DW, Dhong ES, Yoon ES. Precaruncular approach for the reconstruction of medial orbital wall fractures. Ann Plast Surg 2014;72(6):652–656

11 Supraorbital Approach

Phillip A. Bonney, Andrew K. Conner, and Michael E. Sughrue

11.1 Introduction

The supraorbital approach is a frontal approach, which is suitable for the unilateral exposure of the anterior skull base. The surgical route corresponds to the anatomical corridor seated between the inferior aspect of the frontal lobe and the floor of the anterior cranial fossa.

The approach is mainly indicated in case of vascular lesions of the anterior circulation as well as of lesions involving the anterior skull base as well as the parasellar areas.

11.2 Indications

- Anterior circulation aneurysms.
- Anterior skull base meningiomas.
- Parasellar tumors (*e.g.*, craniopharyngiomas).
- Less common: posterior circulation aneurysms, inferior frontal pathology.

11.3 Patient Positioning (Fig. 11.1)

- **Position:** Patient is positioned supine in a 20° of reverse Trendelenburg position.
- **Head:** The head is extended 20°, rotated 5°-15° to the contralateral side for most pathology; for anterior lesions near the midline (e.g., olfactory groove meningiomas) rotation may be up to 60°.
- The **malar eminence** is the highest point in the surgical field.
- Ipsilateral temporary tarsorrhaphy is performed to protect the cornea.

11.4 Skin Incision (Fig. 11.2)

- **Slightly curved incision**
  - ○ **Starting point:** Incision starts just medial to supraorbital notch.

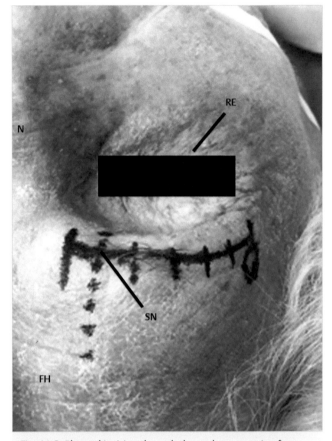

Fig. 11.2 Planned incision through the eyebrow, running from just medial to the supraorbital notch to the edge of the brow. If more medial access is necessary, care should be taken to preserve the supraorbital nerve, which can be found deep to the frontalis muscle.
Abbreviations: FH = forehead; N = nose; RE = right eye; SN = supraorbital notch.

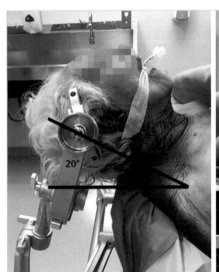
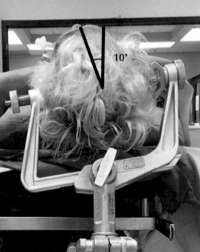

Fig. 11.1 Patient positioning.

○ **Course:** Incision line runs within hair-bearing skin of the eyebrow.
○ **Ending point:** It ends at the lateral edge of the brow (may be extended up to 1 cm).

11.4.1 Critical Structures

• Supraorbital nerve

11.5 Soft Tissue Dissection (Figs. 11.3–11.5)

• **Myofascial and muscular layers**
  ○ The frontal muscle is divided with monopolar electrocautery along the path of the incision.
  ○ Usually this does not need to extend medially to the supraorbital notch.

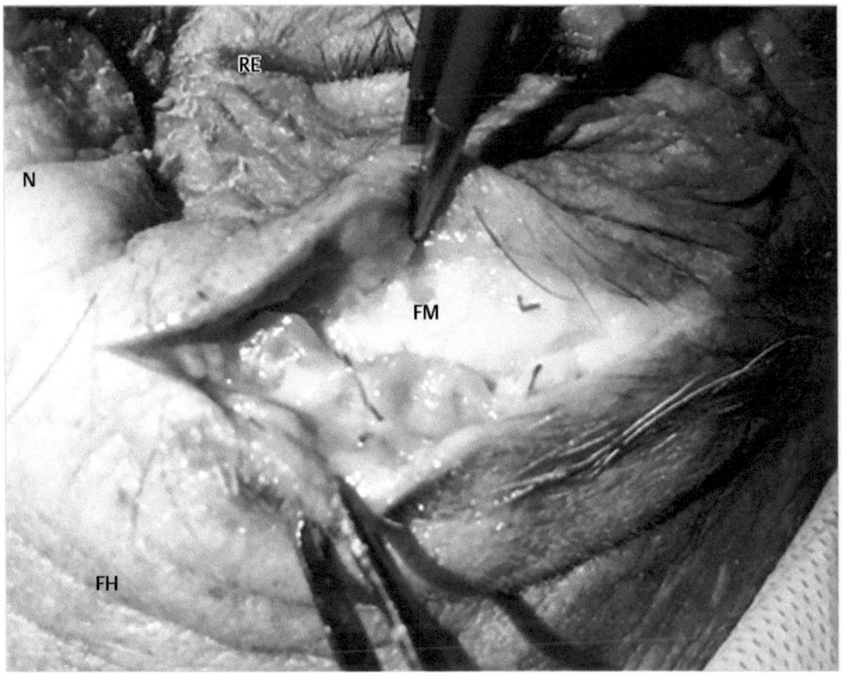

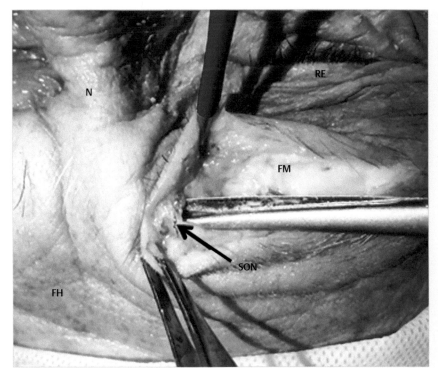

Fig. 11.3 Muscle dissection: frontal muscle is divided in the plane of the incision. Abbreviations: FH = forehead; FM = frontalis muscle; N = nose; RE = right eye.

Fig. 11.4 Muscle dissection: the supraorbital nerve may be identified just deep to the frontalis muscle and carefully retracted medially if required.
Abbreviations: FH = forehead; FM = frontalis muscle; N = nose; RE = right eye; SON = supraorbital nerve.

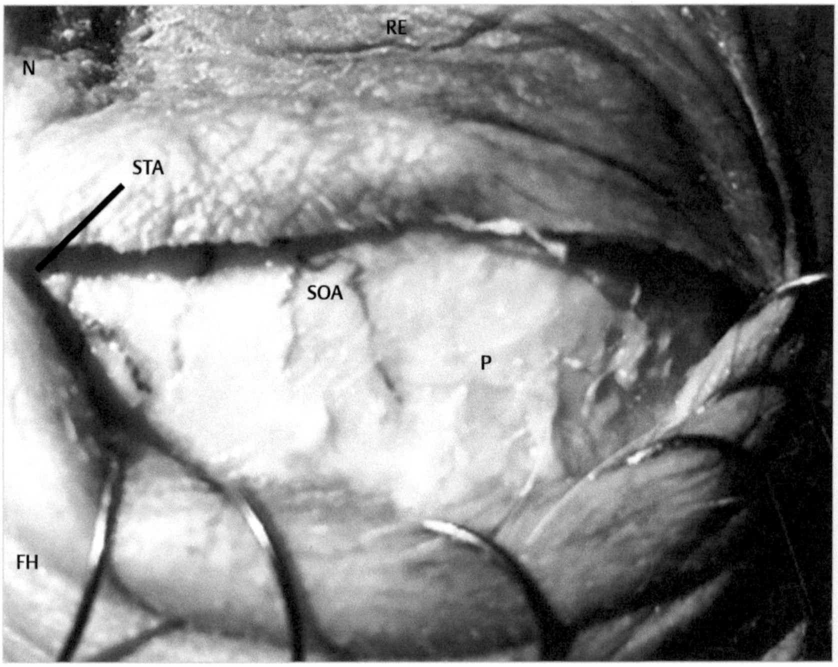

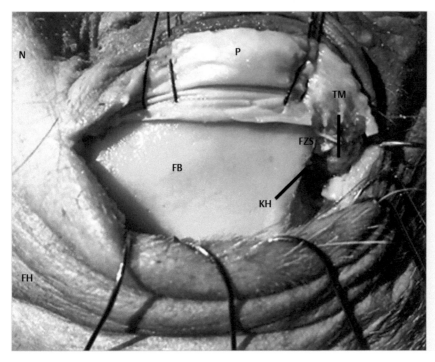

Fig. 11.5 Bone exposure: after scalp hooks are placed to retract the skin superiorly, a pericranial flap is started along the superior edge.
Abbreviations: FH = forehead; N = nose; P = pericranium; RE = right eye; SOA = supraorbital artery; STA = supratrochlear artery.

Fig. 11.6 Bone exposure: the pericranial flap is reflected anteriorly and inferiorly and sutured down along the inferior margin of the flap. The keyhole is exposed utilizing sub-periosteal dissection with the temporal muscle reflected laterally. Care should be taken to avoid dissection superficial to the superficial temporalis fascia to avoid damage to the frontalis branch of the facial nerve.
Abbreviations: FB = frontal bone; FH = forehead; FZS = frontozygomatic suture; KH = keyhole; N = nose; P = pericranium; TM = temporal muscle.

○ The muscle is elevated and reflected superiorly with scalp hooks.
- **Bone exposure**
  ○ The pericranium is cut along the superior edge of the skin incision.
  ○ The medial edge of the temporal muscle is dissected with the pericranium to expose the lateral orbital rim.
  ○ Subperiosteal dissection proceeds until the frontozygomatic suture is visible.
  ○ The pericranial flap is elevated off the bone, reflected inferolaterally, and sutured down.

11.6 Craniotomy (Figs. 11.6, 11.7)

- **Burr hole**
  ○ **I:** The single burr hole is made at the keyhole.
- **Craniotomy landmarks**
  Anatomical landmarks that must be taken into consideration when designing the craniotomy are
  ○ **Medially:** Lateral wall of the frontal sinus or supraorbital nerve.
  ○ **Laterally:** Keyhole.

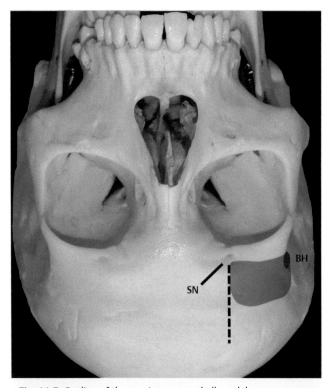

Fig. 11.7 Outline of the craniotomy on skull model.
Abbreviations: BH = burr hole; SN = supraorbital notch.

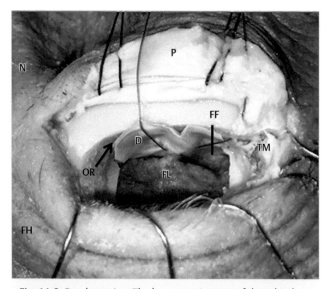

Fig. 11.8 Dural opening. The bony prominences of the orbital roof are drilled flat to the sphenoid wing. If the orbital roof is transgressed, periorbital fat will be evident. A C-shaped dural opening is made.
Abbreviations: D = dura; FF = frontal floor; FH = forehead; FL = frontal lobe; N = nose; OR = orbital rim; P = pericranium; TM = temporal muscle.

  ○ **Superiorly:** Approximately 1.5-2 cm above the frontal floor.
  ○ **Inferiorly:** Orbital roof.
• The craniotomy is made near the frontal floor approximately 2-3 cm wide and 1.5-2 cm high.
• The medial border of the craniotomy should not extend to the frontal sinus.
• Image guidance is helpful to identify the lateral wall of the frontal sinus, which is usually, but not always, medial to the supraorbital notch.

11.6.1 Critical Structures

• Frontal sinus.
• Supraorbital nerve.
• Orbital roof.

11.7 Dural Opening (Fig. 11.8)

• The dura is first separated from the orbital roof and bony prominences are drilled down so that the orbital roof is flush with the sphenoid wing.
• The dural opening is a C-shaped incision based inferiorly.

11.7.1 Critical Structures

• None.

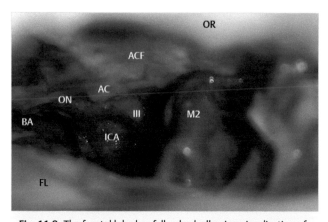

Fig. 11.9 The frontal lobe has fallen back allowing visualization of the suprasellar region.
Abbreviations: AC = anterior clinoid process; ACF = anterior cranial fossa; BA = basilar artery; FL = frontal lobe; ICA = internal carotid artery; III = third cranial nerve; M2 = M2 segment of middle cerebral artery; ON = optic nerve; OR = orbital ridge.

11.8 Intradural Exposure (Fig. 11.9)

• **Parenchymal structures:** Orbital gyrus, pituitary, mammillary bodies, lamina terminalis, brainstem.
• **Arachnoid layer:** Sylvian cistern, opticocarotid cistern, suprasellar cistern, interpeduncular cistern.
• **Cranial nerves:** I, II, III, IV cranial nerves.
• **Arteries:** Internal carotid artery (ICA), middle cerebral artery (MCA), anterior cerebral artery (ACA), anterior

choroidal artery (AChA), posterior communicating artery (PcoA).
- **Veins:** Cavernous sinus, Sylvian fissure veins.

11.9 Pearls

- Having enough room to work requires accessing and draining CSF spaces early. Understanding this concept is the most important aspect of the procedure.
- The 30° endoscope aids in visualizing beyond the field of the microscope. This can be used, for example, when inspecting the sella for residual tumor or assessing the clipping of an aneurysm.

- Optimal cosmetic outcomes can be achieved with a careful attention paid to closure techniques.

References

1. Little AS, Gore PA, Darbar A, et al. Supraorbital eyebrow approach: a less invasive corridor to lesions of the anterior cranial fossa, parasellar region, and ventral brainstem. In: Cappabianca P, Califano L, Iaconetta G, eds. Cranial, craniofacial, and skull base surgery. Milan: Springer; 2010
2. Teo C, Sughrue ME. Principles and practice of keyhole brain surgery. New York, NY: Thieme Medical Publisher; 2014

12 Trans-Ciliar Approach

Khaled M. A. Aziz, Nouman Aldahak, and Mohamed Arnaout

12.1 Introduction

The trans-ciliar approach represents a keyhole approach to the anterior cranial fossa and parasellar region, developed to minimize retraction on the frontal lobes in order to reach the pathology at hand.

As for other keyhole approaches the trauma to the superficial layers is minimal but the final exposure is sufficient to remove large tumors of this area and address selected vascular pathology of the anterior circulation.

12.2 Indications

- Aneurysms of the anterior circulation are the most commonly treated pathology including internal carotid artery, proximal anterior cerebral artery (ACA), anterior communicating artery (AcoA), posterior communicating artery (Pcom), proximal middle cerebral artery (MCA) and basilar tip.
- Tumors of the sellar and parasellar region and anterior skull base.
- Orbital lesions requiring craniotomy for exposure.

12.3 Brain Relaxation

- **Head positioning:** The head is positioned above the heart's level.
- Mannitol, steroids.
- Lumbar drain (optional).

12.4 Patient Positioning (Fig. 12.1)

- **Position:** The patient is positioned supine with the head fixed with a Mayfield head holder.
- **Body:** The body is placed flat at 20° of reverse Trendelenburg position.
- A roll is put below the ipsilateral shoulder.
- **Head:**
  - The head is elevated above the level of the heart (**Fig. 12.1A**.)
  - It is rotated 15-30°according to the lesion approached, opposite to skin incision side (**Fig. 12.1B**.)
  - A slight extension of about 20° toward the floor is provided (**Fig. 12.1C**.)
- **The malar eminence** has to be the highest point in the surgical field.
- **Eye protection techniques:**
  - Lubricant to the ipsilateral eye.
  - Ophthalmology eye shield.
  - Ipsilateral tarsorrhaphy is recommended.

12.5 Skin Incision (Fig. 12.2)

- The incision is placed in the most superior margin of the eyebrow, which can be within a skin fold above the eyebrow (supraciliary).
- **Starting point:** The supraorbital notch can be considered as the medial limit of the incision.
- **Course:** Incision line runs over the eyebrow.

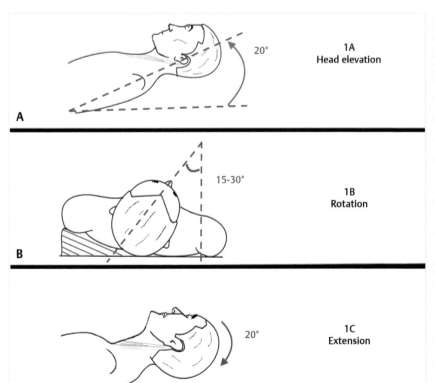

Fig. 12.1 Patient positioning: (**A**) 20° of reverse Trendelenburg position to elevate the head above the level of the heart. (**B**) Rotation 15-30° opposite to skin incision side. (**C**) The head is extended about 20° toward the floor.

20° 1A Head elevation

15-30° 1B Rotation

20° 1C Extension

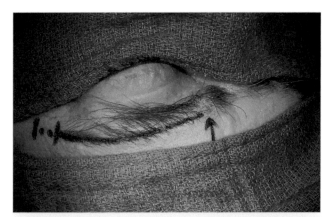

Fig. 12.2 Skin incision. The pointed line reveals the possible lateral extension up to 1 cm, the arrow: the supraorbital notch.

- **Ending point:** Incision ends at the margin point of the tail of the eyebrow, it can be extended up to 1 cm laterally.
- The lateral extension of the incision should be sufficient to reveal the anterior edge of the temporal muscle and, with that, the frontobasal keyhole.

12.5.1 Critical Structures

- The supraorbital neurovascular bundle.

12.6 Soft Tissues Dissection (Fig. 12.3)

- **Myofascial level**
  - Dissection through soft tissues is carried out in the direction of the skin incision.
- **Muscles (Fig. 12.3)**
  - The frontalis muscle is incised along the direction of muscle fibers, parallel to the skin incision.
  - The soft tissue dissection has to be carried out up to 3 cm above the orbital ridge.
  - The temporal fascia and muscle are exposed.
- **Bone exposure**
  - Landmarks for an orbital ridge periosteal incision:
    - Medially: The supraorbital notch.
    - Laterally: The lateral orbital tubercle.
  - The periosteum is incised in U-shaped fashion based on the orbital ridge, then elevated.
  - Elevation of the periosteum across the frontal bone is continued laterally beyond the frontozygomatic junction (**Fig. 12.4**).
  - If an additional orbital osteotomy is planned, the subperiosteal dissection is carried down to orbital roof; the ocular globe should be protected in this step with a malleable retractor.
  - Dissection of the temporal fascia and muscle from the superior temporal line is continued until the extracranial surface of the greater wing of the sphenoid bone is exposed (**Fig. 12.5**).

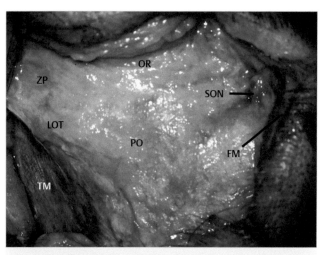

Fig. 12.3 Soft tissue dissection: myofascial dissection and frontal muscle incision.
Abbreviations: FM = frontalis muscle; LOT = lateral orbital tubercle; OR = orbital ridge; PO = periosteum; SON = supraorbital nerve; TM = temporal muscle; ZP = zygomatic process of frontal bone.

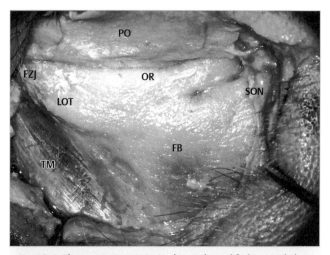

Fig. 12.4 The periosteum is incised in U-shaped fashion and elevated; the subperiosteal dissection is carried out until the fronto zygomatic junction.
Abbreviations: FB = frontal bone; FZJ = frontozygomatic suture; LOT = lateral orbital tubercle; OR = orbital ridge; PO = periosteum; SON = supraorbital nerve; TM = temporal muscle.

12.6.1 Critical Structures

- The supraorbital neurovascular bundle
- The ocular globe

12.6.2 Craniotomy (Fig. 12.6)

- **Burr holes**
  - A fronto-basal keyhole is placed to expose the frontal lobe dura, it can be extended to the extracranial surface of the greater wing of sphenoid bone to expose the temporal pole dura and Sylvian fissure (**Figs. 12.5, 12.6**).
  - Thereafter, the craniotomy is performed and should be large enough to accommodate fully opened bipolar forceps.

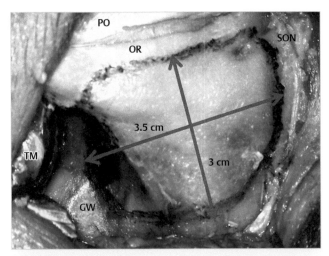

Fig. 12.5 Dissection of the temporal fascia and muscle until the extracranial surface of the greater wing of the sphenoid bone is exposed.
Abbreviations: GW = extracranial surface of the greater wing of sphenoid bone; OR = orbital ridge; PO = periosteum; SON = supraorbital nerve; TM = temporal muscle.

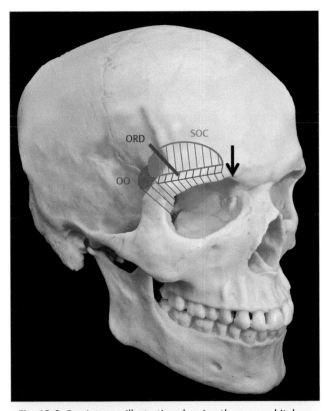

Fig. 12.6 Craniotomy: illustration showing the supraorbital craniotomy and orbital osteotomy.
Colors: green spot = keyhole; green lines = supra orbital craniotomy (SOC); blue lines = the part of the orbital ridge to be drilled and flattened (ORD); red spot = the extension of the keyhole if an orbital osteotomy is needed; red lines = the orbital osteotomy (OO); black arrow = the supraorbital notch.

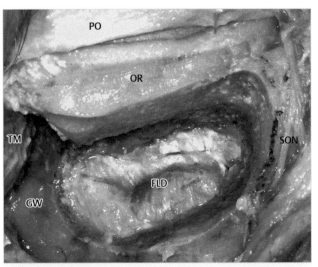

Fig. 12.7 Craniotomy.
Abbreviations: FLD = frontal lobe dura; GW = extracranial surface of the greater wing of sphenoid bone; OR = orbital ridge; PO = periosteum; SON = supraorbital nerve; TM = temporal muscle.

- **Craniotomy landmarks (Figs. 12.5, 12.6)**
  - **Medially:** The supraorbital notch or the frontal sinus if it is lateral to the notch; the neuronavigation is recommended for intraoperative identification of the bony landmarks.
  - **Laterally:** The keyhole.
  - **Superiorly:** Up to 3 cm superior to the supraorbital ridge.
  - **Inferiorly:** The orbital ridge (except if an orbital osteotomy is needed).
  - Since the orbital ridge and the orbital roof are irregular, an extradural drilling to flatten the exposed bony surfaces will enhance the exposure (**Figs. 12.7, 12.8**).
  - Extradural anterior clinoidectomy and optic foraminotomy can be performed as needed.

12.6.3 Critical Structures

- The supraorbital neurovascular bundle
- The ocular globe
- The frontal paranasal sinus

12.7 Dural Opening (Fig. 12.9)

- U-shaped fashion with its flap based inferiorly.

12.8 Intradural Exposure (Figs. 12.10, 12.11)

- **Bony structures:** Anterior and posterior clinoid processes.
- **Parenchymal structures:** Frontal lobe, the temporal lobe can be exposed if needed.
- **Arachnoidal layers:** Optic cistern, carotid cistern, and the proximal Sylvian fissure (if needed).

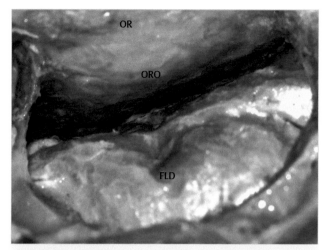

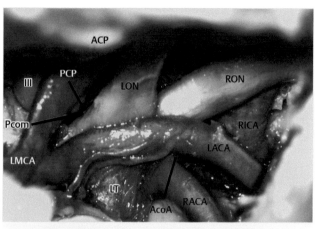

Fig. 12.8 Craniotomy. The orbital ridge and orbital roof are extradurally flattened.
Abbreviations: FLD = frontal lobe dura; OR = orbital ridge; ORO = orbital roof.

Fig. 12.10 Microscopic view: the frontal lobe is retracted. Abbreviations: AcoA = anterior communicating artery; ACP = anterior clinoid process; LACA = left anterior cerebral artery; LMCA = left middle cerebral artery; LON = left optic nerve; LT = lamina terminalis; PCP = posterior clinoid process; Pcom = posterior communicating artery; RACA = right anterior cerebral artery; RICA = right internal carotid artery; RON = right optic nerve; III = oculomotor nerve.

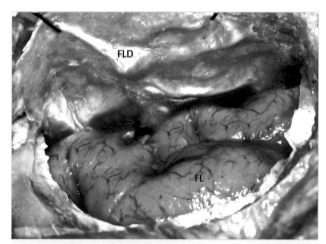

Fig. 12.9 The U-shaped dural opening.
Abbreviations: FL = frontal lobe; FLD: frontal lobe dura.

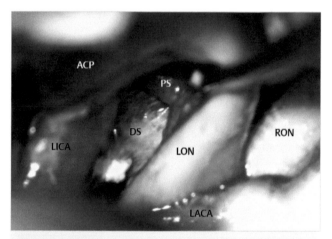

Fig. 12.11 Microscopic view: the pituitary stalk is visualized. Abbreviations: ACP = anterior clinoid process; DS = diaphragma sellae; LACA = left anterior cerebral artery; LICA = left internal carotid artery; LON = left optic nerve; PS = pituitary stalk; RON = right optic nerve.

- **Cranial nerves:** Ipsilateral and contralateral optic nerves, optic chiasm, ipsilateral/contralateral oculomotor nerve.
- **Arteries:** Ipsilateral and contralateral internal carotid artery (ICA), ipsilateral and contralateral ACA, AcoA, ipsilateral Pcom, ipsilateral MCA.
- The pituitary stalk can be visualized.
- Extradural or intradural anterior clinoidectomy and/or bony optic foraminotomy and sectioning the falciform ligament (dural optic foraminotomy) are required to avoid injury of the optic nerve in carotid ophthalmic segment aneurysms, proximal P-com aneurysms and sellar and parasellar lesions.

References

1. Abdel Aziz KM, Bhatia S, Tantawy MH, et al. Minimally invasive transpalpebral "eyelid" approach to the anterior cranial base. Neurosurgery 2011;69(2, Suppl Operative):ons195–ons206, discussion 206–207

2. Jho HD. Orbital roof craniotomy via an eyebrow incision: a simplified anterior skull base approach. Minim Invasive Neurosurg 1997;40(3):91–97

3. Little A, Gore P, Darbar A, et al. Supraorbital eyebrow approach. In: Cappabianca P, Califano L, Iaconetta G, eds. Cranial, craniofacial, and skull base surgery. Milan: Springer; 2010:27–38

4. Perneczky A, Reisch R. Supraorbital approach. In: Perneczky A, Reisch R, eds. Keyhole approaches in neurosurgery. Wien: Springer; 2008:37–95

13 Lateral Orbitotomy

Alfio Spina, Filippo Gagliardi, Michele Bailo, Cristian Gragnaniello, Martina Piloni, Anthony J. Caputy, and Pietro Mortini

13.1 Introduction

Orbital lesions, depending on their location and relationship with the intra-orbital structures, can be approached through different surgical routes (transcranial or trans-orbital).

The lateral orbitotomy, also known as Krönlein approach, and its further modifications allow for an easy reach of intra-orbital lesions located in the superior, lateral, and inferior intraconal compartments as well as pathologies of the lateral aspect of the orbital apex.

Lateral orbitotomy takes advantage of a direct approach to orbital content, avoiding potential complication of a transcranial or direct transorbital route.

13.2 Indications

• Orbital intra-conal and extra-conal lesions.
• Lesions of the lateral aspect of the orbital apex.

13.3 Patient Positioning

• **Position:** The patient is positioned supine with the head fixed with a horseshoe head holder.
• **Body:** The head is slightly elevated, to facilitate the venous backflow.
• **Head:** The head is turned 45° to the contralateral side.
• **Neck:** The neck is slightly extended (about 20°).
• The zygoma must be the highest point in the surgical field.

13.4 Skin Incision

• **Italic "S" skin incision (Fig. 13.1)**
  ○ **Starting point:** Incision starts at the lateral third of the eyebrow, just above the orbital rim.
  ○ **Course:** Incision line runs posteriorly and inferiorly toward the postero-superior (temporal) border of the zygomatic bone.
  ○ **Ending point:** It ends at the zygomatic-temporal suture.

13.4.1 Critical Structures

• Frontal branch of the facial nerve.
• Orbicularis oculi muscle.
• Supraorbital nerve and vessels.
• Lateral canthal ligament.

13.5 Soft Tissue Dissection (Figs. 13.2, 13.3)

• **Temporal fascia and periorbit**
  ○ Superficial temporal muscle fascia is incised, avoiding transecting underlying muscle fibers.
  ○ Periorbit is dissected from the inner surface of the lateral wall of the orbit.

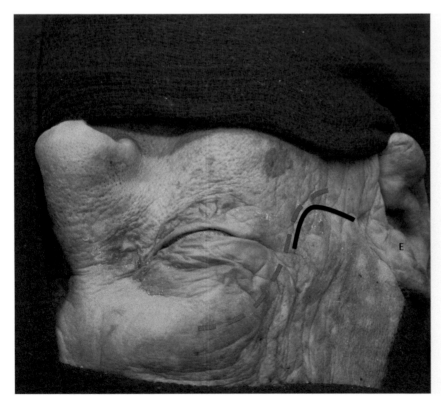

Fig. 13.1 Italic "S" skin incision.
Abbreviations: E = ear.

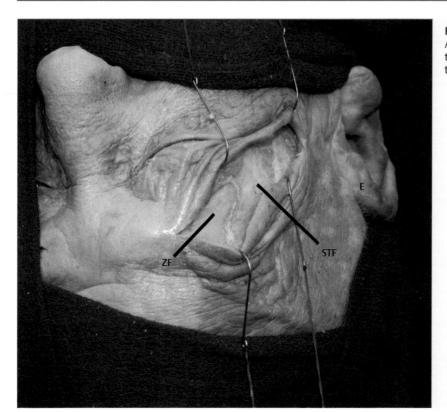

Fig. 13.2 Superficial soft tissue dissection. Abbreviations: E = ear; STF = superficial temporal fascia; ZF = zygomatic process of the frontal bone.

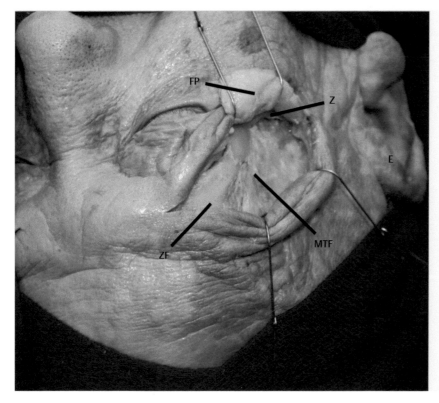

Fig. 13.3 Deep soft tissue dissection. Abbreviations: E = ear; FP = fat pad; MTF = middle temporal fascia; Z = zygoma; ZF = zygomatic process of the frontal bone.

- **Muscle**
  - Interfascial dissection of the temporal muscle is carried out.
  - The superficial layer of temporal fascia together with the fat pad is reflected anteriorly.
  - Temporal muscle fibers are dissected in a subperiosteal fashion and retracted posteriorly.

- **Bone exposure**
  The bone exposure is completed when the following structures come into view:
  - Outer surface of the greater sphenoid wing.
  - Zygomatic process of the frontal bone.
  - Frontal process of the zygomatic bone.
  - Fronto-zygomatic suture.

13.5.1 Critical Structures

- Frontal branch of the facial nerve.
- Zygomatic artery and meningeal branches of the lacrimal artery.
- Periorbit.

13.6 Lateral Orbitotomy (Figs. 13.4, 13.5)

A lateral orbitotomy including the lateral orbital frame is performed.

- **Zygomatic osteotomy (with a reciprocating saw or a C1 without foot attachment)**
  - **I cut:** The first cut is made just above the frontozygomatic suture.

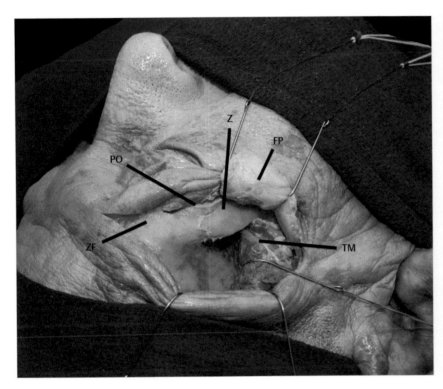

Fig. 13.4 Bone exposure.
Abbreviations: FP = fat pad; PO = periorbit; TM = temporal muscle; Z = zygoma; ZF = zygomatic process of the frontal bone.

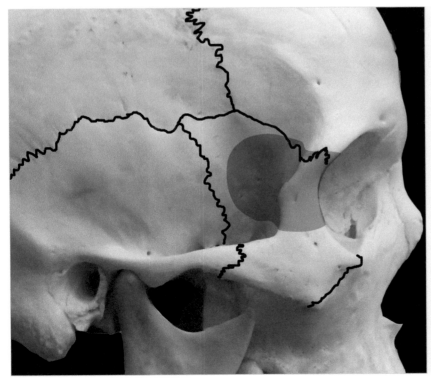

Fig. 13.5 Lateral orbitotomy.

○ **II cut:** The second cut is made at the base of the frontal process of the zygoma.
- **Resection of the lateral orbital wall**
  ○ The greater wing of the sphenoid bone is drilled to expose the periorbit.

13.6.1 Critical Structures

- Periorbit.
- Intra-orbital neurovascular structures.

13.7 Periorbital Opening (Fig. 13.6)

- X-shaped fashion.
- Attention has to be payed not to cut underlying lateral rectus muscle fibers.

13.7.1 Critical Structures

- Optic nerve.
- Ocular muscles.
- Ophthalmic artery and vein.
- Ocular bulb.
- Nasociliary, trochlear, lacrimal and frontal nerves.
- Lacrimal gland.

13.8 Intraorbital Exposure (Fig. 13.7)

- **Parenchymal structures:** Ocular bulb, lacrimal gland, orbital fat, eyelid.
- **Muscles:** Lateral rectus, inferior oblique, inferior rectus, superior oblique muscles.
- **Cranial nerves:** Optic nerve, branches of the third, fourth and fifth cranial nerves.

- **Arteries:** Ophthalmic artery.
- **Veins:** Ophthalmic veins.

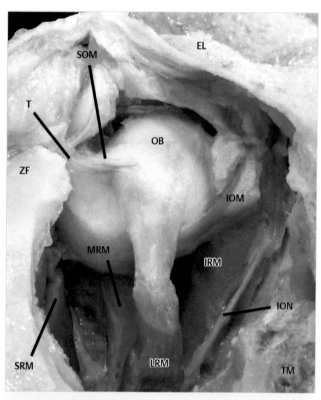

Fig. 13.7 Orbital contents.
Abbreviations: EL = eyelid; IOM = inferior oblique muscle; ION = inferior branch of the oculomotor nerve; IRM = inferior rectus muscle; LRM = lateral rectus muscle; MRM = medial rectus muscle; OB = ocular bulb; SOM = superior oblique muscle; SRM = superior rectus muscle; T = trochlea; TM = temporal muscle; ZF = zygomatic process of the frontal bone.

Fig. 13.6 Exposure of the periorbit.
Abbreviations: FP = fat pad; PO = periorbit; TM = temporal muscle; ZF = zygomatic process of the frontal bone.

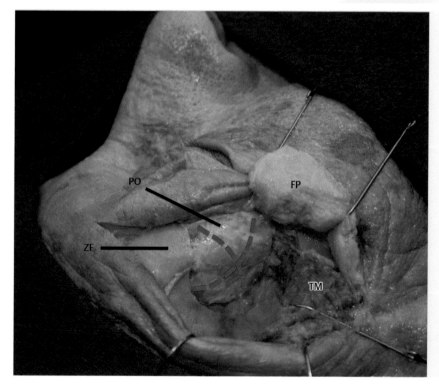

References

1. Krönlein RU. [Zur pathologie und operativen behandlung der dermoidcysten der orbita]. Beitr Klin Chir. 1889; 4:149–163
2. Mohsenipour I. Approaches in neurosurgery: central and peripheral nervous system. New York, NY: Thieme Medical Publisher; 1994
3. Sekhar LN, Fessler RG. Atlas of neurosurgical techniques. Brain. Volume 1. New York, NY: Thieme Medical Publishers; 2016
4. Sindou M. Practical handbook of neurosurgery: from leading neurosurgeons, Volume 1. Wien: Springer-Verlag; 2009

14 Frontal and Bifrontal Approach

Filippo Gagliardi, Alfio Spina, Michele Bailo, Martina Piloni, Cristian Gragnaniello, Anthony J. Caputy, and Pietro Mortini

14.1 Introduction

The unilateral frontal craniotomy and its further extension, the bilateral frontal approach, are extremely versatile procedures, which can be easily tailored according to the existing pathology. The approaches are suitable for the unilateral/bilateral exposure of the lateral and anterior surfaces of the frontal lobe, as well as the most anterior aspect of the interhemispheric fissure.

It is possible to extend the bilateral approach by performing a bilateral orbitotomy to take advantage of the subfrontal anatomical corridor to reach the anterior skull base, as described in detail in **Chapter 30.** The approach is indicated for intra-axial lesions of the frontal lobe, as well as extra-axial tumors of the frontal convexity, of the anterior aspect of the falx and anterior cranial fossa. The approach is also suitable to treat vascular lesions of A2 as well as distal frontal branches of the anterior and middle cerebral artery.

14.2 Indications

- Intra-axial lesions of the frontal lobes.
- Extra-axial lesions of the frontal convexity and anterior third of the falx.
- Vascular lesions of the second segment (A2) and distal frontal branches of the anterior and middle cerebral artery.

14.3 Patient Positioning

- **Position:** The patient is positioned supine with the head fixed in a Mayfield head holder.
- **Body:** The trunk and the head are slightly elevated to facilitate the venous backflow.
- **Head:** The head is placed in neutral position in case of bilateral approach. Alternatively, it can be slightly turned to the opposite side (about 15-20°) in case of unilateral approach.
- **Neck:** The neck is slightly extended (about 20°), to facilitate further brain relaxation after dural opening.

14.4 Skin Incision (Fig. 14.1)

- **Bicoronal skin incision (suggested for the frontal bilateral craniotomy):**
  - **Starting point:** Incision starts 1 cm anterior to the ipsilateral tragus, just above the zygoma.
  - **Course:** The incision line runs to the contralateral side, just behind the hairline over the coronal suture.
  - **Ending point:** It ends 1 cm anterior to the tragus on the contralateral side. Alternatively, it can be taken to the contralateral superior temporal line.
- **Frontotemporal skin incision (suggested for the frontal unilateral craniotomy):**
  - **Starting point:** Incision starts 1 cm anterior to the ipsilateral tragus, just above the zygoma.

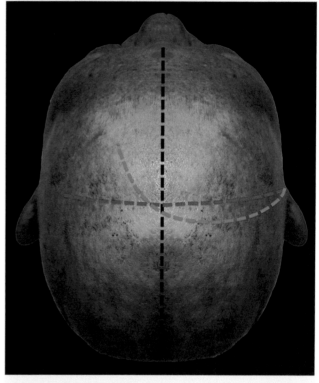

Fig. 14.1 Alternative skin incisions.

- **Course:** The incision line runs slightly curved backward until reaching the coronal suture and then turns toward the contralateral side (2 cm beyond the midline).
- **Ending point:** It ends 2 cm beyond the midline, on the contralateral side just behind the hairline.

14.4.1 Critical Structures

- Superficial temporal artery and its branches.
- Frontal and temporal branches of the facial nerve.

14.5 Soft Tissue Dissection (Figs. 14.2, 14.3)

- **Pericranial layer**
  - Pericranium is smoothly dissected from the bone and the superficial temporal fascia, taking care to preserve its anatomical integrity.
  - It is reflected anteriorly together with the skin flap.
  - Pericranium must be preserved as it may be needed for further reconstruction.
- **Muscle**
  - **Frontal unilateral craniotomy**
    - ❖ Ipsilateral temporal muscle inter-fascial dissection is carried out according to the technique described in **Chapters 6 and 8.**

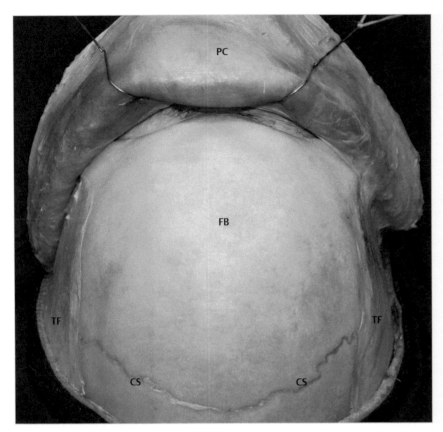

Fig. 14.2 Soft tissue dissection. Abbreviations: CS = coronal suture; FB = frontal bone; PC = pericranium; TF = temporal fascia.

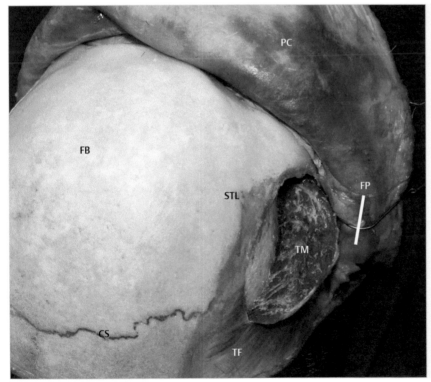

Fig. 14.3 Soft tissue dissection, lateral view. Abbreviations: CS = coronal suture; FB = frontal bone; FP = fat pad; PC = pericranium; STL = superior temporal line; TF = temporal fascia; TM = temporal muscle.

❖ The superficial layer of the temporal fascia together with the fat pad is reflected anteriorly.

❖ The deep layer is dissected from the temporal squama in a subperiosteal fashion and reflected inferiorly, in order to expose the part of temporal squama, located just below the superior temporal line, where burr holes will be made.

○ **Frontal bilateral craniotomy**

❖ The procedure described for the unilateral variant has to be carried out also on the contralateral side.

• **Bone exposure**

The bone exposure is completed, when the following structures come into view:

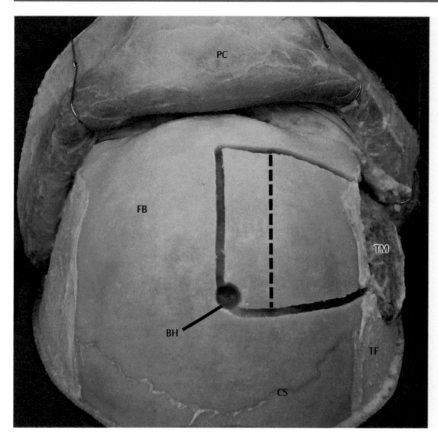

Fig. 14.4 Frontal unilateral approach. Craniotomy landmarks (superior view). Abbreviations: BH = burr hole; CS = coronal suture; FB = frontal bone; PC = pericranium; TF = temporal fascia; TM = temporal muscle.

- Ipsilateral pterion and superior temporal line (bilateral exposure in case of frontal bilateral approach).
- Anterior aspect of the sagittal suture.
- Ipsilateral coronal suture (bilateral exposure in case of frontal bilateral approach).
- Ipsilateral frontal bone (bilateral exposure in case of frontal bilateral approach).
- Orbital rim (bilateral exposure in case of frontal bilateral approach).

14.5.1 Critical Structures

- Frontal branch of the facial nerve.
- Supraorbital nerve, artery and vein.

14.6 Craniotomy (Figs. 14.4–14.7)

14.6.1 Frontal Unilateral Craniotomy, Landmarks (Figs. 14.4, 14.5)

- **Burr holes**
  - **I:** The first burr hole is made at the keyhole on the ipsilateral side.
  - **II:** The second one is placed 4-5 cm posteriorly to the keyhole, just below the superior temporal line for cosmetic reasons to allow it to be covered by temporal muscle.
  - **III:** The third one is made either 1 cm lateral to the midline (in case of a paramedian frontal unilateral craniotomy), or over the superior sagittal sinus (in case of a midline frontal unilateral craniotomy). Posterior extension of the frontal craniotomy has to be tailored according to the pathology, and the planned approach.

- **Cuts**
  - **I:** The first cut is made between the first and second burr hole, taking care not to damage the middle meningeal artery.
  - **II:** The second cut is made from the keyhole toward the midline, taking care not to tear the dura around the area of the pterion.
  - **III:** The third cut is made from median/paramedian hole to the II hole. Craniotome should be directed away from the sinus to minimize the risk of dural tearing and bridging veins damage.
  - **IV:** The fourth cut is made over the sinus.
- **Craniotomy landmarks**
  Anatomical landmarks which have to be taken into consideration in designing the craniotomy are as follows:
  - **Anteriorly:** Ipsilateral orbital rim.
  - **Laterally:** Ipsilateral superior temporal line.
  - **Medially:** Anterior aspect of the sagittal suture.
  - **Posteriorly:** Ipsilateral coronal suture.

14.6.2 Frontal Bilateral Craniotomy, Landmarks (Figs. 14.6, 14.7)

- **Burr holes**
  - **I:** The first burr hole is made at the keyhole on the ipsilateral side.
  - **II:** The second one is made at the keyhole on the contralateral side.
  - **III**: The third one is placed on the midline over the superior sagittal sinus.
- **Cuts**
  - **I:** The first cut is made between the first two holes.
  - **II/III:** The second and third cuts are made from the median hole to the keyholes bilaterally.

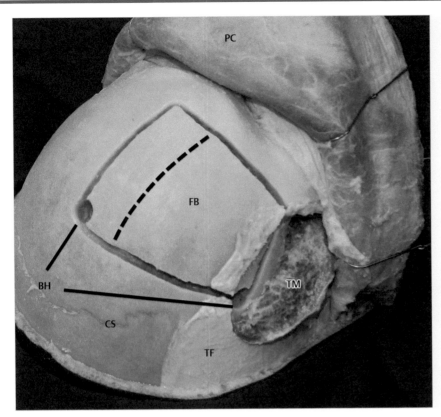

Fig. 14.5 Frontal unilateral approach. Craniotomy landmarks (lateral view). Abbreviations: BH = burr hole; CS = coronal suture; FB = frontal bone; PC = pericranium; TF = temporal fascia; TM = temporal muscle.

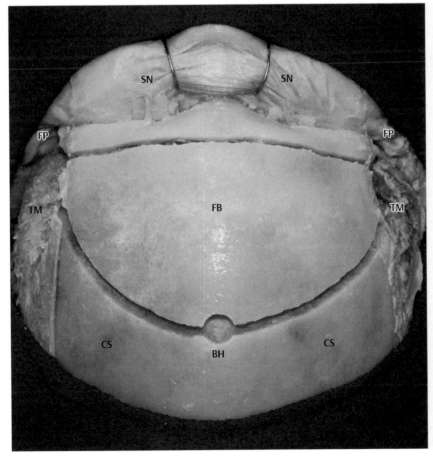

Fig. 14.6 Frontal bilateral approach. Craniotomy landmarks.
Abbreviations: BH = burr hole; CS = coronal suture; FB = frontal bone; FP = fat pad; SN = supraorbital nerve (outlined in green); TM = temporal muscle.

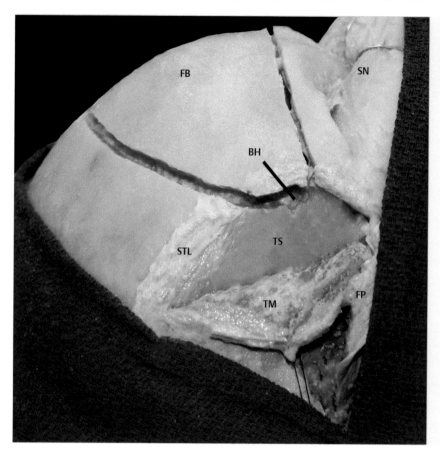

Fig. 14.7 Frontal bilateral approach, lateral view.
Abbreviations: BH = burr hole; FB = frontal bone; FP = fat pad; SN = supraorbital nerve; STL = superior temporal line; TM = temporal muscle; TS = temporal squama.

- **Craniotomy landmarks**
Anatomical landmarks that have to be taken into consideration in designing the craniotomy are as follows:
  - **Anteriorly:** Orbital rims on both sides.
  - **Laterally:** Superior temporal lines on both sides.
  - **Posteriorly:** Coronal suture on both sides.

14.6.3 Variants

- **Inter-hemispheric approach (See Chapter 18)**
  - The craniotomy might be extended contralaterally using an additional burr hole, which has to be placed on the contralateral side of the sinus, in order to completely expose the superior sagittal sinus.
- **Subfrontal approach (See Chapter 30)**
  - A monolateral or bilateral orbitotomy might be performed to allow for a more basal exposure, opening the subfrontal and interhemispheric corridors. The orbitotomy optimizes the surgical access to the floor of the anterior cranial fossa and to the suprasellar area.

14.6.4 Critical Structures

- Superior sagittal sinus.
- **In case of frontal sinus opening a sinus cranialization is suggested according to the following technique (See Chapter 6).**
  - Mucosa must be removed from the walls of the sinus cavity.
  - The posterior wall of the sinus has to be completely removed by using a drill and a rongeur (cranialization).

- The closure of the frontal ostium is obtained by harvesting and positioning a vascularized pericranial flap.

14.7 Dural Opening

- **Frontal unilateral approach**
  - Dura is opened in a C-shaped fashion.
  - The dural flap is based on the superior sagittal sinus and reflected medially.
- **Frontal bilateral approach**
  - Dura is opened into two single flaps, both of them in a C-shaped fashion.
  - Dural flaps are based on the ipsilateral orbital rim, sparing the integrity of the superior sagittal sinus.

14.7.1 Critical Structures

- Cortical draining veins.
- Superior sagittal sinus.

14.8 Intradural Exposure (Figs. 14.8–14.11)

14.8.1 Frontal Unilateral Approach (Figs. 14.8, 14.9)

- **Parenchymal structures:** Anterior and lateral surface of the ipsilateral frontal lobe; in particular middle

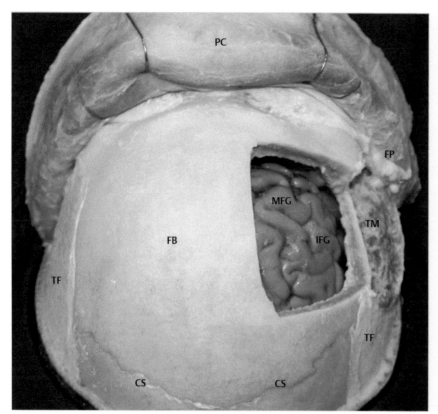

Fig. 14.8 Frontal unilateral approach. Intradural view. Abbreviations: CS = coronal suture; FB = frontal bone; FP = fat pad; IFG = inferior frontal gyrus; MFG = middle frontal gyrus; PC = pericranium; TF = temporal fascia; TM = temporal muscle.

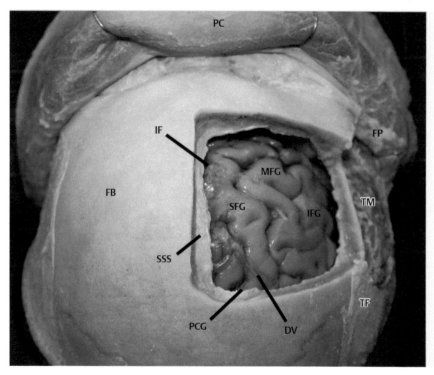

Fig. 14.9 Frontal unilateral approach. Interhemispheric variant. Intradural view. Abbreviations: DV = draining vein; FB = frontal bone; FP = fat pad; IF = interhemispheric fissure; IFG = inferior frontal gyrus; MFG = middle frontal gyrus; PC = pericranium; PCG = precentral gyrus; TF = temporal fascia; TM = temporal muscle; SFG = superior frontal gyrus; SSS = superior sagittal sinus.

and lower frontal gyrus in case of the paramedian frontal unilateral approach, together with the upper frontal gyrus in case of the median frontal unilateral approach.

- **Arachnoidal layer:** Sylvian fissure in case of the paramedian frontal unilateral approach, together with the anterior aspect of the interhemispheric fissure in case of the median frontal unilateral approach.

- **Cranial nerves:** Ipsilateral olfactory and optic nerves if orbitotomy is performed.
- **Arteries:** Frontal branches of the middle cerebral artery in case of the paramedian frontal unilateral approach, together with frontal branches of the anterior cerebral artery in case of the median frontal unilateral approach.
- **Veins:** Interhemispheric vein, frontal cortical draining veins, frontal branches of the superficial middle cerebral vein.

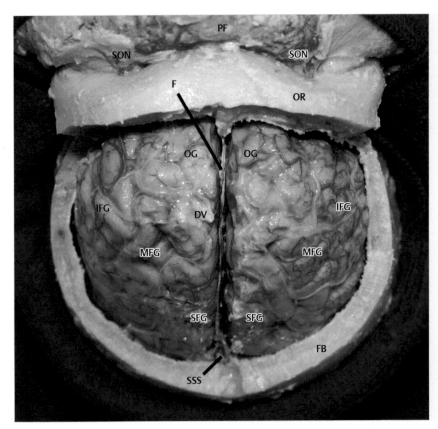

Fig. 14.10 Frontal bilateral approach. Intradural view.
Abbreviations: DV = draining vein; F = falx; FB = frontal bone; IFG = inferior frontal gyrus; MFG = middle frontal gyrus; OG = orbital gyrus; OR = orbital roof; PF = pericranial flap; SFG = superior frontal gyrus; SON = supraorbital nerve; SSS = superior sagittal sinus.

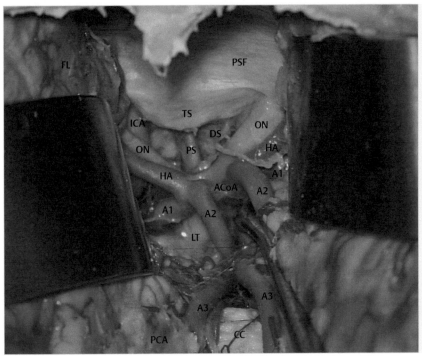

Fig. 14.11 Frontal bilateral approach. Interhemispheric intradural view.
Abbreviations: A1 = A1 segment of the anterior cerebral artery; A2 = A2 segment of the anterior cerebral artery; A3 = A3 segment of the anterior cerebral artery; ACoA = anterior communicating artery; CC = corpus callosum; DS = diaphragma sellae; FL = frontal lobe; HA = Heubner's artery; ICA = internal carotid artery; LT = lamina terminalis; ON = optic nerve; PCA = pericallosal artery; PS = pituitary stalk; PSF = planum sphenoidalis; TS = tuberculum sellae.

14.8.2 Frontal Bilateral Approach (Figs. 14.10, 14.11)

- **Parenchymal structures:** Anterior, medial, basal and lateral surfaces of both the frontal lobes.
- **Arachnoidal layer:** Bilateral exposure of the Sylvian fissure and the anterior aspect of the interhemispheric fissure.

- **Cranial nerves:** Bilateral exposure of olfactory and optic nerves if orbitotomy is performed.
- **Arteries:** Bilateral exposure of both anterior cerebral arteries, of frontal branches of the middle cerebral artery and anterior cerebral artery.
- **Veins:** Bilateral exposure of interhemispheric veins, frontal cortical draining veins, frontal branches of the superficial middle cerebral vein.

References

1. Connolly ES, McKhann GM II, Huang J. Fundamentals of operative techniques in neurosurgery. New York, NY: Thieme Medical Publishers; 2011
2. Fossett D, Caputy AJ. Operative neurosurgical anatomy. New York, NY: Thieme Medical Publisher; 2002
3. Kobayashi S. Neurosurgery of complex vascular lesions and tumors. New York, NY: Thieme Medical Publishers; 2005
4. Sekhar LN, Fessler RG. Atlas of neurosurgical techniques. Brain. Volume 1. New York, NY: Thieme Medical Publishers; 2016
5. Wanibuchi M, Friedman AH, Fukushima T. Photo Atlas of Skull Base Dissection: Techniques and Operative Approaches. New York, NY: Thieme Medical Publishers; 2009

15 Frontotemporal and Pterional Approach

Cristian Gragnaniello, Nicholas J. Erickson, Filippo Gagliardi, Pietro Mortini, and Anthony J. Caputy

15.1 Indications

- Aneurysms.
  - All aneurysms of anterior circulation.
  - Basilar tip aneurysms.
- Parasellar lesions.
- Meningiomas involving the sphenoid wing and the anterior clinoid.

15.2 Patient Positioning

- **Position:** The patient is positioned supine with torso flexed slightly downward and knees slightly flexed to improve venous drainage. Soft gelatin roll placed under the ipsilateral shoulder can be used to reduce neck rotation.
- **Head:** The head is fixed in a Mayfield 3-point head holder. It is rotated to contralateral side such that the pterion area is at 12 o'clock, elevated and slightly extended so that the vertex tilts toward the floor.
- The ipsilateral **zygoma** is the highest point in the surgical field.
- The single pin of the head holder should be placed on the ipsilateral side superior to the mastoid process. On the other arm, one pin is placed superior to the mastoid process on the contralateral side.

15.3 Skin Incision (Fig. 15.1)

- **Starting point**: The incision begins at the zygoma (1 cm anterior to the tragus to avoid damage to frontotemporal branch of facial nerve and frontal branch of superior temporal artery).
- **Run**: The incision extends cephalad crossing the superficial temporal artery while coursing posterior to the hairline.
- **Ending point**: The incision terminates at widow's peak.
- The base of the skin incision should equal its height to avoid necrosis of the margin. Hemostatic clips are attached to skin edge and galea to keep vascularity.
- The **superficial temporal artery** is preserved in every case, especially if the surgeon anticipates the potential for bypass.

15.3.1 Critical Structures

- Frontal branch of the facial nerve.
- Superficial temporal artery.

15.4 Soft Tissue Dissection

- **Myofascial level (Fig. 15.2)**
  - Yasargil first described the interfascial dissection of the temporal muscle that serves to preserve the frontotemporal

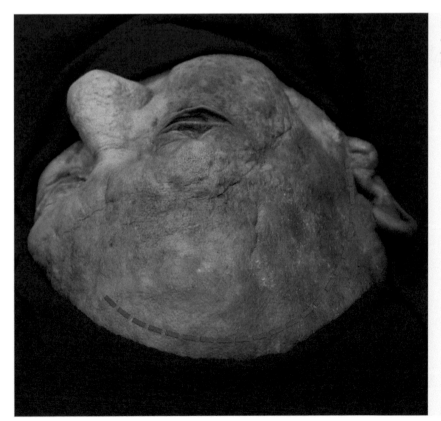

Fig. 15.1 Skin incision. The incision begins at the zygoma, 1 cm anterior to the tragus and extends cephalad posterior to the hairline ending at the widow's peak.

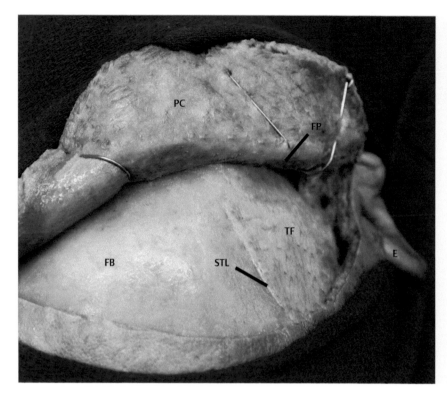

Fig. 15.2 Soft tissue dissection. After the skin flap, pericranium and fat pad are reflected anteriorly, the frontal bone along with the temporal fascia and its insertion at the superior temporal line are visualized. Abbreviations: E = ear; FB = frontal bone; FP = fat pad; PC = pericranium; STL = superior temporal line; TF = temporal fascia.

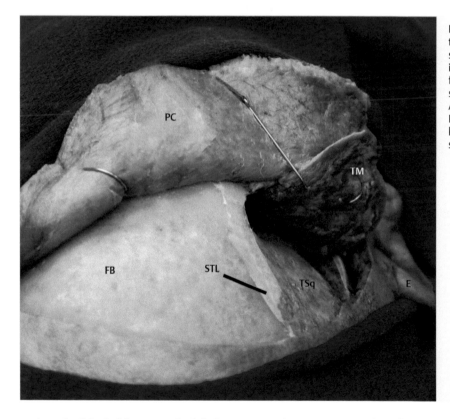

Fig. 15.3 Temporal muscle detachment. The temporal muscle is elevated away from the squamous portion of the temporal bone and is reflected in the same manner as the skin flap. A small cuff of fascia is left along the superior temporal line.
Abbreviations: E = ear; FB = frontal bone; PC = pericranium; STL = superior temporal line; TM = temporal muscle; TSq = temporal squama.

branch of the facial nerve and minimize postoperative cosmetic changes **(see Chapters 6 and 8).**

○ The temporal muscle is covered by a superficial fascia. This dissection should be made vertically starting from the superior temporal line, 1.5 to 2 cm from the superior rim of the orbit to the posterior portion of the zygomatic arch using a cold scalpel and Metzenbaum scissors.

○ The reflection of the skin and superficial fascia along with its underlying fat pad is completed with the use of hooks or sutures and elastic bands as per surgeon's preference.

• **Muscles (Fig. 15.3)**

○ The dissection and detachment of the temporal muscle is done in two stages. A vertical incision is made perpendicularly to the zygoma posteriorly and a transverse incision

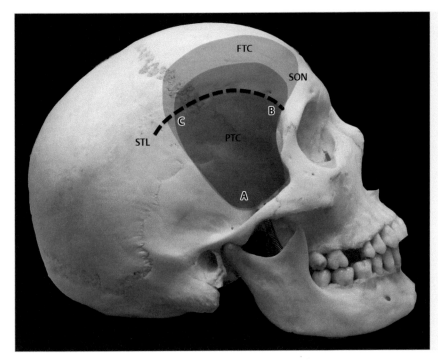

Fig. 15.4 Craniotomy. After the keyhole (**B**) is made, a second burr hole is made posteriorly in the squamous portion of the temporal bone just above the posterior root of the zygoma (**A**). In older patients, a third burr hole (**C**) may be necessary as strenuous attachment of the dura to the bone is expected. Different sizes of the craniotomy are shown, tailoring for the different types of exposure that may be needed. Abbreviations: FTC = fronto-temporal craniotomy; PTC = pterional craniotomy; SON = superior orbital notch; STL = superior temporal line.

parallel to the superior
temporal line, leaving a superior strap attached to the skull.

○ Using a Cushing's elevator, the detachment of the deep muscular fascia of the skull is started on its posterior superior portion using horizontal movements with the tip of the elevator.

○ Using three hooks or elastic bands, the temporal muscle is reflected anteriorly and inferiorly.

15.4.1 Critical Structures

• Frontal branch of the facial nerve.

15.5 Craniotomy/Craniectomy (Figs. 15.4, 15.5)

• **Burr holes**
  ○ Usually **two burr holes** are sufficient, placed at points **A** and **B** to easily cross the sphenoid wing.
  ○ Point **A** is located in the squamous portion of the temporal bone just above the posterior root of the zygoma.
  ○ Point **B** is called "keyhole" and is located at the intersection of the zygomatic bone, the superior temporal line and the supraorbital edge. The drill must be positioned posteriorly and inferiorly to prevent entering the orbit.
  ○ A third burr hole at point **C** is recommended in older patients where the dura mater is firmly attached to the bone.
• **Cuts**
  ○ A pneumatic craniotome with continuous irrigation is then used to cut a bone flap **starting** at point **B** and extending **anteriorly** across the anterior margin of the superior temporal line and then following it posteriorly to the extent of the bony exposure ending at point **A.**

○ It is important to stay as low as possible on the orbit to avoid having to rongeur bone, which can be cosmetically unappealing as will be covered by thin skin and reconstructed by large burr hole cover that could further create issues over time.

○ **Starting** again at point **B**, the craniotomy is taken **posteriorly** across the sphenoid wing until the drill hangs up due to the presence of the greater wing of the sphenoid.

○ Starting at point **A**, the craniotomy is taken **anteriorly** across the sphenoid wing until the drill hangs up.

○ The bone between the two points, where the drill hangs up, is then drilled with a large burr.

○ The length and height of drilling and resulting size of the bone flap will vary depending on the aim of surgery.

○ The bone flap is removed using periosteal elevators and holes are drilled in the bone and bone flap for placing dural retention sutures.

○ The sphenoid ridge is removed with a high-speed drill to the lateral margin of the superior orbital fissure. The temporal bone is removed with a rongeur so that it is flush with the floor of the middle fossa. These steps are crucial to achieve adequate intradural exposure.

15.5.1 Variants (See Chapter 17)

• Orbitozygomatic osteotomy

15.6 Dural Opening (Fig. 15.6)

• A curvilinear incision in the dura and the flap is pediculated towards the greater sphenoid wing.
• The dural flap is sutured to the base of the temporal muscle.

15.6.1 Critical Structures

• Middle meningeal artery.

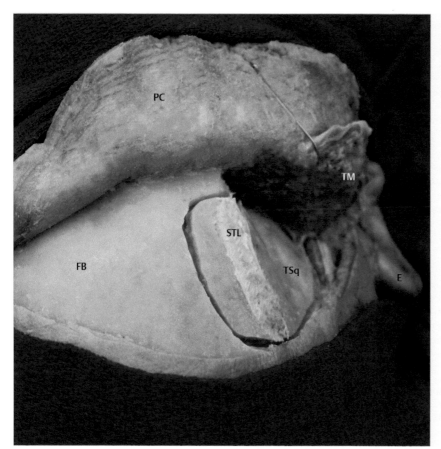

Fig. 15.5 Superior view of the craniotomy in place.
Abbreviations: E = ear; FB = frontal bone; PC = pericranium; STL = superior temporal line; TM = temporal muscle; TSq = temporal squama.

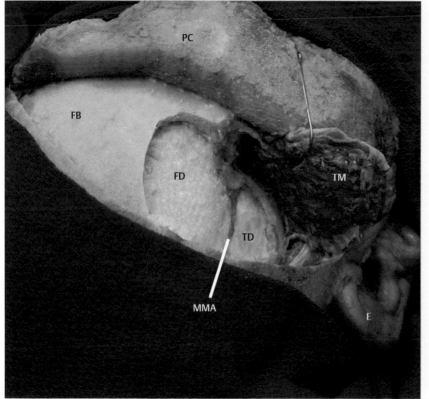

Fig. 15.6 Dural exposure. The frontal and temporal dura delineated by the middle meningeal artery.
Abbreviations: E = ear; FB = frontal bone; FD = frontal dura; MMA = middle meningeal artery; PC = pericranium; TD = temporal dura; TM = temporal muscle.

15.7 Intradural Exposure (Figs. 15.7, 15.8)

- **Parenchymal structures**: Sylvian fissure, inferior frontal gyrus, superior temporal gyrus and middle temporal gyrus are exposed.
- **Arachnoidal layer**: Optic and carotid cisterns.
- **Cranial nerves**: Second and third cranial nerves, optic chiasm.
- **Arteries**: Internal carotid artery, M1 segment of middle cerebral artery, A1 segment of anterior cerebral artery, basilar artery.
- **Veins**: Superficial Sylvian veins, vein of Labbè.
- Two 15-mm retractors are placed on the frontal and temporal lobes, each covered with a protective coating of non-adherent dressing.
- The surgeon will section veins of the temporal lobe that enter the sphenoparietal sinus as necessary to open the Sylvian fissure and gain subfrontal and pre-temporal exposure.
- The arachnoid of the optic and carotid cisterns is incised and CSF is aspirated.
- The two 15-mm retractors stretch the arachnoid of the Sylvian fissure such that it can be cut and the Sylvian fissure opened.
- Brain relaxation techniques and patience are important to prevent retraction-induced venous stasis and arterial compression.

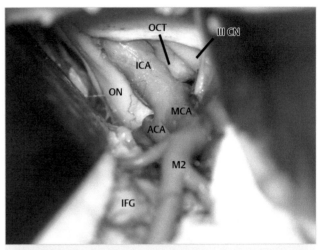

Fig. 15.8 Intradural exposure after dissection of the Sylvian fissure. The internal carotid artery (ICA) is seen with its bifurcation and anterior cerebral artery (ACA) running antero-medially to cross the optic nerve (ON) and the middle cerebral artery (MCA) that bifurcates to give rise to the two M2 segments. It can be appreciated that the superior division of M2 bifurcates soon after the MCA bifurcation to give rise to an anterior branch.
Abbreviations: ACA = anterior cerebral artery; ICA = internal carotid artery; IFG = inferior frontal gyrus; III CN = third cranial nerve; MCA = middle cerebral artery; OCT = oculomotor-carotid triangle; ON = optic nerve.

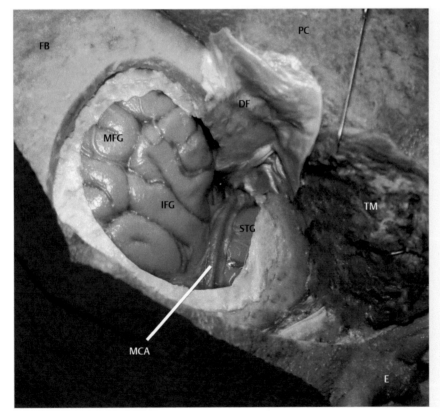

Fig. 15.7 Intradural exposure. The dura has been opened in a semicircular fashion, with the flap based and reflected anteriorly. The middle frontal gyrus, inferior frontal gyrus and superior temporal gyrus along with the middle cerebral artery are visualized upon reflection of the dural flap.
Abbreviations: DF = dural flap; E = ear; FB = frontal bone; IFG = inferior frontal gyrus; MCA = middle cerebral artery; MFG = middle frontal gyrus; PC = pericranium; STG = superior temporal gyrus; TM = temporal muscle.

References

1. Fossett D, Caputy AJ. Operative neurosurgical anatomy. New York, NY: Thieme Medical Publisher; 2002
2. Greenberg MS. Handbook of neurosurgery. New York, NY: Thieme Medical Publishers; 2010
3. Sekhar LN, Fessler RG. Atlas of neurosurgical techniques. Brain. Volume 1. New York, NY: Thieme Medical Publishers; 2016
4. Yasargil MG, Antic J, Laciga R, Jain KK, Hodosh RM, Smith RD. Microsurgical pterional approach to aneurysms of the basilar bifurcation. Surg Neurol 1976;6(2):83–91

16 Mini-Pterional Approach

Chad A. Glenn, Joshua D. Burks, Phillip A. Bonney, and Michael E. Sughrue

16.1 Introduction

The mini-pterional approach is a lateral approach, which enables access to the trans-sylvian corridor through a minimally invasive craniotomy.

The approach is indicated for vascular pathology involving the anterior circulation, for extra-axial lesions of the anterior skull base and parasellar area, as well as intra-axial lesions of the inferior aspect of the frontal lobe.

16.2 Indications

- Anterior circulation aneurysms
- Anterior skull base meningiomas
- Parasellar tumors (*e.g.,* craniopharyngiomas)
- Less common: Inferior frontal and fronto-orbital pathology

16.3 Patient Positioning (Fig. 16.1)

- **Position:** The patient is positioned supine with torso flexed slightly downward.
- **Head:** The head is extended 20°, rotated 5° to contralateral side for most pathologies.
- The ipsilateral **malar eminence** is the highest point in the surgical field.
- The single pin should be placed on the ipsilateral side superior to the mastoid process. On the two-pin arm, one pin is placed superior to the mastoid process on the contralateral side and the other superiorly over the parietal bone.

16.4 Skin Incision (Fig. 16.2)

- **Small, lightly curved incision**
  - **Starting point:** Incision starts just inside the sideburn, 2 fingerbreadths anterior to the pinna.
  - **Course:** Incision runs along the hairline in a downward arc.
  - **Ending point:** It curves anteriorly making a cut no longer than 6-7 cm.

16.4.1 Critical Structures

- Superficial temporal artery.
- Frontal branch of the facial nerve.

16.5 Soft Tissue Dissection (Figs. 16.3, 16.4)

- **Myofascial and muscular layers**
  - The scalp is reflected antero-inferiorly and postero-superiorly to expose the superficial temporoparietal fascia.
  - Temporal fascia is elevated in a sub-fascial incision and retracted to protect the frontal branch of the facial nerve.
  - A "T-cut" is made in the upper posterior corner of the temporal muscle, and spread away from the inferior edge.
- **Bone exposure**
  - Subperiosteal dissection proceeds until the sphenoid wing is exposed.

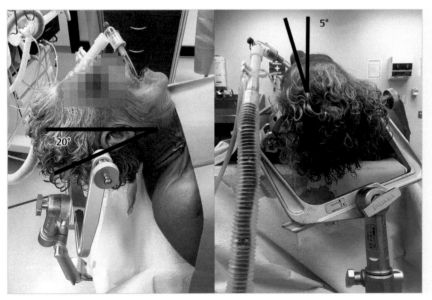

Fig. 16.1 Patient positioning. Care must be taken to extend the neck in order to allow gravity to aid in retraction of the frontal lobe in relation to the floor of the anterior fossa. Rotation of the head is variable and is used in order to garner access to more medial or more lateral trajectories.

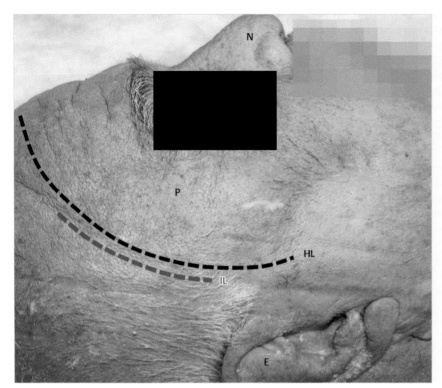

Fig. 16.2 Planned incision along the hairline, running over the temporal fossa. Care must be taken to preserve the frontal branch of the facial nerve.
Abbreviations: E = ear; HL = hairline; IL = incision line; N = nose; P = pterion.

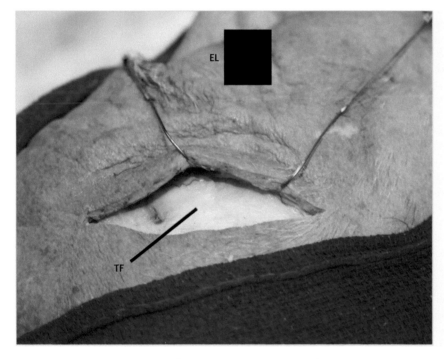

Fig. 16.3 Muscles dissection. Skin incision revealing temporal muscle below within superficial fascia.
Abbreviations: EL = eyelid; TF = temporal fascia.

16.6 Craniotomy (Figs. 16.5, 16.6)

- **Burr hole**
  - **I:** A single burr hole can be made anywhere behind the wing of the sphenoid.
- **Craniotomy landmarks**
  - **Superiorly/Inferiorly:** Small frontotemporal craniotomy below the temporal muscle.
  - **Medially:** Bone work as necessary to flatten the lesser wing of the sphenoid to the meningo-periorbital band (which is skeletonized).
  - **Anteriorly:** Orbital roof is accessed as needed for exposure.

16.6.1 Variants

- **Dolenc Approach**
  - Possible with well-planned craniotomy.
  - Cavernous sinus is accessible with gentle retraction of temporal lobe.

16.6.2 Critical Structures

- Optic nerve
- Cavernous sinus
- Middle meningeal artery (MMA)

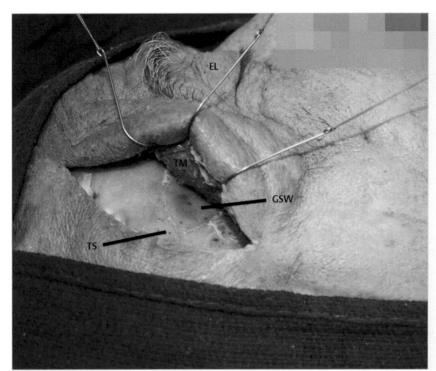

Fig. 16.4 Muscles dissection. The temporalis is divided most anteriorly for better access to anterior structures.
Abbreviations: EL = eyelid; GSW = greater sphenoid wing; TM = temporal muscle; TS = temporal squama.

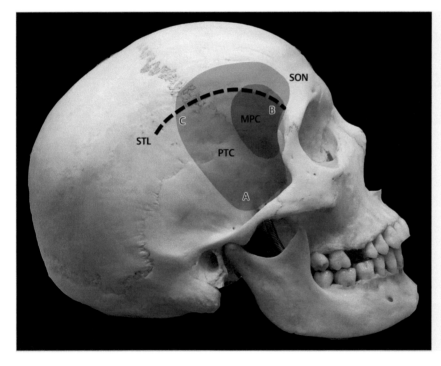

Fig. 16.5 Schematic picture showing the difference between pterional (PTC) and mini-pterional craniotomy (MPC). A, B, C: burr holes sites for standard pterional approach.
Abbreviations: MPC = mini-pterional craniotomy; PTC = pterional craniotomy; SON = superior orbital notch; STL = superior temporal line.

16.7 Dural Opening (Fig. 16.7)

- The dural opening is a C-shaped incision.
- The dural flap is then retracted using sutures toward the orbit and sphenoid ridge.

16.7.1 Critical Structures

- Superficial middle cerebral veins located temporally.
- Orbito-meningeal band entering superior orbital fissure.
- Cavernous sinus.

16.8 Intradural Exposure (Fig. 16.8)

- **Parenchymal structures:** Pars orbitalis of the frontal lobe, superior temporal gyrus.
- **Arachnoid layer:** Sylvian cistern, opticocarotid cistern, suprasellar cistern.

16.9 Pearls

- This approach can be tailored as needed for more frontal and/or temporal exposure.

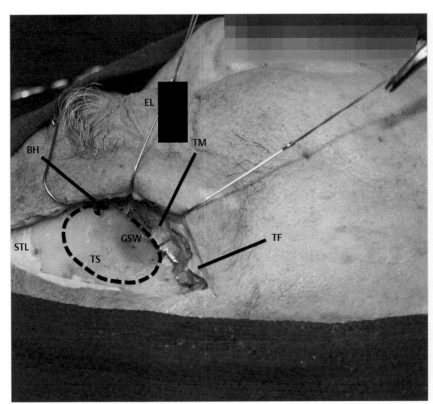

Fig. 16.6 Craniotomy. Burr hole is above the fronto-sphenoidal suture and anterior to the fronto-parietal suture where the temporal muscle is reflected.
Abbreviations: BH = burr hole; EL = eyelid; GSW = greater sphenoid wing; STL = superior temporal line; TF = temporal fascia; TM = temporal muscle; TS = temporal squama.

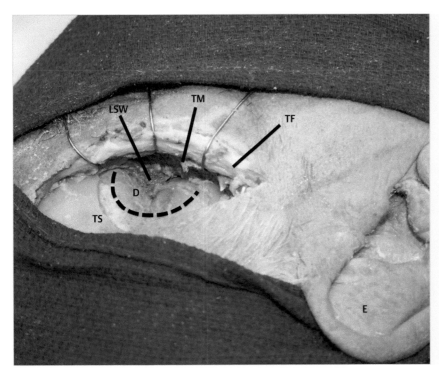

Fig. 16.7 Craniotomy is made medially above the lateral canthus and extends laterally beyond the spheno-temporal suture.
Abbreviations: D = dura; E = ear; LSW = lesser sphenoid wing; TF = temporal fascia; TM = temporal muscle; TS = temporal squama.

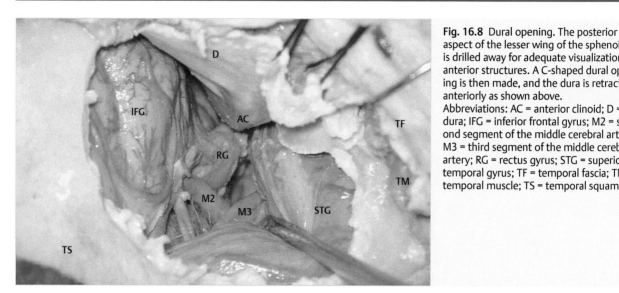

Fig. 16.8 Dural opening. The posterior aspect of the lesser wing of the sphenoid is drilled away for adequate visualization of anterior structures. A C-shaped dural opening is then made, and the dura is retracted anteriorly as shown above.
Abbreviations: AC = anterior clinoid; D = dura; IFG = inferior frontal gyrus; M2 = second segment of the middle cerebral artery; M3 = third segment of the middle cerebral artery; RG = rectus gyrus; STG = superior temporal gyrus; TF = temporal fascia; TM = temporal muscle; TS = temporal squama.

References

1. Iaconetta G, Ferrer E, Galino AP, et al. Frontotemporal approach. In: Cappabianca P, Califano L, Iaconetta G, eds. Cranial, craniofacial, and skull base surgery. Milan: Springer; 2010

2. Teo C, Sughrue ME. Principles and practice of keyhole brain surgery. New York, NY: Thieme Medical Publishers; 2014

17 Combined Orbito-Zygomatic Approaches

Pietro Mortini, Alfio Spina, Michele Bailo, Anthony J. Caputy, Cristian Gragnaniello, and Filippo Gagliardi

17.1 Introduction

The Fronto-orbito-zygomatic (FOZ) approach represents one of the workhorses of skull base surgery. Through this approach, it is possible to provide a wide exposure and a direct access to different tumoral and cerebrovascular pathology of the anterior and middle cranial fossa, sellar and suprasellar area, and anterior upper brainstem. In addition, the orbitozygomatic osteotomy provides the benefit of the extradural unroofing of the optic canal.

17.2 Indications

- Sellar, suprasellar, presellar and parasellar lesions.
- Lesions of the third ventricle.
- Lesions of the anterior surface of the upper brainstem.
- Aneurisms of circle of Willis.

17.3 Patient Positioning

- **Position:** The patient is positioned supine with head fixed with a Mayfield head holder.
- **Body:** The chest should be elevated to facilitate venous return.

- **Head:** The head is rotated 30° to the contralateral side, and extended about 20°.
- The **zygomatic process** must represent the highest point of the surgical field.
- Pin holders must be positioned **as distant as possible** to the planned skin incision.

17.4 Skin Incision

17.4.1 Extended Coronal Skin Incision (Figs. 17.1)

- **Starting point:** Incision starts less than 1 cm anterior to the tragus on the side of the approach.
- **Course:** Incision runs toward the midline and to the contralateral side, just behind the hairline.
- **Ending point:** It ends at the junction between the lateral and middle third of the coronal line.

17.4.2 Critical Structures

- Superficial temporal artery and its distal branches.
- Peripheral branches of the facial nerve.

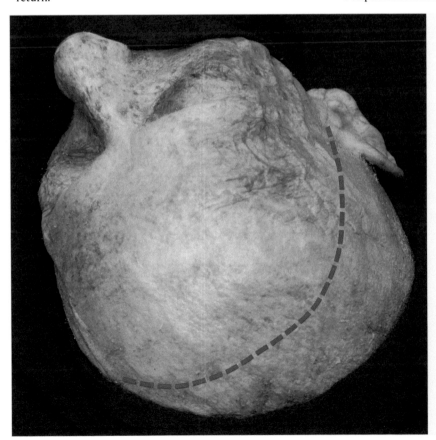

Fig. 17.1 Bicoronal skin incision.

17.5 Soft Tissue Dissection

- **Pericranial layer**
  - The pericranial flap is reflected together with the skin flap, up to the orbital rim.
- **Muscle** (Figs. 17.2, 17.3)
  - Interfascial dissection of the temporal muscle is carried out **(see Chapters 6 and 8).**

- The subperiosteal dissection of the temporal muscles is performed to the frontal process of the zygoma; the body of the zygomatic bone and the temporal fossa are exposed.
- Temporal muscle is reflected inferiorly.
- **Bone exposure** (Fig. 17.4)
  - Zygomatic process of the frontal bone, frontal process of the zygomatic bone, temporal fossa (greater wing of the sphenoid, temporal squama).

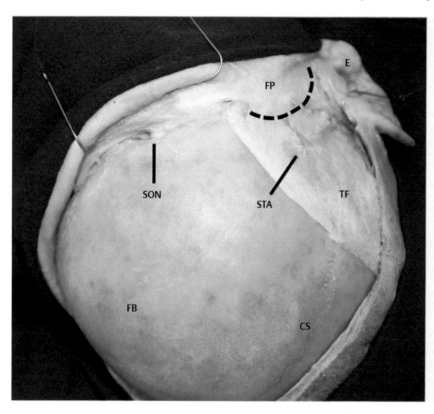

Fig. 17.2 Superficial soft tissue dissection. Abbreviations: CS = coronal suture; E = ear; FB = frontal bone; FP = fat pad; SON = supraorbital nerve; STA = superficial temporal artery; TF = temporal fascia.

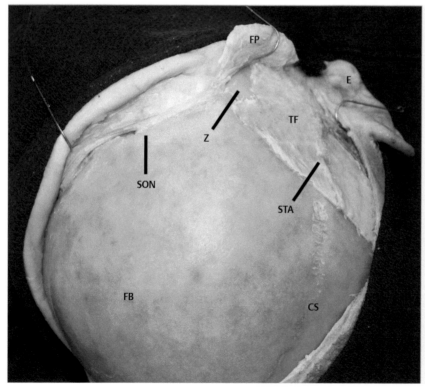

Fig. 17.3 Superficial soft tissue dissection: Interfascial dissection.
Abbreviations: CS = coronal suture; E = ear; FB = frontal bone; FP = fat pad; SON = supraorbital nerve; STA = superficial temporal artery; TF = temporal fascia; Z = zygomatic process of the frontal bone.

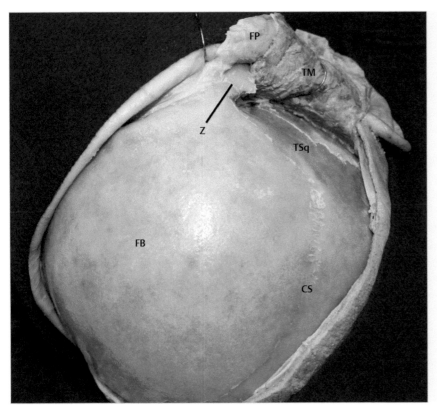

Fig. 17.4 Bone exposure.
Abbreviations: CS = coronal suture; FB = frontal bone; FP = fat pad; TM = temporal muscle; Tsq = temporal squama; Z = zygomatic process of the frontal bone.

○ Supraorbital foramen is opened avoiding injury to the supraorbital nerve, artery and vein **(see Chapter 6).**
• **Orbital contents**
○ Periorbit is subperiostally dissected from the roof and the lateral wall of the orbit, 3 cm deep from the orbital rim.

17.5.1 Critical Structures

• Frontal branch of the facial nerve.
• Supraorbital nerve, artery and vein.

17.6 Craniotomy

17.6.1 Frontotemporal Craniotomy (Figs. 17.5, 17.6)

• **Burr holes**
○ **I:** The first burr hole is made at the keyhole, just posterior to the frontozygomatic suture.
○ **II:** The second burr hole is placed behind the spheno-squamous suture of the temporal squama.
• **Craniotomy landmarks**
○ **Anteriorly:** A basal exposure is performed from the key-hole to the medial third of the orbital rim.
○ **Laterally:** The burr holes are connected by drilling the lesser sphenoid wing with a high-speed drill.
○ **Medially:** Craniotomy runs parallel to the superior sagittal sinus.
○ **Posteriorly:** The posterior cut is made from the second burr hole to the medial limit of the craniotomy in the frontal bone.

17.6.2 Variants

• **One and half craniotomy**
○ The craniotomy crosses the midline toward the contralateral frontal bone.
○ One and half craniotomy provides the exposure of the superior sagittal sinus, the interhemispheric fissure, and the contralateral frontal lobe.

17.6.3 Critical Structures

• Middle meningeal artery.
• Superior sagittal sinus.

17.7 Orbitozygomatic Osteotomy (Figs. 17.7, 17.8)

The roof and the lateral wall and the orbit are exposed by elevating the dura from the frontal and the temporal bone.

17.7.1 Osteotomies cuts

• **I:** The first cut is made at the medial third of the superior orbital rim.
• **II:** The second cut is made at the lateral orbital rim, just superiorly to the body of the zygomatic bone at the fronto-zygomatic suture, and it is directed toward the inferior orbital fissure.
• **III:** The two cuts are connected starting from the inferior orbital fissure, always keeping the saw anterior to the superior orbital fissure.
• **IV:** The remaining part of the orbital roof, located close to the orbital apex, is removed.

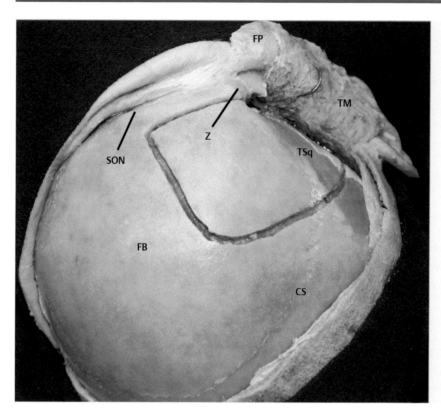

Fig. 17.5 Craniotomy.
Abbreviations: CS = coronal suture;
FB = frontal bone; FP = fat pad; SON =
supraorbital nerve; TM = temporal muscle;
Tsq = temporal squama; Z = zygomatic
process of the frontal bone.

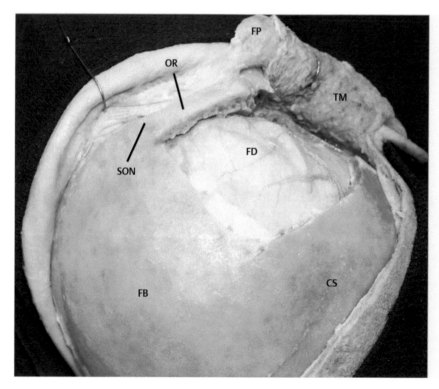

Fig. 17.6 Dural exposure.
Abbreviations: CS = coronal suture; FB =
frontal bone; FD = frontal dura; FP = fat pad;
OR = orbital ridge; SON = supraorbital nerve;
TM = temporal muscle.

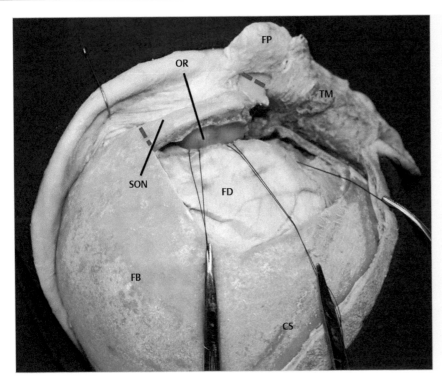

Fig. 17.7 Exposure of the orbital roof. Red dotted lines depict the cuts of orbitotomy. Abbreviations: CS = coronal suture; FB = frontal bone; FD = frontal dura; FP = fat pad; OR = orbital roof; SON = supraorbital nerve; TM = temporal muscle.

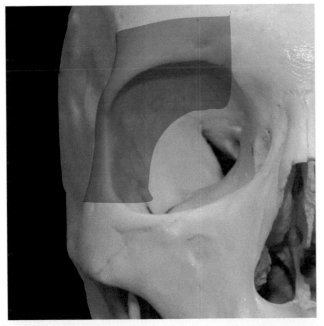

Fig. 17.8 Orbitotomy.

17.7.2 Variants

- **Zygomatic osteotomies** (**Fig. 17.9**)
  - **I:** The posterior cut can be made across the root of the zygomatic process.
  - **II:** The anterior cut can be made obliquely at the level of the maxillary process of the zygomatic bone.
- **Unroofing of the optic canal**
  - Unroofing of the optic canal is required in case of pre-operative compressive optic neuropathy.
  - The technique consists in drilling of the superior, lateral and medial surface of the optic canal.

17.7.3 Critical Structures

- Supraorbital neurovascular bundle.
- Superior orbital fissure.
- Optic nerve.

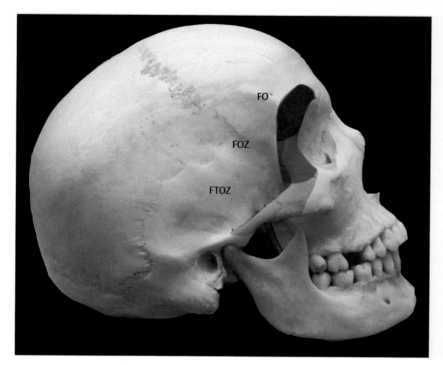

Fig. 17.9 Main variants of orbitotomies. Abbreviations: FO = fronto-orbital approach; FOZ = fronto-orbito-zygomatic approach; FTOZ = complete fronto-temporal-orbito-zygomatic approach.

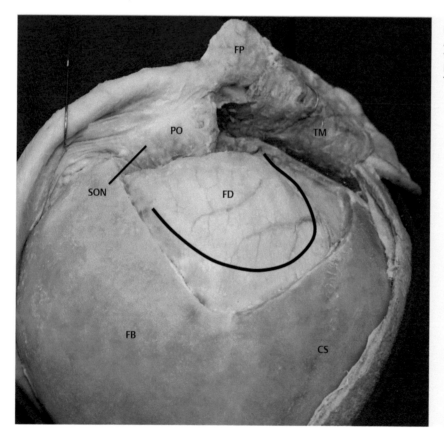

Fig. 17.10 Dural opening. Abbreviations: CS = coronal suture; FB = frontal bone; FD = frontal dura; FP = fat pad; PO = periorbit; SON = supraorbital nerve; TM = temporal muscle.

17.8 Dural Opening (Fig. 17.10)

- Dura mater is incised in a C-shape.
- Dural flap is reflected anteriorly above the periorbit and suspended to the skin flap.

- After dural opening the lateral surface of the frontal and temporal lobe as well as the Sylvian fissure come into view.

17.9 Intradural Exposure
(Figs. 17.11–17.14)

- **Parenchymal structures:** Orbital and Sylvian surfaces of the frontal and temporal lobes.
- **Arachnoidal layer:** Sylvian fissure, carotid and optic-chiasmatic cisterns.
- **Cranial nerves:** Olfactory and optic nerves.
- **Arteries:** Internal carotid, posterior communicating, anterior choroidal, anterior cerebral, anterior communicating, middle cerebral, posterior cerebral, and superior cerebellar arteries.
- **Veins:** Sylvian, frontal and temporal cortical veins.
- **Intra-cavernous space:** Internal carotid artery, oculomotor, trochlear, abducens, first and second branch of the trigeminal nerve.

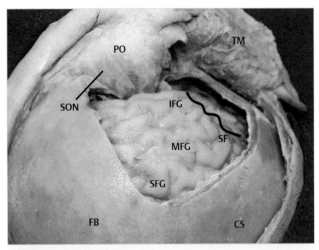

Fig. 17.11 Intradural exposure.
Abbreviations: CS = coronal suture; FB = frontal bone; FP = fat pad; IFG = inferior frontal gyrus; MFG = middle frontal gyrus; PO = periorbit; SF = Sylvian fissure; SFG = superior frontal gyrus; SON = supraorbital nerve; TM = temporal muscle.

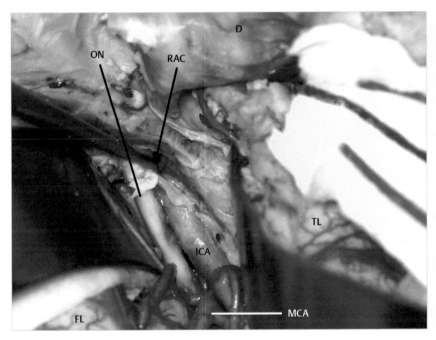

Fig. 17.12 Intradural clinoidectomy.
Abbreviations: D = dura; FL = frontal lobe; ICA = internal carotid artery; MCA = middle cerebral artery; ON = optic nerve; RAC = resected anterior clinoid; TL = temporal lobe.

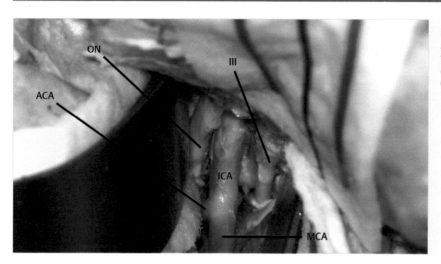

Fig. 17.13 Intradural view.
Abbreviations: ACA = anterior cerebral artery; ICA = internal carotid artery; III = third cranial nerve; MCA = middle cerebral artery; ON = optic nerve.

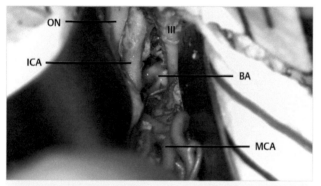

Fig. 17.14 Intradural view.
Abbreviations: BA = basilar artery; ICA = internal carotid artery; III = third cranial nerve; MCA = middle cerebral artery; ON = optic nerve.

References

1. Fossett D, Caputy AJ. Operative neurosurgical anatomy. New York, NY: Thieme Medical Publisher; 2002
2. Mortini P, Gagliardi F, Boari N, Roberti F, Caputy AJ. The combined interhemispheric subcommissural translamina-terminalis approach for large craniopharyngiomas. World Neurosurg 2013;80(1–2):160–166
3. Mortini P, Losa M, Pozzobon G, et al. Neurosurgical treatment of craniopharyngioma in adults and children: early and long-term results in a large case series. J Neurosurg 2011;114(5):1350–1359

18 Midline Interhemispheric Approach

Marzia Medone, Filippo Gagliardi, Cristian Gragnaniello, Anthony J. Caputy, Pietro Mortini, and Remi Nader

18.1 Introduction

The interhemispheric approach is a midline transcranial approach, which provides access through this anatomical corridor to the corpus callosum and the ventricular system. The craniotomy can be easily tailored according to the pathology and to the venous anatomy, which is one of the main limiting factor of surgical maneuverability.

Callosotomy provides access to the lateral ventricle and to the third ventricle, either through the foramen of Monro or through the choroidal fissure.

The approach is indicated for extra-axial tumors involving the interhemispheric fissure, as well as intra-axial lesions located in the anterior aspect of the third ventricle and lateral ventricles.

18.2 Indications

- Vascular and neoplastic lesions located in the anterior aspect of the third ventricle, including lesions extending out of the third ventricle into the lateral ventricles.
  - Tumors of the third ventricle including gliomas, ependymomas, choroid plexus papillomas, meningiomas, craniopharyngiomas.
  - Colloid cysts.
  - Vascular malformations.
- Extra-axial tumors of the interhemispheric fissure (i.e., falx or parasagittal meningiomas).

18.3 Patient Positioning

- **Position:** The patient is positioned supine or lateral decubitus with the head fixed with a Mayfield head holder.
- **Body:** The body is lined horizontally.
- **Head:** The head is flexed 15 to 30°, depending on the location of the lesion.

18.4 Skin Incision (Fig. 18.1)

- **U-shaped unilateral incision**
  - An area of approximately 5x5 cm centered on the **bregma** is shaved, prepped and draped.
  - A U-shaped horseshoe scalp incision is made with the open end of the "U" pointing laterally.
  - **Starting point:** The incision starts just behind the hairline, 5 cm lateral from the midline.
  - **Course:** It runs 1/3 anterior and 2/3 posterior to the coronal suture.
  - **Ending point:** Incision ends the same as the starting but more posterior.
- **Linear ¾ Suttar or bicoronal incision**
  - **Starting point:** The incision starts just above the pinna.
  - **Course:** It runs along the coronal suture.

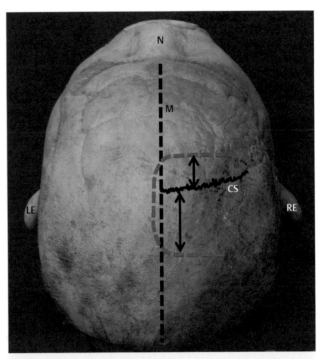

Fig. 18.1 Skin incision (*red dotted line*).
Abbreviations: CS = coronal suture; LE = left ear; M = midline; N = nose; RE = right ear.

  - **Ending point:** Incision ends at the superior attachment of the temporal muscle controlaterally.

18.4.1 Critical Structures

- Superficial temporal artery.
- Auriculo-temporal nerve.

18.5 Soft Tissues Dissection

- **Myofascial level**
  - The myofascial level is incised according to skin incision.
  - It is important to preserve the **pericranial** layer, for further reconstruction.
- **Muscles**
  - Although the temporal muscle is exposed by the skin incision, there is no need to incise it, thus it is preserved.
- **Bone exposure**
  - The bone exposure is completed when the frontal and parietal bony surface are exposed for about 5x5 cm.
  - Antero-posterior extension of the bone exposure has to run 1/3 anterior and 2/3 posterior to the coronal suture.
  - Lateral exposure extends up to the temporal muscle attachment on the ipsilateral side.
  - The sagittal suture has to be exposed on the midline.

18.6 Craniotomy/ Craniectomy (Figs. 18.2, 18.3)

Midline coronal craniotomy
- **Burr holes**
  - ○ **I:** The first burr hole has to be placed along the midline about 2 to 3 cm anterior to the coronal suture.
  - ○ **II:** The second burr hole is made along the midline about 3 to 4 cm posterior to the coronal suture.
- **Cuts**
  - ○ The first cut is made between the two burr holes, laterally in a U-shaped fashion with a lateral extension reaching the superior temporal line.
  - ○ The second cut is made along the sagittal sinus.

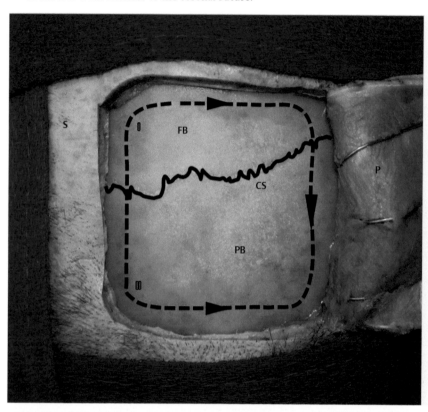

Fig. 18.2 Craniotomy landmarks (*black dotted line*).
Abbreviations: CS = coronal suture; FB = frontal bone; I = first burr hole; II = second burr hole; P = pericranium; PB = parietal bone; S = skin.

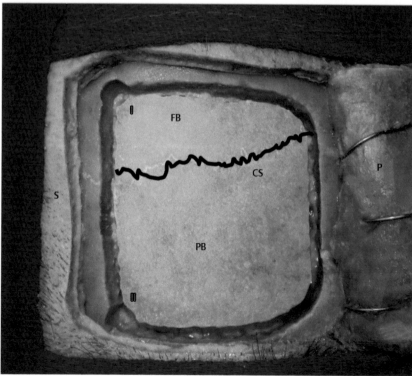

Fig. 18.3 Craniotomy.
Abbreviations: CS = coronal suture; FB = frontal bone; I = first burr hole; II = second burr hole; P = pericranium; PB = parietal bone; S = skin.

- **Craniotomy landmarks**
  - **Medially:** The sagittal suture on the midline.
  - **Laterally:** The superior temporal line.
  - **Rostrally:** An ideal line parallel to the coronal plane, which runs 2 cm anterior to coronal suture.
  - **Caudally:** An ideal line parallel to the coronal plane, which runs 3 to 4 cm posterior to coronal suture.

18.6.1 Variants

- **Burr holes**
  - Four burr holes, straddling the superior sagittal sinus may alternatively be made.
  - Two of them are made anteriorly and the remaining two posteriorly.
  - This technical variant aims to increase safety in and avoid injuring the sinus, and it is mostly advised in elderly patients.
  - An extra burr hole might be made laterally, in cases where the dura is tightly adherent to the bone in order to achieve a better dural dissection.

18.6.2 Critical Structures

- Superior sagittal sinus.
- Dural venous lakes.
- Motor cortex below the dura and posterior to the coronal suture.

18.7 Dural Opening (Fig. 18.4)

- The dura is opened in a C-shaped fashion.
- The edges of dural incision are based on the superior sagittal sinus.

- The flap is reflected along the midline.
- The ends of the dural incision have to be kept close to, but not violating the sagittal sinus.

18.7.1 Critical Structures

- Superior sagittal sinus.
- Venous lakes.
- Parasagittal draining veins.
- Motor cortex.

18.8 Intradural Exposure (Figs. 18.5, 18.6)

- **Parenchymal structures:** Fronto-parietal cortex, cingulate gyrus, corpus callosum.
- **Arachnoidal layer:** Interhemispheric fissure and cistern.
- **Arteries:** Callosomarginal and pericallosal arteries, distal anterior cerebral artery (ACA).
- **Veins:** Bridging cortical veins, superior sagittal sinus.

18.8.1 Details of Intradural Exposure

- Brain retractors are placed on the ipsilateral cerebral hemisphere in the interhemispheric fissure and gentle retraction is applied.
- A gentle dissection with gradual advancement of the retractors is used to visualize the corpus callosum.
- Care must be taken to accurately define the corpus callosum and to avoid injury to the pericallosal arteries.

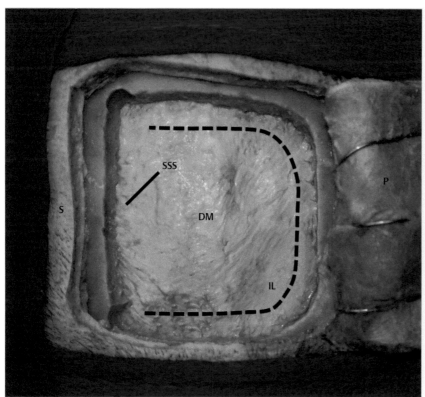

Fig. 18.4 Dural opening. Abbreviations: DM = dura mater; IL = incision line; P = pericranium; S = skin; SSS = superior sagittal sinus.

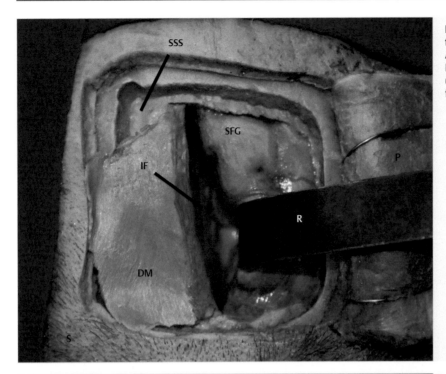

Fig. 18.5 Brain retraction and opening of the interhemispheric fissure. Abbreviations: DM = dura mater; IF = interhemispheric fissure; P = pericranium; R = retractor; S = skin; SFG = superior frontal gyrus; SSS = superior sagittal sinus.

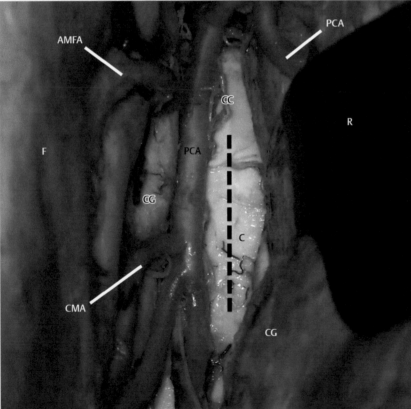

Fig. 18.6 Exposure of the corpus callosum. Callosotomy (*black dotted line*). Abbreviations: AMFA = anterior medial frontal artery; C = callosotomy; CC = corpus callosum; CG = cingulate gyrus; CMA = callosomarginal artery; F = falx; PCA = pericallosal artery; R = retractor.

18.9 Intraventricular Exposure (Fig. 18.7)

18.9.1 Approach to the Lateral Ventricle

- A 1 cm midline incision is made along corpus callosum fibers.
- The incision is kept less than 2 cm to decrease the risk of disconnection syndrome.

- The retractors should now be advanced in order to visualize the choroidal fissure.
- The choroidal fissure is opened between the thalamus and the fornix and might be split by opening the tela choroidea.
- The fornix is displaced allowing visualization of the third ventricle.

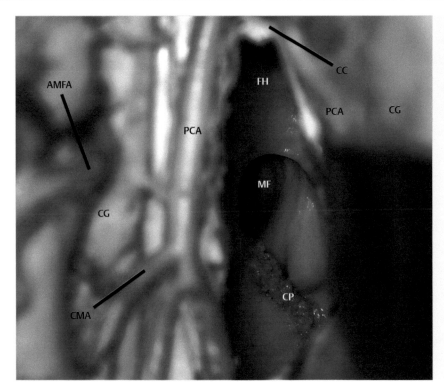

Fig. 18.7 Callosotomy and opening of the third ventricle.
Abbreviations: AMFA = anterior medial frontal artery; CC = corpus callosum; CG = cingulate gyrus; CMA = callosomarginal artery; CP = choroid plexus; FH = frontal horn; MF = Monro foramen; PCA = pericallosal artery; R = retractor.

18.9.2 Approaches to the Third Ventricle

- **Transforaminal approach**
  - The choroid plexus is followed anteriorly to the foramen of Monro.
  - Monro foramen is usually enlarged in case of hydrocephalus, improving surgical maneuverability.
  - When it is unclear which ventricle is entered, the laterally placed thalamostriate vein will assist the surgeon with the orientation.
  - The choroid plexus is cauterized, to minimize the chance of bleeding.
  - At the end of the procedure the septum pellucidum should be opened to prevent univentricular hydrocephalus.
- **Subchoroidal approach**
  - The choroidal fissure, which is in continuity with the superior part of the tela choroidea is exposed.
  - The terminal branch of the thalamostriate (preferentially) or septal vein may be sacrificed in order to enter the third ventricle after division of the choroidal fissure.
  - When the septal vein is divided, additional separation of the internal cerebral veins is necessary, whereas when the thalamostriate vein is sacrificed separation of the internal cerebral veins is not needed.
- **Interforniceal approach**
  - A wide dissection of the septum pellucidum is performed.
  - The first lateral ventricle is entered.
  - Interforniceal dissection is carried out under direct vision of both fornices.
  - The internal cerebral veins are widely separated and the tela choroidea is dissected.

18.9.3 Critical Structures

- Thalamus as well as the surrounding large veins including the thalamostriate vein during the deep portion of the approach.
- Corpus callosum (disconnection syndrome or mutism)
- Fornix (memory loss).

References

1. Connolly ES, McKhann GM II, Huang J. Fundamentals of operative techniques in neurosurgery. New York, NY: Thieme Medical Publishers; 2011
2. Fossett D, Caputy AJ. Operative neurosurgical anatomy. New York, NY: Thieme Medical Publisher; 2002
3. Greenberg MS. Handbook of neurosurgery. New York, NY: Thieme Medical Publishers; 2010
4. Sekhar LN, Fessler RG. Atlas of neurosurgical techniques. Brain. Volume 1. New York, NY: Thieme Medical Publishers; 2016

19 Temporal Approach and Variants

Cristian Gragnaniello, Nicholas J. Erickson, Filippo Gagliardi, Marzia Medone, Pietro Mortini, and Anthony J. Caputy

19.1 Indications

- Temporal lobectomy for epilepsy (amygdalo-hippocampectomy).
- Tumors and vascular malformations of the lateral and middle temporal lobe.
- Temporal lobe open brain biopsy.

19.2 Patient Positioning

- **Position:** The patient is positioned supine with the head fixed with a Mayfield head holder.
- **Body:** The body is kept in neutral position slightly rotated toward the contralateral side and a roll is placed under the ipsilateral shoulder.
- **Head:** The head is rotated of about 60° toward the contralateral side and tilted up to 30° toward the floor.
- The zygoma should be kept as the highest point of the surgical field.
- The frontotemporal region has to be kept on a horizontal plane, parallel to the floor.

19.3 Skin Incision

- **Question-mark shaped unilateral incision** (**Fig. 19.1**)
  - **Starting point:** The incision starts just above the zygomatic arch, 1 cm in front of the tragus, in order to preserve the frontal branches of the facial nerve and it makes a small "V" in front of the tragus itself to allow for a more cosmetic closure result.

  - **Run:** Incision line curves first posteriorly around the top of the pinna for 6 to 9 cm, then turns superiorly along the superior temporal line, turning anteriorly toward the forehead.
  - **Ending point:** The surgical incision ends at the hairline.
- **Linear unilateral incision**
  Linear incision is mostly used for minimally invasive keyhole temporal approaches.
  - **Starting point:** The linear incision does begin in the same position as the question-mark-shaped one, 1 cm above the zygomatic arch and 1 cm anterior to the tragus.
  - **Run:** It runs superiorly for about 6 cm at the level of the temporal muscle.
  - **Ending point:** Incision line ends at the superior temporal line.

19.3.1 Critical Structures

- Frontal branch of the facial nerve.
- Superficial temporal artery.

19.4 Soft Tissues Dissection

- **Myofascial level** (**Fig. 19.2, 19.3**)
  - Interfascial dissection of the temporal muscle is carried out according to the technique described in **Chapters 6 and 8.**
  - The masseter muscle is carefully detached from the inferior margin of the zygomatic arch.
  - The superficial temporal fascia is incised according to the skin incision.

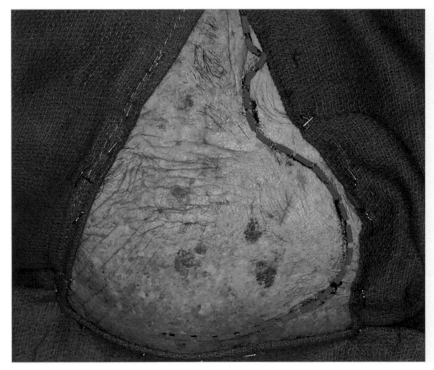

Fig. 19.1 Skin incision. Starting just above the zygomatic arch and anterior to the tragus, the incision curves posteriorly around the top of the pinna and continues superiorly and anteriorly along the superior temporal line towards the forehead.

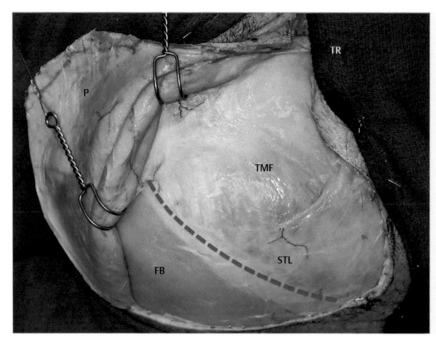

Fig. 19.2 Myofascial level. The skin flap along with the pericranium plane is reflected anteriorly and inferiorly to expose the temporal fascia and its attachment to the frontal bone along the superior temporal line.
Abbreviations: FB = frontal bone; P = pericranium; STL = superior temporal line; TMF = temporal muscle fascia; TR = projection of the tragus.

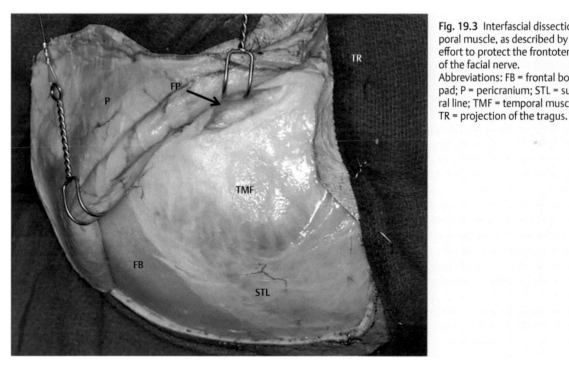

Fig. 19.3 Interfascial dissection of the temporal muscle, as described by Yasargil, is an effort to protect the frontotemporal branch of the facial nerve.
Abbreviations: FB = frontal bone; FP = fat pad; P = pericranium; STL = superior temporal line; TMF = temporal muscle fascia; TR = projection of the tragus.

- **Zygomatic osteotomy** (**Fig. 19.4**)
  The zygoma is cut to gain a direct access to the middle fossa floor, reaching a more basal exposure, which enables to open the intradural, subtemporal corridor.
  - The **first cut** is made anteriorly at the temporal process of the zygomatic bone, just behind the zygomaticofacial foramen.
  - The **second cut** is made posteriorly at the zygomatic process of the temporal bone, just anterior to the mandibular fossa.
- **Muscles** (**Fig. 19.5**)
  - The temporal muscle is incised in a curvilinear manner along the superior temporal line, leaving a cuff of about 7-10 mm at its insertion at the superior temporal line.
  - Muscle fibers are then detached from the temporal squama, starting from the superior temporal line in a subperiosteal manner.
  - The muscle together with the zygomatic arch is reflected downward.
- **Bone exposure**
  - Bone exposure is completed when the temporal squama, as well as the outer surface of the greater wing of the sphenoid bone until the pterion are exposed.
  - The skull base is exposed as far as the inferior orbital fissure.

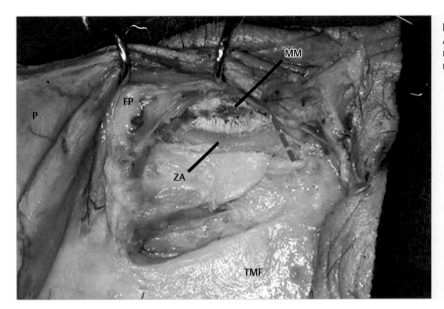

Fig. 19.4 Zygomatic osteotomy. Abbreviations: FP = fat pad; MM = masseter muscle; P = pericranium; TMF = temporal muscle fascia; ZA = zygomatic arch.

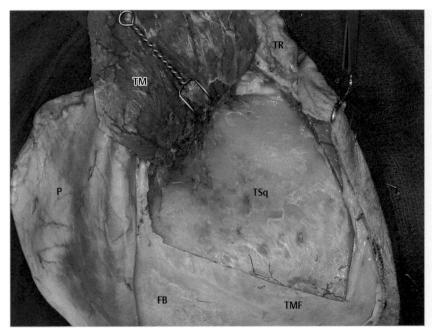

Fig. 19.5 Temporal muscle detachment. The temporal muscle is incised in a curvilinear manner along the temporal line, leaving a cuff of muscle and fascia. Muscle fibers are then detached from the temporal squama. Abbreviations: FB = frontal bone; P = pericranium; TM = temporal muscle; TMF = temporal muscle fascia; TR = tragus; TSq = temporal squama.

19.4.1 Critical Structures

- Frontal branch of the facial nerve.
- Inferior orbital fissure.

19.5 Craniotomy/Craniectomy (Figs. 19.6, 19.7)

- **Burr holes**
  - **I:** The first burr hole is made at the squamosal portion of the temporal bone, just behind the spheno-temporal suture and under the temporal muscle for cosmetic reason, at the McCarty point **(see Chapter 6).**
  - **II:** The second hole is placed about 3 cm posteriorly from the squamosal suture in the parietal bone, just below the superficial temporal line at the posterior limit of the bone exposure.
  - **III:** The third hole is made on the temporal squama just above the posterior root of the zygomatic arch.
  - **IV:** An additional, fourth hole is suggested in elderly patient along the superior temporal line, to facilitate dural detachment from the inner calvaria.
- **Craniotomy landmarks (Figure 6)**
  - **Anteriorly:** The pterion and the outer surface of the greater wing of the sphenoidal bone.
  - **Superiorly:** The superior temporal line.
  - **Inferiorly:** The zygomatic process of the temporal bone posteriorly and the temporal process of the zygomatic bone anteriorly, which were both previously divided.
  - **Posteriorly:** The posterior aspect of the temporo-parietal suture.

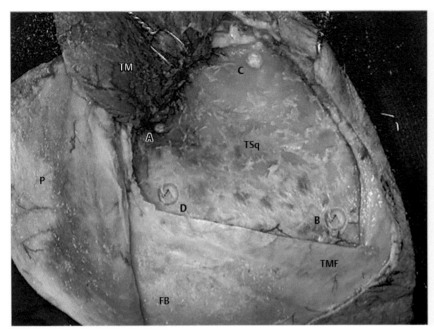

Fig. 19.6 Craniotomy. The first burr hole (A) is made at the squamosal portion of the temporal bone, just behind the spheno-temporal suture. The second (B) is placed about 3 cm posteriorly from the squamosal suture in the parietal bone at the posterior limit of the bone exposure. The third (C) is made on the temporal squama just above the posterior root of the zygomatic arch. The fourth (D) is placed along the superior temporal line to help with dissection of the dura.
Abbreviations: FB = frontal bone; P = pericranium; TM = temporal muscle; TMF = temporal muscle fascia; TSq = temporal squama.

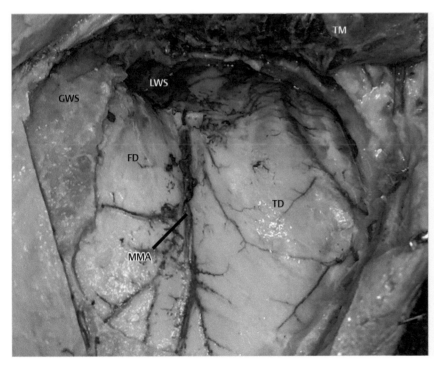

Fig. 19.7 Dural Exposure. Branches of the middle meningeal artery can be seen after the craniotomy is performed.
Abbreviations: FD = frontal dura; GWS = greater wing of the sphenoid; LWS = lesser wing of the sphenoid; MMA = middle meningeal artery; TD = temporal dura; TM = temporal muscle.

19.5.1 Variants

• The extradural subtemporal approach **(see Chapter 21).**

19.6 Dural Opening

• "Cruciate/stellate" or a "horseshoe" - shaped fashion.
• **Horseshoe-shaped fashion**

   ○ The basal edge of the horseshoe is based on the sphenoid ridge.
   ○ Dural flap is reflected antero-inferiorly.

19.6.1 Critical Structures

• Middle meningeal artery.
• Underlying superficial temporal veins (superficial Sylvian veins, vein of Labbé).

19.7 Intradural Exposure (Fig. 19.8)

• **Parenchymal structures:** Lateral aspect of the superior, middle, and inferior temporal gyrus, superior and inferior temporal sulcus, inferior frontal gyrus, and temporal-mesial

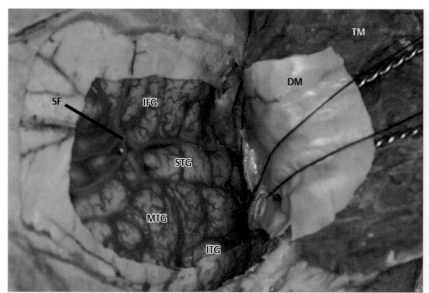

Fig. 19.8 Intradural Exposure. The lateral aspect of the superior, middle and inferior temporal gyri, inferior frontal gyrus and superficial Sylvian veins are visualized after the dura is reflected.
Abbreviations: DM = dura mater; IFG = inferior frontal gyrus; ITG = inferior temporal gyrus; MTG = middle temporal gyrus; SF = Sylvian fissure; STG = superior temporal gyrus; TM = temporal muscle.

aspect of the temporal lobe (amygdalo-hippocampal structures, parhyppocampal gyrus, lateral and medial temporal-occipital gyrus).

- **Arachnoidal layer:** Sylvian cistern, temporal horn of the ipsilateral ventricle, ambiens and crural cisterns (in case of surgical access to the medial part of the temporal lobe).
- **Cranial nerves:** Third cranial nerve, fourth cranial nerve just below the tentorial incisura, Gasserian ganglion (in case of surgical access to the medial part of the temporal lobe).
- **Arteries:** Middle cerebral artery and its branches (anterior and posterior temporal branches).
- **Veins:** Superficial Sylvian veins, vein of Labbè.

References

1. Fossett D, Caputy AJ. Operative neurosurgical anatomy. New York, NY: Thieme Medical Publisher;2002
2. Jandial R, McCormick P, Black PM. Core techniques in operative neurosurgery. Philadelphia, PA: Elsevier Health Sciences;2011
3. Nader R, Gragnaniello C, Berta SC, et al, Eds. Neurosurgery Tricks of the Trade: Cranial. New York, NY: Thieme Medical Publisher;2014
4. Sekhar LN, Fessler RG. Atlas of neurosurgical techniques. Brain. Volume 1. New York, NY: Thieme Medical Publishers; 2016

20 Intradural Subtemporal Approach

Erin McCormack, Isabella Esposito, Filippo Gagliardi, Pietro Mortini, Anthony J. Caputy, and Cristian Gragnaniello

20.1 Introduction

The subtemporal approach is a lateral approach that provides access to the middle cranial fossa through a single burr hole craniotomy. This approach can be used to access peri-peduncular segments of the posterior cerebral artery (as demonstrated here), as well as for aneurysms of the superior cerebellar and basilar arteries and tumors found within this neuroanatomical location. This approach also provides extensive access to the temporal lobe for epilepsy surgery.

20.2 Indications

- Basilar apex aneurysm.
- Posterior cerebral artery aneurysm.
- Superior cerebellar and basilar artery aneurysm.
- Anteromedial tentorial meningiomas.
- Petroclival tumors.
- Posterior cavernous sinus lesion.
- Epilepsy surgery.

20.3 Patient Positioning

- Either the lateral or supine position can be used for this approach.
- The Authors prefer the full lateral as it is felt that gravity can be used to have the temporal lobe "fall away" more with less retraction needed to reach its undersurface.

20.3.1 Full Lateral

- **Position:** The patient is positioned in the full lateral position with the dependent arm and shoulder superior to the edge of the operating table supported in a sling. The axilla is cushioned with a roll. The superior shoulder is gently displaced inferiorly. The recumbent malleolus is padded.
- **Head:** The head is pinned in the anterior-posterior direction in the Mayfield clamp. The head is tilted 90° to be parallel with the floor. The head is then tilted 10° toward the floor.
- A 2 cm wide strip is shaved along the planned incision.

20.3.2 Supine

- **Position:** The patient is positioned supine with the ipsilateral shoulder supported with a shoulder roll.
- **Head:** The head is pinned in the anterior-posterior direction in the Mayfield clamp. The head is tilted 90° to be parallel with the floor. The head is then tilted 20° toward the floor with the zygoma as the most superior point in the surgical field.

20.4 Skin Incision (Fig. 20.1)

Different skin incisions are possible. Our preference is to use a straight vertical incision as it is easier to reconstruct and cosmetically more acceptable with less chances of skin breakdown.
- **Vertical incision**
  - **Starting point:** Incision starts at the superior temporal line.
  - **Course:** Incision line runs perpendicular to the zygoma and extends inferiorly to the level of the zygomatic arch, anterior to the tragus.
  - **Ending point:** It ends at the level of the zygomatic arch.
- **Horseshoe incision**
  - **Starting point:** Incision starts at the root of the zygoma anterior to the tragus.
  - **Course:** Incision line runs superiorly to the superior temporal line and then extends posteriorly above the pinna curving 2 cm behind the mastoid.
  - **Ending point:** It ends at the level of the mastoid.

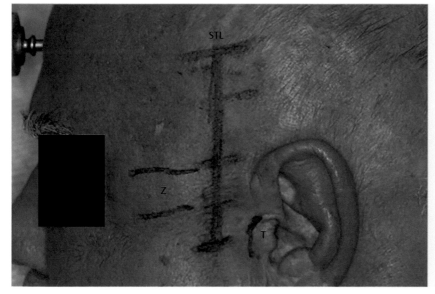

Fig. 20.1 Skin incision.
Abbreviations: STL = superior temporal line; T = tragus; Z = zygoma.

20.4.1 Critical Structures

• Superficial temporal artery.
• Upper branch of the facial nerve at the level of the zygomatic arch.

20.5 Soft Tissue Dissection (Figs. 20.2–20.4)

• **Myofascial and muscular layers**
   ○ The skin is incised to the layer of the galea aponeurotica to expose the superficial temporal artery; both are cut to expose the temporal fascia (**Figs. 20.2, 20.3**).
   ○ The temporal fascia is incised in a subfascial T-shaped incision with the horizontal portion superior and the vertical portion extending inferiorly towards the zygoma.
   ○ The temporal muscle is dissected from the zygoma in a subperiosteal plane and the muscle fibers are reflected anterior-superiorly, posterior-superiorly, and laterally (**Fig. 20.4**).
• **Bone exposure**
   ○ Subperiosteal dissection is continued until the squamous temporal bone is exposed (**Fig. 20.5**).

20.6 Craniotomy (Fig. 20.6)

• **Burr hole**
   ○ A single burr hole is made anterior to the tragus at the root of the zygoma.
• **Craniotomy landmarks** (**Fig. 20.6**)
   ○ **Superiorly:** Superficial temporal line.
   ○ **Inferiorly:** Superior to the zygoma (temporo-basal line).
   ○ **Anteriorly:** The anterior edge of the craniotomy is tailored to the location and extent of the pathology that is being treated.
   ○ **Posteriorly:** Plane of the external auditory canal.

20.7 Dural Opening (Fig. 20.7)

• The dura is opened in a C-shaped incision.
• The dural flaps are reflected anterior-inferiorly and posterior-inferiorly and tacked with sutures.

20.7.1 Critical Structures

• Temporal cortical veins.
• Vein of Labbé if approaching the dominant hemisphere.

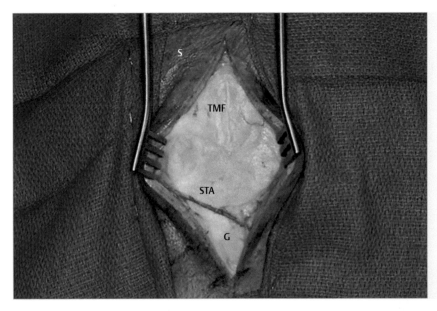

Fig. 20.2 Soft tissue dissection. Abbreviations: G = galea aponeurotica; S = skin; STA = superficial temporal artery; TMF = temporal muscle fascia.

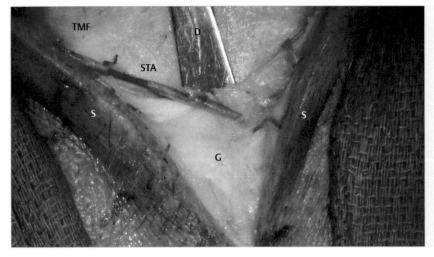

Fig. 20.3 Myofascial and muscle dissection. Abbreviations: D = dissector; G = galea aponeurotica; S = skin; STA = superficial temporal artery; TMF = temporal muscle fascia.

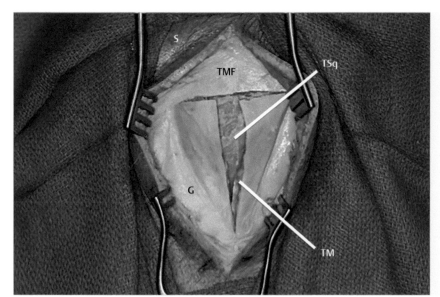

Fig. 20.4 Temporal muscle incision. Abbreviations: G = galea aponeurotica; S = skin; TM = temporal muscle; TMF = temporal muscle fascia; TSq = temporal squama.

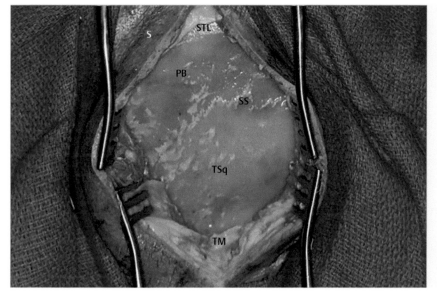

Fig. 20.5 Bone exposure. Abbreviations: PB = parietal bone; S = skin; SS = squamosal suture; STL = superior temporal line; TM = temporal muscle; TSq = temporal squama.

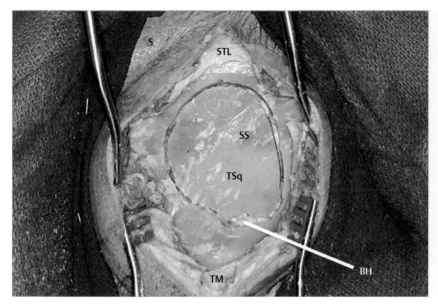

Fig. 20.6 Craniotomy. Abbreviations: BH = burr hole; S = skin; SS = squamosal suture; STL = superior temporal line; TM = temporal muscle; TSq = temporal squama.

20.8 Intradural Exposure (Figs. 20.8, 20.9)

- **Parenchymal structures:** Temporal lobe (superior, inferior and middle temporal gyri), lateral surface of the midbrain.
- **Dural layer:** Free edge of the tentorium.
- **Arachnoidal layer:** Ambiens and cruralis cisterns.
- **Cranial nerves:** Trochlear nerve is visible at the free edge of the tentorium as it crosses over the basilar artery superior to the superior cerebellar artery and inferior to the posterior cerebral artery and posterior communicating artery.

- **Arteries:** Posterior communicating artery (PCom), superficial cerebellar arteries, P2 segment of the posterior cerebral artery (PCA), P3 segment of the posterior cerebral artery, superior cerebellar artery (SCA) with its arachnoid sheath, origin of the lateral posterior choroidal artery (LPChA), and the quadrigeminal artery.
- **Veins:** Lateral ponto-mesencephalic vein and basal vein of Rosenthal.

20.9 Pearls

- Craniotomy can be adjusted for further visualization of the brainstem and posterior fossa.

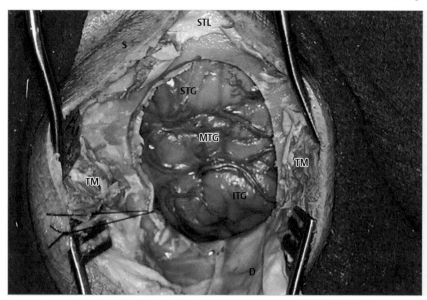

Fig. 20.7 Dural opening. Abbreviations: D = dura; ITG = inferior temporal gyrus; MTG = middle temporal gyrus; S = skin; STG = superior temporal gyrus; STL = superior temporal line; TM = temporal muscle.

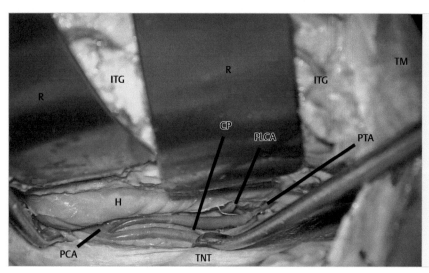

Fig. 20.8 Intradural exposure. **Step 1.** Abbreviations: CP = cerebral peduncle; H = hyppocampus; ITG = inferior temporal gyrus; PCA = posterior cerebral artery; PLCA = posterior lateral choroidal artery; PTA = posterior temporal artery; R = retractor; TM = temporal muscle; TNT = tentorium.

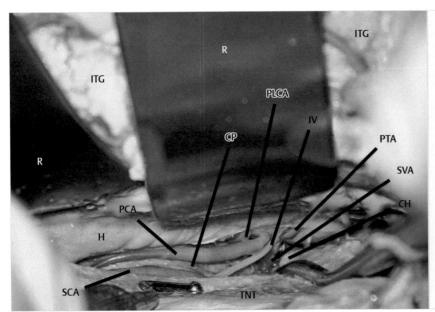

Fig. 20.9 Intradural exposure. **Step 2.** Abbreviations: CH = cerebellar hemisphere; CP = cerebral peduncle; H = hyppocampus; ITG = inferior temporal gyrus; IV = trochlear nerve; PCA = posterior cerebral artery; PLCA = posterior lateral choroidal artery; PTA = posterior temporal artery; R = retractor; SCA = superior cerebellar artery; SVA = superior vermian artery; TNT = tentorium.

References

1. Fossett D, Caputy AJ. Operative neurosurgical anatomy. New York, NY: Thieme Medical Publisher; 2002

2. Nader R, Gragnaniello C, Berta SC, et al, eds. Neurosurgery Tricks of the Trade: Cranial. New York, NY: Thieme Medical Publisher; 2014

21 Extradural Subtemporal Transzygomatic Approach

Filippo Gagliardi, Cristian Gragnaniello, Nicola Boari, Anthony J. Caputy, and Pietro Mortini

21.1 Introduction

The subtemporal transzygomatic approach combines some of the nuances of a classic subtemporal exposure with the possibilities of a pure skull base approach, suitable for the treatment of extradural tumors of the middle-upper clivus extending into the ipsilateral paraclival area and middle fossa.

Sectioning of the mandibular branch (V3) of the trigeminal nerve and petrous apicectomy can further enlarge the surgical exposure as well as the maneuverability area and improve vascular control on the internal carotid artery.

21.2 Indications

- Extradural lesions of middle-upper clivus with lateral extension.

21.3 Patient Positioning

- **Position:** The patient is positioned supine with the head fixed by a Mayfield head holder.
- **Body:** The body is rotated 30°.
- **Head:** The head is extended 20°, rotated 60° to the contralateral side and tilted 10° toward the floor.

- **Shoulder:** A roll is placed under the ipsilateral shoulder.
- Please note that the zygoma has to be the highest point in the surgical field.

21.4 Skin Incision (Fig. 21.1)

Two main options are available for the skin flap.
- **Question-mark shaped unilateral temporal incision**
  - ○ **Starting point:** Incision starts 1 cm in front of the tragus at the level of the zygoma.
  - ○ **Course:** Incision line runs posteriorly around the superior margin of the ear; turns anteriorly after reaching the posterior aspect of the pinna.
  - ○ **Ending point:** It ends on the midline, just behind the hairline.
- **Coronal bilateral incision**
  - ○ **Starting point:** Incision starts 1 cm in front of the tragus at the level of the zygoma.
  - ○ **Course:** Incision line runs medially, parallel and behind the hairline.
  - ○ **Ending point:** It ends at the contralateral superior temporal line.

21.4.1 Critical Structures

- Superficial temporal artery.
- Frontal and temporal branches of the facial nerve.

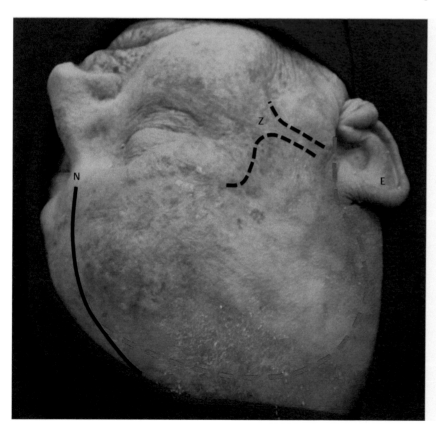

Fig. 21.1 Question-mark shaped unilateral temporal incision.
Abbreviations: Incision (*red dotted line*); midline (*black continuous line*); zygomatic profile (*black dotted line*). E = ear; N = nasion; Z = zygoma.

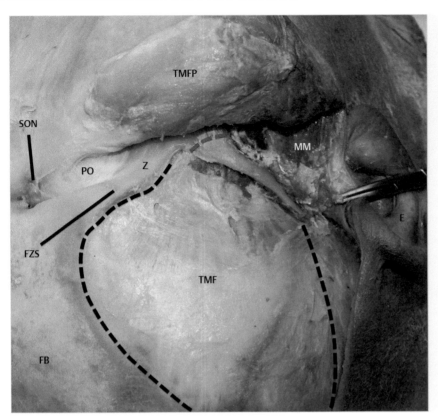

Fig. 21.2 Soft tissue dissection. Abbreviations: Temporal muscle insertion incision (*black dotted line*); Limits of zygomatic osteotomy (*red dotted lines*); E = ear; FB = frontal bone; FZS = fronto-zygomatic suture; MM = masseter muscle; PO = periorbit; SON = supraorbital nerve; TMF = temporal muscle fascia; TMFP = temporal muscle fat pad; Z = zygoma.

21.5 Soft Tissue Dissection and Zygomatic Osteotomy (Figs. 21.2, 21.3)

- **Myofascial level**
  - ○ The myofascial level is incised parallel to the course of the skin incision.
  - ○ The flap is reflected anteriorly with the skin.
- **Muscles: Step 1**
  - ○ *Temporal muscle:* inter-fascial dissection is carried out as it is already described **(see Chapters 6 and 8).**
  - ○ Deep temporal muscle fascia is detached from the inner surface of the zygoma.
  - ○ *Masseter muscle* is detached from the inferior margin of the zygoma.

21.5.1 Zygomatic Osteotomy

- **Cuts**
  - ○ **I:** Posterior cut is made in front of the mandibular fossa.
  - ○ **II:** Anterior cut is made at the basis of the zygomatic temporal process.
- **Muscles: Step 2**
  - ○ *Temporal muscle* is incised posteriorly along the posterior margin of the skin incision.
  - ○ *Temporal muscle* insertion is cut along the superior temporal line.

- **Bone exposure**
  The bone exposure is completed, when the following structures come into view:
  - ○ Temporal squama, outer surface of sphenoid greater wing, pterion, inferior aspects of frontal and parietal bone located below the superior temporal line.

21.5.2 Critical Structures

- Frontal branch of the facial nerve.

21.6 Craniotomy/Craniectomy (Fig. 21.4)

A temporal, low-positioned craniotomy, including the greater sphenoid wing and the squamosal part of the temporal bone is performed.

21.6.1 Temporal Craniotomy

- **Burr holes**
  - ○ **I:** At the McCarty keyhole.
  - ○ **II:** At the posterior aspect of temporal squama just below the superior temporal line.
  - ○ **III:** At the greater wing of the sphenoid bone at the zygomatic level.

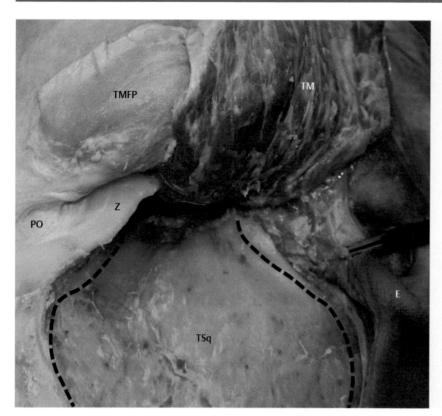

Fig. 21.3 Bone exposure after zygomatic osteotomy and temporal muscle reflection. Abbreviations: Craniotomy margins (*black dotted line*); E = ear; PO = periorbit; TM = temporal muscle; TMFP = temporal muscle fat pad; TSq = temporal squama; Z = zygoma.

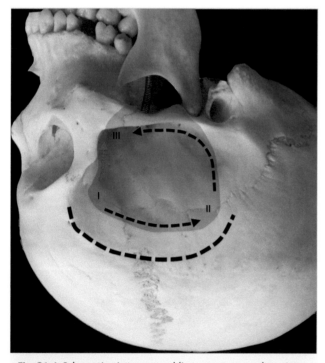

Fig. 21.4 Schematic picture resembling osteotomy and craniotomy landmarks. I, II, III: sequential order of the craniotomy cuts. Arrows indicate direction of the craniotomy cuts. Black dotted line = superior temporal line. Red dotted line = connection of the burr holes by drilling the greater wing of the sphenoid bone with a high-speed drill.

- **Craniotomy landmarks**
  - **Anteriorly:** Anterior margin of spheno-temporal fossa.
  - **Posteriorly:** External auditory canal.
  - **Superiorly:** Superior temporal line.
  - **Inferiorly:** Middle fossa floor.

21.6.2 Further Osteotomies

- Lateral orbitotomy.
- Extradural clinoidectomy.

21.6.3 Middle Fossa Floor Drilling

The temporal dura is gently separated from middle fossa floor, which is drilled using a diamond burr.

- **Sequential exposure of anatomical landmarks (Fig. 21.5)**
  - **I:** Arcuate eminence.
  - **II:** Greater superficial petrosal nerve (GSPN).
  - **III:** Middle meningeal artery (MMA) and foramen spinosum.
  - **IV:** Mandibular nerve (V3) and foramen ovale.
  - **V:** Maxillary nerve (V2) and foramen rotundum.
  - **VI:** Superior orbital fissure.
- **Surgical steps of middle fossa dissection (Figs 21.6, 21.7)**
  - GSPN division (to protect the geniculate ganglion from mechanical and thermal injury).
  - MMA division, on the dural side, distal and away from the foramen, to avoid retraction of the artery inside the foramen, which may lead to difficult to control bleeding.
  - Skeletonization of the foramen rotundum and ovale.

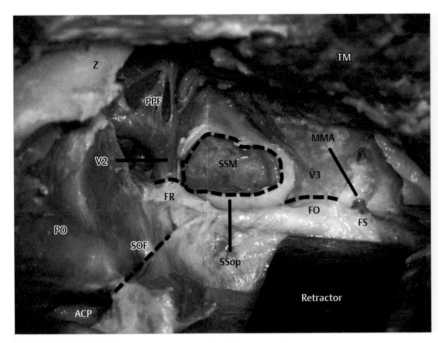

Fig. 21.5 Middle fossa floor drilling. Skeletonization of V2, V3 and middle meningeal artery, further opening of the sphenoid sinus.
Abbreviations: ACP = anterior clinoid process; FO = foramen ovale; FR = foramen rotundum; FS = foramen spinosum; MMA = middle meningeal artery; PPF = pterygopalatine fossa; PO = periorbit; SOF = superior orbital fissure; SSM = sphenoid sinus mucosa; SSop = sphenoid sinus opening; TM = temporal muscle; V2 = second branch of trigeminal nerve; V3 = third branch of trigeminal nerve; Z = zygoma.

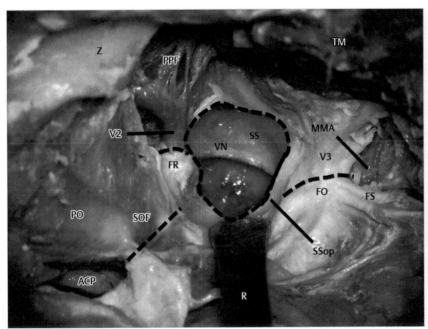

Fig. 21.6 Middle fossa floor drilling. Skeletonization of the Vidian nerve.
Abbreviations: ACP = anterior clinoid process; FO = foramen ovale; FR = foramen rotundum; FS = foramen spinosum; MMA = middle meningeal artery; PPF = pterygopalatine fossa; PO = periorbit; R = retractor; SOF = superior orbital fissure; SS = sphenoid sinus; SSop = sphenoid sinus opening; TM = temporal muscle; V2 = second branch of trigeminal nerve; V3 = third branch of trigeminal nerve; VN = Vidian nerve; Z = zygoma.

○ Sphenoid sinus opening (medially and rostrally to the vidian nerve).
○ Vidian canal skeletonization (between V2 and V3).
○ Eustachian tube isolation (laterally and caudally to the vidian nerve).
○ V2 division at the foramen rotundum.
○ V3 division at the foramen ovale.
○ Pituitary and ipsilateral carotid prominences skeletonization.
○ Middle clival dura exposure.
○ Skeletonization of the contralateral carotid, V2 and V3.

21.6.4 Petrous apicectomy (Fig. 21.8)

This maneuverer allows for exposure of posterior fossa dura and for internal carotid artery (ICA) mobilization
• ICA is freed from the carotid sulcus trough the resection of the petrolingual ligament.
• Petrous bone apex is drilled.
• ICA is mobilized posteriorly and laterally.
• Gives access to a blind corner located at the lateral edge of the middle clivus, medial to the horizontal segment of the ICA.

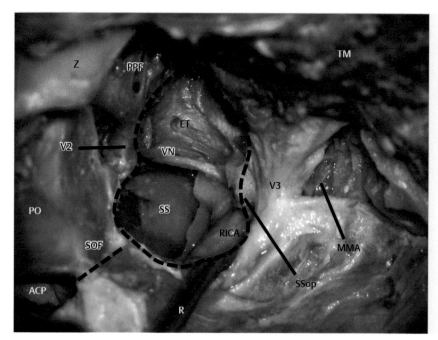

Fig. 21.7 Middle fossa floor drilling. Skeletonization of the carotid canal and the Eustachian tube.
Abbreviations: ACP = anterior clinoid process; ET = Eustachian tube; MMA = middle meningeal artery; PPF = pterygopalatine fossa; PO = periorbit; R = retractor; RICA = right internal carotid artery; SOF = superior orbital fissure; SS = sphenoid sinus; SSop = sphenoid sinus opening; TM = temporal muscle; V2 = second branch of trigeminal nerve; V3 = third branch of trigeminal nerve; VN = Vidian nerve; Z = zygoma.

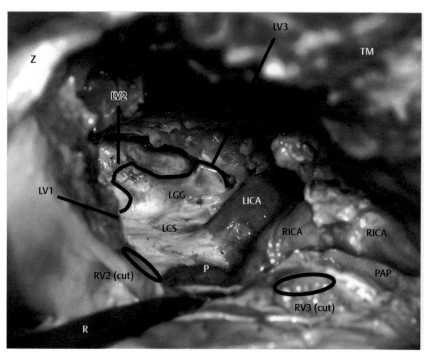

Fig. 21.8 Final dural exposure (Eustachian tube and pterygopalatine fossa are not in view).
Abbreviations: LCS = left cavernous sinus; LGG = left Gasserian Ganglion; LICA = left internal carotid artery; LV1 = left first branch of the trigeminal nerve; LV2 left second branch of trigeminal nerve; LV3 = left third branch of trigeminal nerve; P = pituitary; PAP = petrous apex; R = retractor; RICA = right internal carotid artery; RV2 = right second branch of trigeminal nerve; RV3 = right third branch of trigeminal nerve; TM = temporal muscle; Z = zygoma.

21.6.5 Critical Structures

- Ipsilateral superior orbital fissure.
- Ipsilateral and contralateral V2.
- Ipsilateral and contralateral V3.
- Ipsilateral and contralateral ICA.
- Ipsilateral Eustachian tube.

References

1. al-Mefty O, Anand VK. Zygomatic approach to skull-base lesions. J Neurosurg 1990;73(5):668–673

2. Sekhar LN, Janecka IP, Jones NF. Subtemporal-infratemporal and basal subfrontal approach to extensive cranial base tumours. Acta Neurochir (Wien) 1988;92(1–4):83–92

3. Sekhar LN, Schramm VL Jr, Jones NF. Subtemporal-preauricular infratemporal fossa approach to large lateral and posterior cranial base neoplasms. J Neurosurg 1987;67(4):488–499

22 Occipital Approach

Alan Siu, Filippo Gagliardi, Cristian Gragnaniello, Pietro Mortini, and Anthony J. Caputy

22.1 Introduction

The medial occipital approach and its further paramedian extension provide access to pathologies involving the occipital region, ranging from dural-based to intraparenchymal lesions, as well as pathologies involving the posterior aspect of the interhemispheric fissure.

22.2 Indications

- Occipital convexity meningiomas.
- Small posterior tentorial meningiomas.
- Occipital parenchymal lesions.

22.3 Patient Positioning

- **Position**: The patient is positioned prone, and the head is fixed with a Mayfield head holder.
- **Body**: The bed is placed in reverse Trendelenburg position and knees are flexed. The shoulders are tucked against the body.
- **Head**: The head is slightly flexed, with two-finger breadths from chin to sternum and it can be either placed in neutral position, or slightly turned laterally, according to the location of the pathology, which must be treated.
- In the neutral position, the inion should be the highest point of the surgical field.

22.4 Skin Incision (Fig 22.1)

- **Horseshoe incision**
  - **Starting point:** The starting point is located on the midline at the inion.
  - **Course:** Incision runs upward, progressively turning first laterally and then inferiorly in a U-shaped fashion.
  - **Ending point:** Incision line ends just posterior to the mastoid.
- **Linear incision**
  Linear incision might be placed along the midline or laterally, parallel to the midline, according to the pathology, which must be treated, tailoring the length of the incision accordingly.

22.4.1 Critical Structures

- Occipital artery.
- Greater occipital nerve.

22.5 Soft Tissue Dissection (Figs. 22.2, 22.3)

- **Myocutaneous level**
  - Muscles are incised according to the skin incision.
  - A myocutaneous flap is raised.

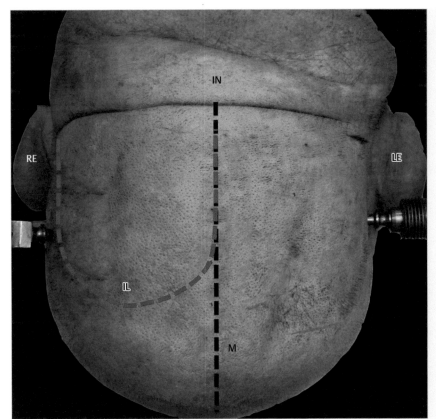

Fig. 22.1 Skin incision, which starts at the inion.
Abbreviations: IL = incision line; IN = inion; LE = left ear; M = midline; RE = right ear.

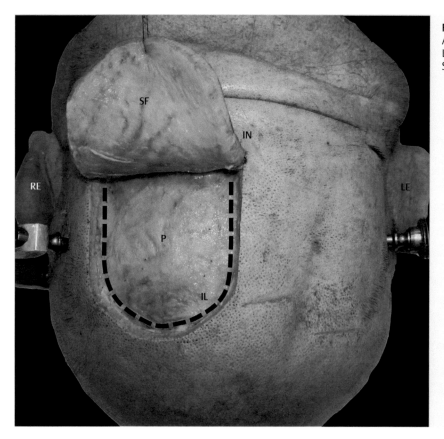

Fig. 22.2 Skin flap.
Abbreviations: IL = incision line; IN = inion; LE = left ear; P = pericranium; RE = right ear; SF = skin flap.

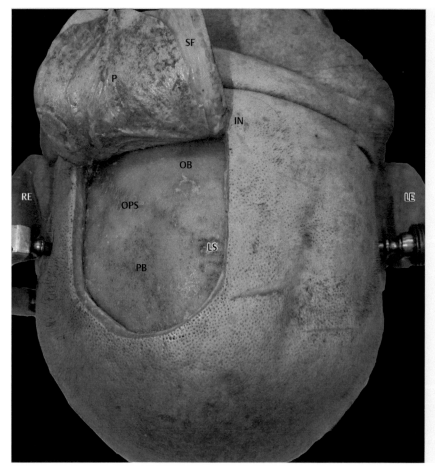

Fig. 22.3 Pericranium reflected to expose the skull, composed of the occipital and parietal bones. The lambdoid suture is also seen.
Abbreviations: IN = inion; LS = lambdoid suture; P = pericranium; LE = left ear; OB = occipital bone; OPS = occipito-parietal suture; PB = parietal bone; RE = right ear; SF = skin flap.

- **Periosteum Level**
  - o A periosteal flap can be raised separately and preserved for further reconstruction.

22.6 Craniotomy (Fig. 22.4)

22.6.1 Median occipital approach

- **Burr holes**
  - o **I:** The first burr hole is placed lateral and superior to the transverse sinus.
  - o **II:** An optional lateral burr hole can be placed on the parietal bone.
  - o **III:** Inferior aspect of the superior sagittal sinus.
  - o **IV:** Superior aspect of the superior sagittal sinus.
- **Cuts**
  - o **I and II:** The first and second cuts should be directed from the holes previously made on the midline, to the lateral one.
  - o **III:** The last cut is performed on the midline, just over the superior sagittal sinus.

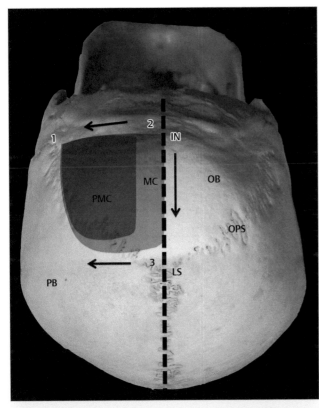

Fig. 22.4 Burr holes are placed in the order demarcated by the numbers. Craniotomy will then follow the arrows, which are parallel to the superior sagittal and transverse sinuses. The median (MC) and paramedian (PMC) craniotomy variants are illustrated.
Abbreviations: IN = inion; LS = lambdoid suture; MC = median craniotomy; OB = occipital bone; OPS = occipito-parietal suture; PB = parietal bone; PMC = paramedian craniotomy.

22.6.2 Paramedian Occipital Approach

- **Burr holes**
  - o **I:** The first burr hole is placed at the lateral aspect of the planned craniotomy.
  - o **II and III:** The second and third burr holes are made paramedian, along the median margin of the planned craniotomy.
- **Cuts**
  - o **I and II:** The first and second cuts should be directed from the medial holes to the lateral one.
  - o **III:** The last cut is performed parallel to the midline, connecting the paramedian holes.
- **Craniotomy landmarks for both the variants**
  Anatomical landmarks which must be taken into consideration in designing the craniotomy are as follows:
  - o **Medially:** Midline, corresponding to the superior sagittal sinus.
  - o **Inferiorly:** Just above the transverse sinus.
  - o **Superiorly:** Lambdoid suture.
  - o **Laterally:** Occipito-parietal suture.

22.6.3 Critical Structures

- Superior sagittal sinus.
- Transverse sinus.

22.7 Dural Opening (Fig. 22.5)

- Dura might be incised either in a curvilinear or in a cruciate fashion.
- Curvilinear incision is directed from superomedial to inferolateral, and split in half superolateral to inferomedial.

22.7.1 Critical Structures

- Superior sagittal sinus.
- Transverse sinus.

22.8 Intradural Exposure (Figs. 22.6, 22.7)

- **Parenchymal Structures:** The inferior, superior and lateral occipital gyrus.
- **Arachnoidal layer:** The posterior aspect of the interhemispheric cistern.
- **Veins:** The occipital cortical veins, the vein of Labbé, the vein of Trolard, the superior sagittal sinus and the transverse sinus.
- **Dura mater:** Tentorium and falx.

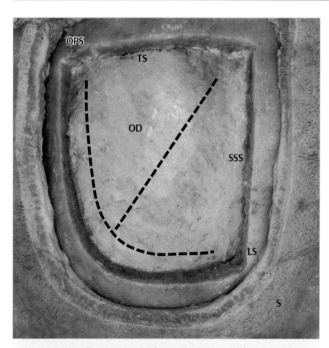

Fig. 22.5 Dural opening, which consists of a semi-lunar opening, that is then cut in a stellate fashion.
Abbreviations: LS = lambdoid suture; OD = occipital dura; OPS = occipito-parietal suture; S = skin; SSS = superior sagittal sinus; TS = transverse sinus.

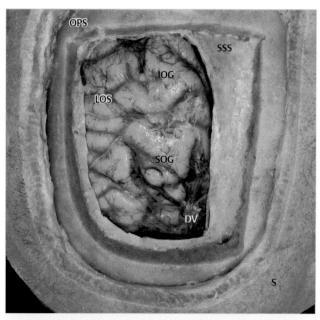

Fig. 22.6 Dura reflected, which exposes the superior and inferior occipital gyri with the intervening lateral occipital sulcus.
Abbreviations: DV = draining veins; IOG = inferior occipital gyrus; LOS = lateral occipital sulcus; OPS = occipito-parietal suture; SOG = superior occipital gyrus; SSS = superior sagittal sinus.

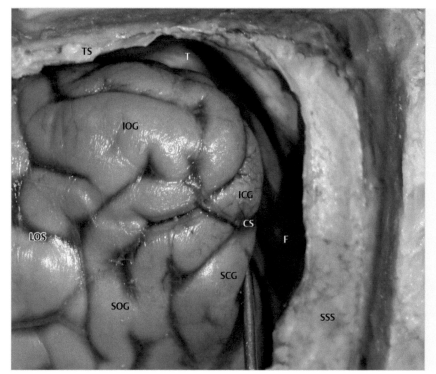

Fig. 22.7 Retraction of the occipital lobe medially will expose the tentorium cerebelli and falx cerebri posteriorly. Care should be taken to avoid retraction of the calcarine sulcus (CS).
Abbreviations: CS = calcarine sulcus; F = falx; ICG = inferior calcarine gyrus; IOG = inferior occipital gyrus; LOS = lateral occipital sulcus; SCG = superior calcarine gyrus; SOG = superior occipital gyrus; SSS = superior sagittal sinus; T = tentorium; TS = transverse sinus.

References

1. Boockvar JA, Stiefel M, Malhotra N, Dolinskas C, Dwyer-Joyce C, LeRoux PD. Dural cavernous angioma of the posterior sagittal sinus: case report. Surg Neurol 2005; 63(2):178–181, discussion 181

2. Martin NA, Wilson CB. Medial occipital arteriovenous malformations. Surgical treatment. J Neurosurg 1982; 56(6):798–802

23 Supracerebellar Infratentorial Approach

Pablo González-López, Javier Abarca Olivas, Iván Verdú-Martínez, and Sananthan Sivakanthan

23.1 Introduction

The supracerebellar infratentorial approach is suitable for the bilateral exposure of the pineal region as well as the posterior surface of the midbrain, and it allows access to the posterior part of the third ventricle.

The surgical route corresponds to the anatomical corridor seated between the tentorial surface of both cerebellar hemispheres and the inferior surface of the tentorial fold.

The approach can be varied according to the pathology, in a midline and a paramedian variant. The complex venous vascular anatomy of the pineal region must be taken into consideration in the surgical planning.

The approach is indicated for lesions of the pineal gland, tectal part of the mesencephalon as well as of the posterior aspect of the third ventricle.

23.2 Indications

- Pineal gland tumors.
- Superior and inferior colliculi tumors and cavernous malformations.
- Tumors of the third ventricle.
- Midbrain and cerebellar peduncles tumors and cavernous malformations.

23.3 Patient Positioning (Fig. 23.1)

- **Sitting position**
  - **Position:** The patient is positioned in a sitting position with the head fixed with a Mayfield head holder.
  - **Head:** The head is flexed as much as possible, to get the tentorium parallel to the floor.
  - **Body:** The body must be elevated about 60° from the horizontal. Care should be taken not to flex the head too much in order not to compromise the venous backflow.
  - **Legs:** The legs are flexed about 20-30° and the knees elevated.
- **Prone (Concorde) position**
  - **Position:** The patient is positioned in prone position with the head fixed with a Mayfield head holder.
  - **Head:** Patient's head is elevated at a higher level as compared to the heart to facilitate venous backflow. The head has to be flexed as much as possible to get the tentorium perpendicular to the floor.
  - **Body:** The chest is elevated about 30° from the horizontal.
  - **Legs:** The legs are flexed 15° by using pillows.

23.4 Skin Incision (Fig. 23.2)

- **Linear incision (midline approach)**
  - **Starting point:** The incision starts 2 cm above the inion on the midline.
  - **Course:** It runs inferiorly on the midline toward the cervical spinous processes.
  - **Ending point:** It ends at the spinous process of C3 on the posterior cervical midline.
- **Linear incision (paramedian approach)**
  - **Starting point:** The incision starts 4 cm above the ideal line connecting the inion and the posterior root of zygoma.
  - **Course:** The incision line runs inferiorly in a vertical direction, perpendicular to the course of the transverse sinus.
  - **Ending point:** It ends 8 cm below the ideal line connecting the inion and the posterior root of zygoma.

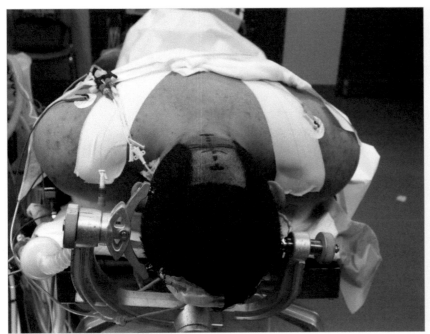

Fig. 23.1 Patient positioning. Prone (Concorde) position and sitting position. The sitting position is generally preferred for the supracerebellar approach because it facilitates cerebellar retraction, reduces venous bleeding and pooling in the operative field. The main disadvantage is related to the risk of air embolism. Alternatively, the supracerebellar approach can be performed in "Concorde" position, as shown by the figure.

23.4.1 Critical Structures

- Greater occipital nerve.
- Occipital artery.

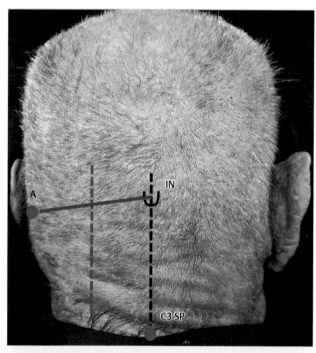

Fig. 23.2 Skin incision. Midline and paramedian approach.
Midline approach (black dotted line). Linear incision starts 2 cm above the external occipital protuberance and runs downward to C3 spinous process.
Paramedian approach (red dotted line). Linear incision runs perpendicular to the line (blue line) connecting the inion and the posterior root of the zygoma.
Abbreviations: A = asterion; C3 SP = C3 spinous process; IN = inion.

23.5 Soft Tissues Dissection (Fig. 23.3)

- **Myofascial level**
  - The myofascial level is incised according to the course of the skin incision.
- **Muscles** (**Figs. 23.3, 23.4, 23.5**)
  - **Superficial muscle layer**
    - ❖ The fascia covering the trapezius, splenius and semispinalis capitis is exposed.
    - ❖ The muscles of the superficial layers are divided at the tendinous midline, or '*linea alba*', reaching the periosteal layer.
    - ❖ In the **paramedian approach**, all suboccipital muscles are divided following the course of the skin incision.
  - **Deep muscle layer**
    - ❖ The rectus capitis posterior minor and major, the inferior oblique as well as the semispinalis cervicis are exposed at the level of the atlas (C1) and axis (C2).
    - ❖ The vertebral artery and its venous plexus are not necessarily exposed.
- **Bone exposure**
  - **Midline approach:** A subperiosteal dissection is carried out. Soft tissues are bilaterally detached from the posterior arch of C1, as well as from the occipital bone, starting from the midline toward the asterion. The foramen magnum might be exposed.
  - **Paramedian approach:** The subperiosteal dissection is unilaterally performed from the inion to the asterion. The foramen magnum region is not necessarily exposed.

23.5.1 Critical Structures

- Vertebral artery and surrounding venous plexus.
- First cervical (C1) nerve rootlet.

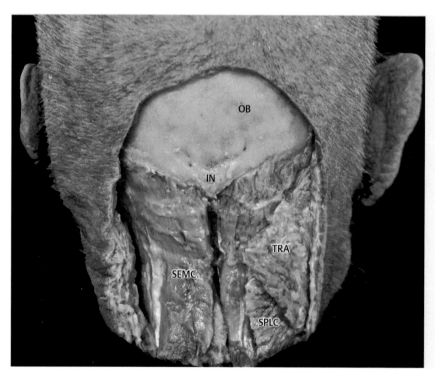

Fig. 23.3 Muscles dissection. After dissecting the superficial fascia, the underlying superficial suboccipital muscles are exposed. Abbreviations: IN = inion; OB = occipital bone; SEMC = semispinalis capitis; SPLC = splenius capitis; TRA = trapezius.

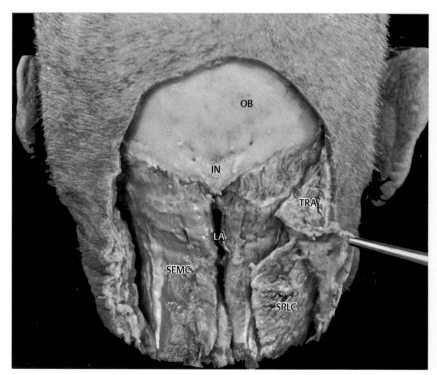

Fig. 23.4 Muscles dissection. The trapezius and splenius capitis are detached and transposed laterally exposing the semispinalis capitis, which is divided on the midline from the linea alba.
Abbreviations: IN = inion; LA = linea alba; OB = occipital bone; SEMC = semispinalis capitis; SPLC = splenius capitis; TRA = trapezius.

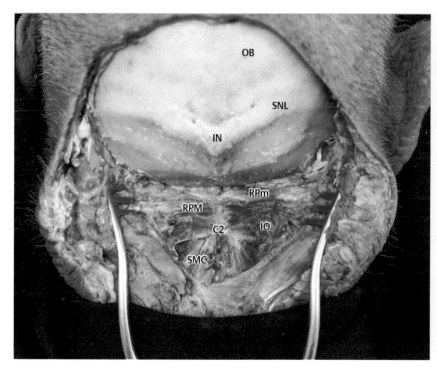

Fig. 23.5 Muscles dissection. The suboccipital bone is largely exposed above the deep muscular layer, exposing the rectus capitis posterior minor and major. The inferior oblique as well as the semispinalis cervicis are exposed at the level of C1 and C2.
Abbreviations: C2 = C2 spinous process; IN = inion; IO = inferior oblique; OB = occipital bone; RPm = rectus capitis posterior minor; RPM = rectus capitis posterior major; SMC = semispinalis cervicis; SNL = superior nuchal line.

23.6 Craniotomy/Craniectomy (Fig. 23.6)

23.6.1 Bilateral Suboccipital Craniotomy, Landmarks

- **Burr holes**
  - **I:** The first burr hole is made on the midline, just above the inion.
  - **II and III:** Following burr holes have to be made on both sides, 4 cm laterally from the inion.
- **Craniotomy landmarks**
  - **Laterally:** The lateral limits correspond to the asterion.
  - **Superiorly:** The superior margin of the craniotomy is located 2 cm above the superior nuchal line.
  - **Inferiorly:** The inferior limit of the craniotomy is the foramen magnum.

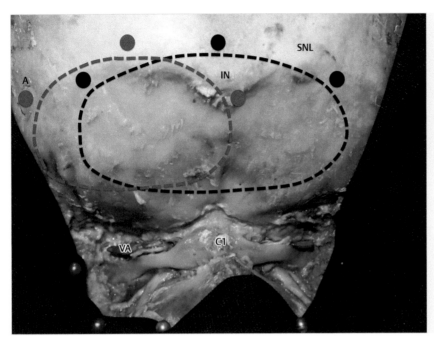

Fig. 23.6 Alternative craniotomies. Midline craniotomy (*black dotted line*) performed through three burr holes (*black circles*), which are placed superior to the inion and bilaterally posterior to the asterion. Paramedian craniotomy (*red dotted line*) performed through three burr holes (*red circles*) inferior to the inion, just posterior to the asterion and just above the superior nuchal line. Abbreviations: A = asterion; C1 = C1 posterior arch; IN = inion; SNL = superior nuchal line; VA = vertebral artery.

23.6.2 Paramedian Suboccipital Craniotomy, Landmarks

- **Burr holes**
  - **I:** The first burr hole is placed 2 cm above the superior nuchal line, at the midpoint of the line connecting the asterion to the inion.
  - **II:** The second burr hole is made just lateral to the external occipital crest, below the inion.
  - **III:** The third burr hole is placed at the asterion.
- **Craniotomy landmarks**
  - **Medially:** The medial margin of the craniotomy corresponds to the external occipital crest (inion).
  - **Laterally:** The craniotomy extends laterally toward the asterion.
  - **Superiorly:** The superior bone cut is made 2 cm above the superior nuchal line.
  - **Inferiorly:** The inferior limit of the craniotomy is the foramen magnum.

23.6.3 Critical Structures

- Vertebral artery.
- Torcula.
- Transverse-sigmoid sinus junction.

23.7 Dural Opening (Figs. 23.7, 23.8)

23.7.1 Midline Approach

- Dura is opened in a U-shaped fashion. The flap is based on both the transverse sinuses and the torcula and reflected antero-superiorly.
- Occipital sinus has to be ligated in order to avoid venous bleeding.

23.7.2 Paramedian Approach

- Dura is opened in a U-shaped fashion. The flap is based on the ipsilateral transverse sinus and reflected antero-superiorly.

23.7.3 Critical Structures

- Sigmoid and transverse venous sinuses junction.
- Occipital sinus.
- Torcula.

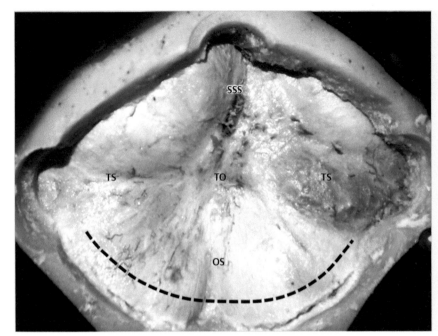

Fig. 23.7 Dural opening. Midline exposure showing the U-shaped durotomy. Abbreviations: OS = occipital sinus; SSS = superior sagittal sinus; TO = torcular; TS = transverse sinus.

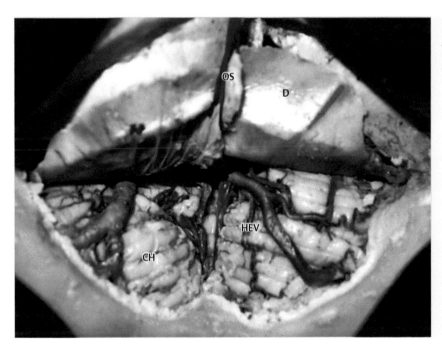

Fig. 23.8 Dural opening. Intradural view. Abbreviations: CH = cerebellar hemisphere; D = dura; HEV = hemispheric vein; OS = occipital sinus.

23.8 Intradural Exposure (Figs. 23.9–23.15)

- **Parenchymal structures:** Cerebellar suboccipital and tentorial surfaces, corpora quadrigemina, pineal gland, pulvinar thalami, posterolateral mesencephalic tegmental aspect and the splenium of the corpus callosum.

- **Arachnoidal layer:** Quadrigeminal and ambient cisterns.
- **Cranial nerves:** Fourth cranial nerve.
- **Arteries:** Posterior inferior cerebellar artery (PICA), superior cerebellar artery (SCA), and posterior cerebral artery (PCA).
- **Veins:** Superior hemispheric and vermian veins, internal occipital veins, basal veins of Rosenthal, vein of the cerebello-mesencephalic fissure or precentral cerebellar veins, and great Galen veins.

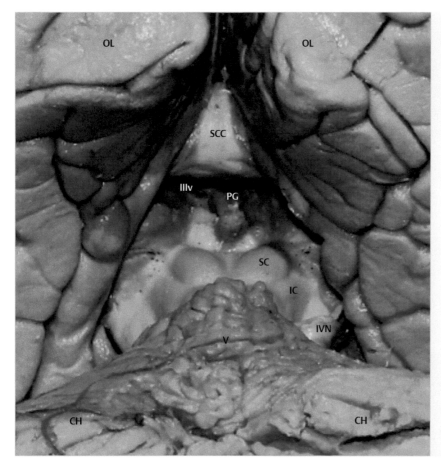

Fig. 23.9 Parenchymal structures involved in the supracerebellar infratentorial approach. Abbreviations: CH = cerebellar hemisphere; IC = inferior colliculus; IIIv = third ventricle; IVN = fourth cranial nerve; OL = occipital lobule; PG = pineal gland; SC = superior colliculus; SCC = splenium of the corpus callosum; V = vermis.

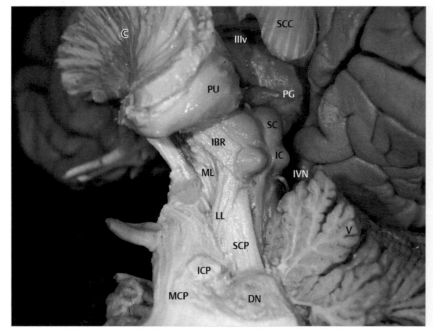

Fig. 23.10 Parenchymal structures involved in the supracerebellar infratentorial approach.
Abbreviations: DN = dentate nucleus; IBR = inferior brachium; IC = inferior colliculus; C = internal capsule; ICP = inferior cerebellar peduncle; IIIv = third ventricle; IVN = fourth cranial nerve; LL = lateral lemniscus; MCP = middle cerebellar peduncle; ML = medial lemniscus; PG = pineal gland; PU = pulvinar thalami; SC = superior colliculus; SCC = splenium of the corpus callosum; SCP = superior cerebellar peduncle; V = vermis.

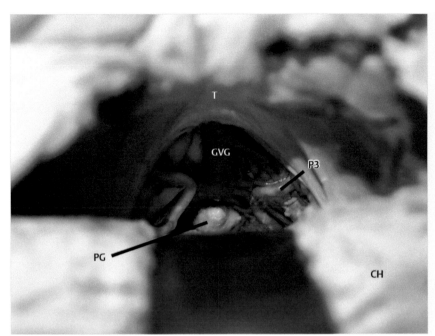

Fig. 23.11 Intra-cisternal structures exposed by the supracerebellar infratentorial approach. Midline approach, microscopic view. Abbreviations: CH = cerebellar hemisphere; GVG = great vein of Galen; P3 = P3 segment of posterior cerebral artery; PG = pineal gland; T = tentorium.

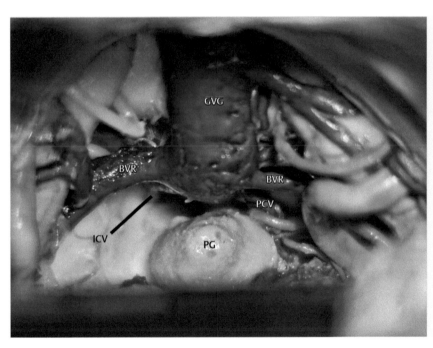

Fig. 23.12 Intra-cisternal structures exposed by the supracerebellar infratentorial approach. Midline approach, microscopic view. Abbreviations: BVR = basal vein of Rosenthal; GVG = great vein of Galen; ICV = internal cerebral vein; PCV = precentral cerebellar vein; PG = pineal gland.

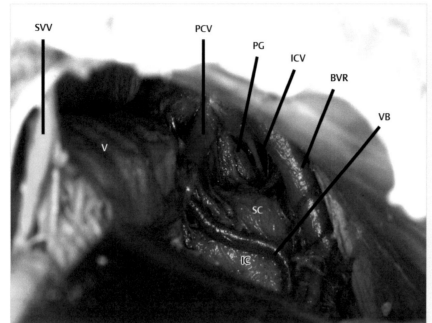

Fig. 23.13 Intra-cisternal structures exposed by the supracerebellar infratentorial approach. Paramedian approach.
Abbreviations: BVR = basal vein of Rosenthal; IC = inferior colliculus; ICV = internal cerebral vein; PCV = precentral cerebellar vein; PG = pineal gland; SC = superior colliculus; SVV = superior vermian vein; V = vermis; VB = vermian branches of the superior cerebellar artery.

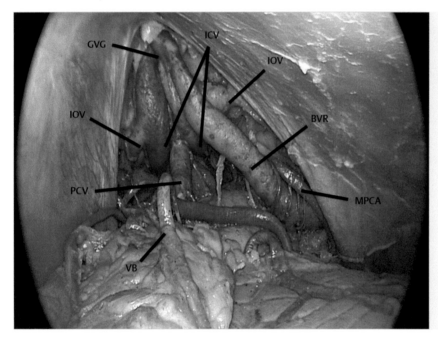

Fig. 23.14 Intra-cisternal structures exposed by the supracerebellar infratentorial approach. Paramedian approach, endoscopic view.
Abbreviations: BVR = basal vein of Rosenthal; GVG = great vein of Galen; ICV = internal cerebral vein; IOV = internal occipital vein; MPCA = medial posterior choroidal artery; PCV = precentral cerebellar vein; VB = vermian branches of the superior cerebellar artery.

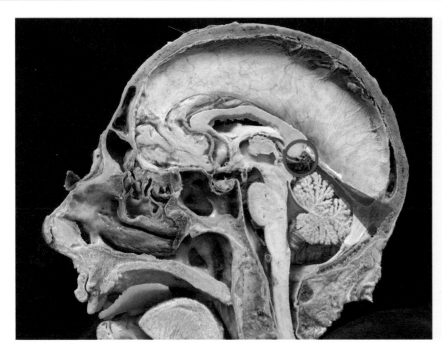

Fig. 23.15 Supracerebellar infratentorial route to the pineal region.

References

1. Kawashima M, Rhoton AL Jr, Matsushima T. Comparison of posterior approaches to the posterior incisural space: microsurgical anatomy and proposal of a new method, the occipital bi-transtentorial/falcine approach. Neurosurgery 2002;51(5):1208–1220, discussion 1220–1221

2. Rey-Dios R, Cohen-Gadol AA. A surgical technique to expand the operative corridor for supracerebellar infraten-torial approaches: technical note. Acta Neurochir (Wien) 2013;155(10):1895–1900

3. Sekhar LN, Goel A. Combined supratentorial and infraten-torial approach to large pineal-region meningioma. Surg Neurol 1992;37(3):197–201

4. Türe U, Harput MV, Kaya AH, et al. The paramedian supracere-bellar-transtentorial approach to the entire length of the me-diobasal temporal region: an anatomical and clinical study. Laboratory investigation. J Neurosurg 2012; 116(4):773–791

24 Endoscopic Approach to Pineal Region

Hasan A. Zaidi and Peter Nakaji

24.1 Introduction

The endoscope-controlled supracerebellar infratentorial approach for pineal region pathology is a potentially powerful approach that can minimize surgical approach-related morbidity.

Patients are positioned in a sitting position, with the secondary surgeon holding the endoscope while the primary surgeon, who maintains bimanual dexterity, visualizes the screen. This is an ergonomic position that can facilitate surgery.

A small vertical incision is made in the scalp with a small craniotomy, which is large enough to accommodate the endoscope and microsurgical instruments.

24.2 Indications

- Pineal tumors of any size or pathology, though germinoma could be considered for biopsy and radiation instead.
- Large, symptomatic pineal cysts.
- Tectal or anterosuperior vermian tumors.
- Tentorial incisura tumors.
- Many supratentorial tumors can also be approached trans-tentorially.
- Pineal tumors that are predominantly in the anterior or mid-part of the third ventricle or the aqueduct should not be approached in this way.

24.3 Patient Positioning (Fig. 24.1)

- **Position:** The patient is placed in sitting position with the head fixed with a Mayfield head holder.
- **Body:** Body lies sitting 45° from the horizontal.
- **Head:** The head is flexed an additional 45°, rotated 10° to the contralateral side, not tilted.
- **Shoulder position:** Shoulders are adequately padded in the sitting slouch position.
- **Anti-decubitus device:** Backrest should be at the level of the mid-scapula or lower.
- **The inion** should be facing straight back toward the surgeon, who is standing behind.
- **Image guidance** is very helpful; the midline tentorium should be as close to level with the floor as possible.

24.4 Skin Incision (Fig. 24.2)

- **Linear vertical unilateral incision**
  - **Starting point:** Incision starts 1 cm above the line between the inion and the top of the zygoma, 25 mm from midline.
  - **Course:** Incision line runs inferiorly from this point for 2.5 cm.
  - **Ending point:** It ends 3.5 mm from the top of the incision, ending in the muscles.

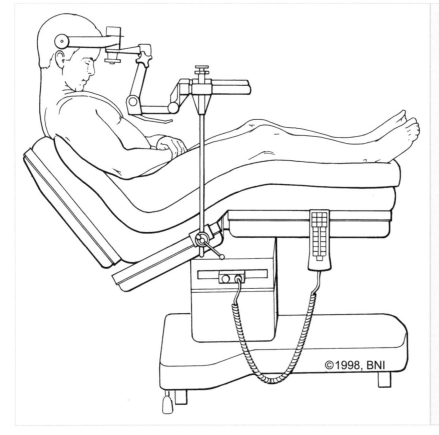

Fig. 24.1 Patient positioning. (Used with permission from Barrow Neurological Institute, Phoenix, AZ.)

©1998, BNI

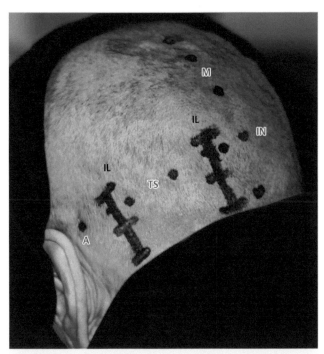

Fig. 24.2 Alternative skin incisions are outlined; paramedian incision and extreme lateral excision. (Used with permission from Barrow Neurological Institute, Phoenix, AZ.)
Abbreviations: A = asterion; IL = incision line; IN = inion; M = midline; TS = transverse sinus.

24.4.1 Critical Structures

- Occipital artery
- Greater and lesser occipital nerves

24.5 Soft Tissues Dissection (Fig. 24.3)

- **Myofascial level**
  - Incised according to skin incision.
- **Muscles**
  - Layers of the splenius capitis muscle and semispinalis capitis muscle are visualized at the inferior aspect of the incision.
  - These are incised along the length of the incision and retracted medially and laterally.
- **Bone exposure**
  - Subperiosteal dissection of occipital bone overlying the lower part of the transverse sinus and the upper cerebellum, lateral to the torcular, is performed.

24.5.1 Critical Structures

- Transverse sinus.

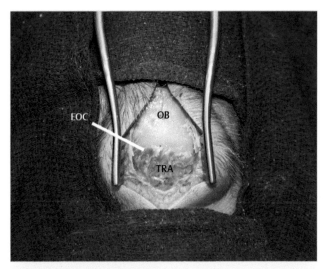

Fig. 24.3 Soft tissue dissection.
Abbreviations: EOC = external occipital crest; OB = occipital bone; TRA = trapezius.

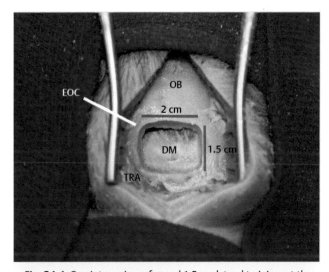

Fig. 24.4 Craniotomy is performed 1.5 cm lateral to inion, at the inferior edge of transverse sinus.
Abbreviations: DM = dura mater; EOC = external occipital crest; OB = occipital bone; TRA = trapezius.

24.6 Craniotomy/Craniectomy (Fig. 24.4)

24.6.1 Paramedian suboccipital craniotomy landmarks

- **Burr holes**
  - **Option 1:** A single oval burr hole is made at the level of the inferior edge of the transverse sinus.
  - **Option 2:** One medial upper corner burr hole is placed over bottom edge of transverse sinus and one 2.5 cm lateral to this at the same height.

- **Craniotomy landmarks**
  - ○ **Medially:** 1.5 cm lateral to inion.
  - ○ **Laterally:** 2.5 cm lateral to medial side.
  - ○ **Superiorly:** Inferior edge of transverse sinus, at level of the line from the inion to the upper edge of the zygoma.
  - ○ **Inferiorly:** 1.5 to 2.0 cm below top edge, over the cerebellar hemisphere.

24.6.2 Variants

- **Extreme lateral supracerebellar infratentorial (SCIT) approach (Fig. 24.5)**
  - ○ Exposure of the transverse sinus-sigmoid sinus junction.
  - ○ Longer reach for lesions located in the pineal region.

24.6.3 Critical Structures

- Transverse sinus.
- Sigmoid sinus.

24.7 Dural Opening (Fig. 24.6)

- Trap-door incision is ideal.
- Edges are based on dural venous sinuses.
- Flaps are reflected toward the sinus, stich is placed close to the sinus and tied to the bone itself to maximize visualization.

24.7.1 Critical Structures

- Sigmoid and transverse venous sinuses.
- Bridging veins from the cerebellum to dura.

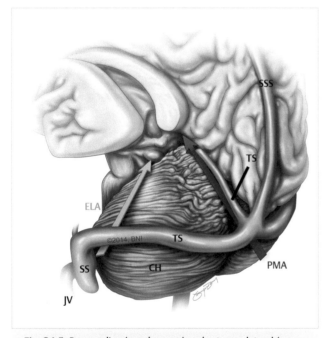

Fig. 24.5 Paramedian (*purple arrow*) and extreme lateral (*green arrow*) SCIT approaches to the pineal region. (Used with permission from Barrow Neurological Institute, Phoenix, AZ.)
Abbreviations: CH = cerebellar hemisphere; ELA = extreme lateral approach; JV = jugular vein; PMA = paramedian approach; SS = sigmoid sinus; SSS = superior sagittal sinus; TS = transverse sinus.

24.8 Intradural Exposure (Figs. 24.6–24.8) (See Chapter 23)

- **Parenchymal structures:** Superior aspect of the cerebellar cortex, vermis, pineal gland, pulvinar, superior and inferior colliculi.
- **Arachnoidal layer:** Cerebellopontine cistern.
- **Cranial nerves:** Fourth cranial nerve.
- **Arteries:** Superior cerebellar artery, posterior cerebral artery.
- **Veins:** Bridging cerebellar veins, great vein of Galen, basal vein of Rosenthal, internal cerebral vein.

24.9 Pearls

- Bridging veins are more commonly encountered with the midline approach, and we typically avoid this approach and minimize sacrifice of bridging veins.

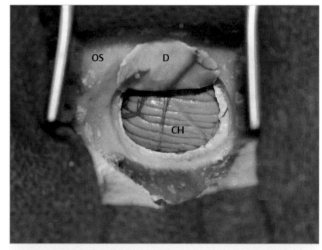

Fig. 24.6 Dural opening, shown here in a trapdoor fashion with the pedicle at the transverse sinus.
Abbreviations: CH = cerebellar hemisphere; D = dura; OS = occipital squama.

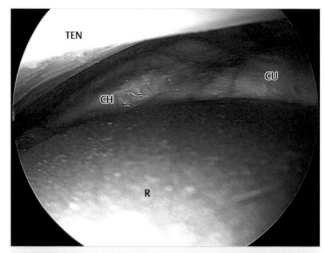

Fig. 24.7 After dural opening, the superior surface of cerebellar hemisphere comes into view. (Used with permission from Barrow Neurological Institute, Phoenix, AZ.)
Abbreviations: CH = cerebellar hemisphere; CU = culmen; R = retractor; TEN = tentorium.

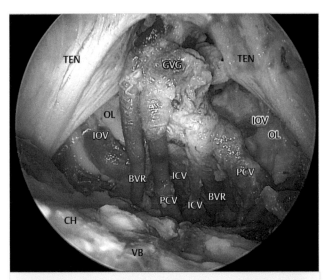

Fig. 24.8 Arachnoid dissection of the cisterna magna relaxes the cerebellum and allows for visualization of pineal region structures. The gland is covered by the venous structures.
Abbreviations: BVR = basal vein of Rosenthal; CH = cerebellar hemisphere; GVG = great vein of Galen; ICV = internal cerebral vein; IOV = internal occipital vein; OL = occipital lobule; PCV = precentral cerebellar vein; VB = vermian branches of the superior cerebellar artery; TEN = tentorium.

- The endoscope should help follow the instruments in and out of the intracranial cavity. This requires dynamic visualization, similar to endoscopic pituitary surgery.
- Three-dimensional endoscopes are typically much easier to use for the microsurgical surgeon, and helps to ease the transition to the endoscopic supracerebellar infratentorial approach.

References

1. Ammirati M, Bernardo A, Musumeci A, Bricolo A. Comparison of different infratentorial-supracerebellar approaches to the posterior and middle incisural space: a cadaveric study. J Neurosurg 2002;97(4):922–928

2. Cardia A, Caroli M, Pluderi M, et al. Endoscope-assisted infratentorial-supracerebellar approach to the third ventricle: an anatomical study. J Neurosurg 2006;104(6, Suppl):409–414

3. Zaidi HA, Elhadi AM, Lei T, Preul MC, Little AS, Nakaji P. Minimally invasive endoscopic supracerebellar-infratentorial surgery of the pineal region: anatomical comparison of four variant approaches. World Neurosurg 2015;84(2):257–266

25 Midline Suboccipital Approach

S. Alexander König, Veronika Messelberger, and Uwe Spetzger

25.1 Introduction

The suboccipital approach is a midline approach to the posterior cranial fossa, which gives direct access to the suboccipital surface of the cerebellar hemispheres.

By opening the inferior medullary velum, the fourth ventricle as well as the brainstem can be accessed. The surgical approach can be tailored to accommodate the relevant pathology. Options include, supratentorial extension as well as the removal of the posterior arch of the atlas (C1).

25.2 Indications

- Parenchymal lesions of the lower cerebellum (*e.g.,* hemorrhages, metastases, von Hippel-Lindau angiomas).
- Parenchymal lesions of the upper cerebellum and lesions in the pineal region (supracerebellar infratentorial approach).
- Lesions of the fourth ventricle (*e.g.,* ependymomas).
- Dorsal brainstem lesions (*e.g.,* cavernomas).
- Meningiomas of the medial posterior fossa.
- Posterior inferior cerebellar artery (PICA) aneurysms.
- Dorsal meningiomas of the foramen magnum.
- Chiari malformation.

25.3 Patient Positioning (Figs. 25.1, 25.2)

- **Position**: The patient is positioned prone. The head is flexed and fixed to a Mayfield clamp.
- **Body:** The body is placed in a slight 'Concorde' position with 10 to 20° of reverse Trendelenburg.

- **Head:** The head is maintained straight and flexed, leaving a space of about 2 cm between the chin and the chest.
- **Shoulders:** Shoulders are slightly pulled down for a safe position of the arms on the armrests.
- The spinous process of the third dorsal vertebra (T3) should be the highest point of patient´s body.
- The inion is the highest point in the surgical field.

25.4 Skin Incision

- **Straight skin incision on the midline**
  - **Starting point:** Incision starts 3 cm above the inion on the midline.
  - **Course:** Incision line runs exactly along the midline.
  - **Ending point:** It ends at the spinous process of the axis (C2).

25.4.1 Critical Structures

- None

25.5 Soft Tissues Dissection (Figs. 25.3–25.5)

- **Myofascial level**
  - The myofascial level is incised along the midline, according to the course of the skin incision (**Fig. 25.3**)
- **Muscles**
  - Origins of both **trapezius muscles** are detached from the occipital bone and reflected laterally (**Figs. 25.3, 25.4**).

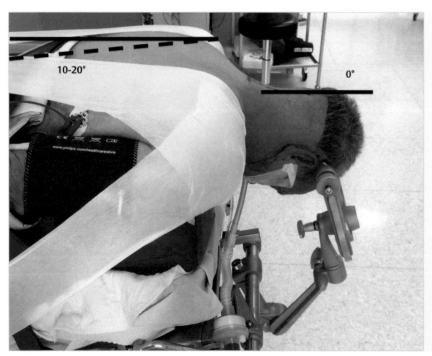

Fig. 25.1 Patient positioning. The head is inclined ventrally and fixed by a Mayfield clamp, while the patient is in prone position.

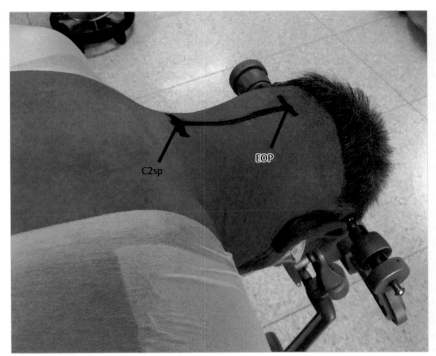

Fig. 25.2 Patient positioning. Skin incision.
Abbreviations: C2sp = spinous process of C2;
EOP = external occipital protuberance.

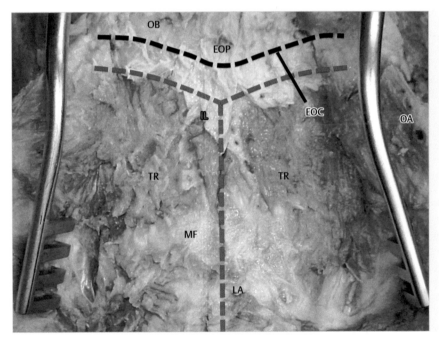

Fig. 25.3 Muscles dissection and bone
exposure. By reflecting the skin inferior
to the superficial muscle layer will merge.
The trapezius muscle is detached from the
occipital bone and the nuchal ligament in
the midline (red lines).
Abbreviations: EOC = external occipital crest;
EOP = external occipital protuberance;
IL = incision line; LA = linea alba; MF = muscle
fascia; OA = occipital artery; OB = occipital
bone; TR = trapezius muscle.

- Further incision of the **nuchal ligament** along the midline is carried out.
- *Semispinalis capitis* is detached and reflected laterally (**Fig. 25.4**).
- *Rectus capitis posterior minor* and *rectus capitis posterior major* are detached and reflected laterally (**Fig. 25.5**).
- **Bone exposure**
  - Subperiosteal dissection of the occipital squama laterally from the midline to both sides is performed (**Fig. 25.5**).
  - Subperiosteal dissection of the posterior arch of the C1 vertebra is carried out.

- **Vertebral arteries**
  - The vertebral arteries are identified by dissecting the muscle layer laterally from the posterior atlanto-occipital membrane (blunt dissection) at the cranial edge of the C1 lamina.

25.5.1 Critical Structures

- Vertebral arteries.
- Greater occipital nerve (dorsal ramus of the second cervical nerve root) close to the external occipital protuberance.

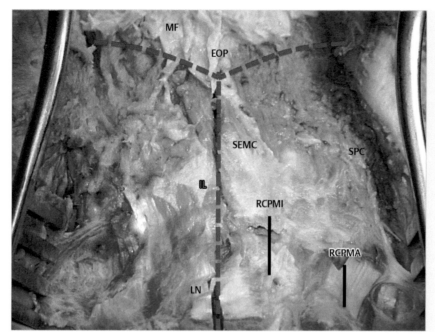

Fig. 25.4 Exposure of the deep muscle layer. The semispinalis capitis muscle is detached from the occipital bone and the nuchal ligament in the midline (red lines). After detaching the semispinalis capitis muscle both posterior rectus capitis muscles are detached.
Abbreviations: EOP = external occipital protuberance; IL = incision line; LN = ligamentum nuchae; MF = muscle fascia; RCPMA = rectus capitis posterior major muscle; RCPMI = rectus capitis posterior minor muscle; SEMC = semispinalis capitis muscle; SPC = splenius capitis muscle.

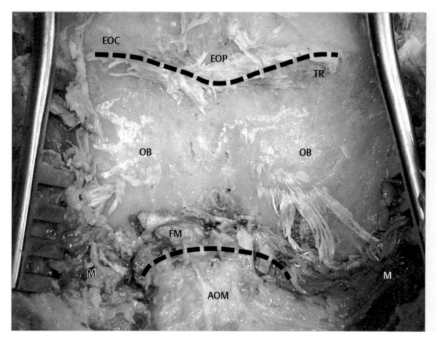

Fig. 25.5 Exposure of the occipital bone over the posterior fossa.
Abbreviations: AOM = atlanto-occipital membrane; EOC = external occipital crest; EOP = external occipital protuberance; FM = foramen magnum; M = retracted muscles; OB = occipital bone; TR = trapezius muscle.

25.6 Craniotomy/Craniectomy (Figs. 25.6, 25.7)

25.6.1 Suboccipital Craniotomy Landmarks (Fig. 25.6)

- **Burr holes**
  - **I and II:** The first two burr holes are placed about 1 cm paramedian and about 1 cm below the superior nuchal line.
  - **III and IV:** Following burr holes are placed about 3 cm below the previous two holes, at the extreme lateral aspect of the surgical field on both sides.

- **Craniotomy landmarks**
  - **Laterally:** Craniotomy extends about 3.5 cm paramedian at the level of the inferior nuchal line.
  - **Superiorly:** Bone cut runs 1 cm below the superior nuchal line.
  - **Inferiorly:** Inferior margin of sub-occipital craniotomy is the magnum foramen.

25.6.2 Variants (Figs. 25.7, 25.8)

- **Optional C1 laminectomy (Fig. 25.7)**
  - C1 laminectomy is indicated for surgical decompression in Chiari malformation.
  - By resecting the posterior arch of C1 a special emphasis should be put on the course of the vertebral arteries.

- **Supracerebellar infratentorial approach (Krause's approach) (Fig. 25.8)**
  - Krause's approach is indicated for lesions of the upper cerebellum and of the pineal region **(see Chapter 23).**

- Patient is placed in a sitting position.
- Two burr holes are placed directly over the transverse sinuses as lateral as possible; one optional burr hole is made directly over the superior sagittal sinus, and two paramedian burr

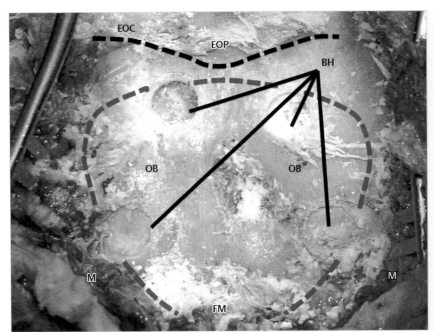

Fig. 25.6 Median suboccipital craniectomy and laminectomy of C1. Placement of four burr holes over the posterior fossa. Craniotomy (*red lines*) from 1 cm below the superior nuchal line and down to the posterior edge of the foramen magnum.
Abbreviations: BH = burr holes; EOC = external occipital crest; EOP = external occipital protuberance; FM = foramen magnum; M = retracted muscles; OB = occipital bone.

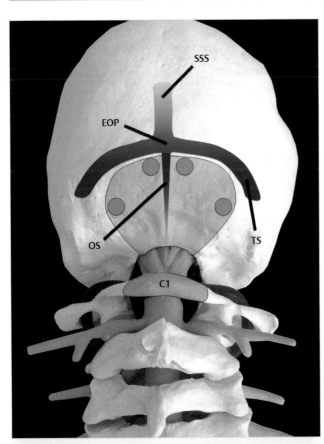

Fig. 25.7 Median suboccipital craniotomy/craniectomy.
Abbreviations: C1 = atlas; EOP = external occipital protuberance; OS = occipital sinus; SSS = superior sagittal sinus; TS = transverse sinus.

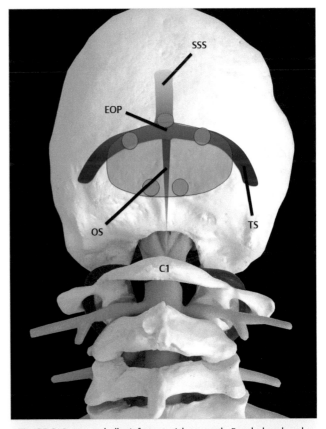

Fig. 25.8 Supracerebellar infratentorial approach. Burr holes placed directly over the venous sinuses for optimum dura dissection and bleeding control if necessary.
Abbreviations: C1 = atlas; EOP = external occipital protuberance; OS = occipital sinus; SSS = superior sagittal sinus; TS = transverse sinus.

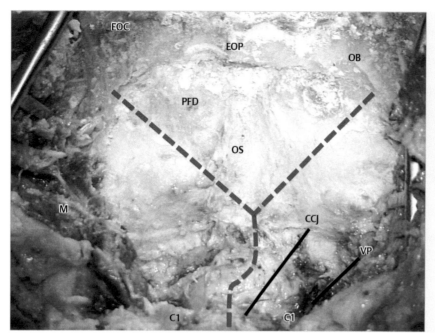

Fig. 25.9 Median suboccipital craniectomy and laminectomy of C1. Completed craniectomy with resection of the posterior C1 arch. Y-shaped dural opening. Paramedian incision (red line) for better control of the occipital sinus.
Abbreviations: C1 = C1 remnants after laminectomy; CCJ = craniocervical junction; EOC = external occipital crest; EOP = external occipital protuberance; M = retracted muscles; OB = occipital bone; OS = occipital sinus; PFD = dura of the posterior fossa; VP = vertebral plexus.

holes over the posterior fossa (**Fig. 25.8**). Perforator drivers of modern drilling systems leave an "eggshell" of bone on the dura, especially by drilling directly over the venous sinuses.
○ Blunt dissection of the dura from the internal table with a curved dissector before completing the craniotomy must be performed.

25.6.3 Critical Structures

• Vertebral arteries (laminectomy of C1)
• Transverse and superior sagittal sinuses (supracerebellar infratentorial approach)

25.7 Dural Opening (Fig. 25.9)

• Dura is opened in a Y-shaped fashion.
• Lower margin corresponds to the upper edge of the C2 lamina.
• Triangular flaps are based on the superior and lateral edges of the craniotomy.
• Connection of the three cuts are not exactly in the midline to avoid heavy bleeding from the occipital sinus.
• Flaps are reflected laterally and superiorly.

25.7.1 Critical Structures

• Occipital sinus.
• Transverses sinuses in case of a supracerebellar infratentorial approach.

25.8 Intradural Exposure (Fig. 25.10)

• **Parenchymal structures:** Cerebellar hemispheres, vermis, cerebellar tonsils, medulla oblongata.

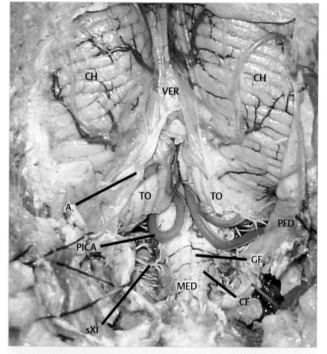

Fig. 25.10 Intradural exposure.
Abbreviations: A = arachnoid of the cerebello-medullary cistern; CH = cerebellar hemisphere; CF = cuneate fasciculus; GF = gracile fasciculus; MED = medulla oblongata; PFD = dura of the posterior fossa; PICA = posterior inferior cerebellar artery; sXI = spinal roots of accessory nerve (XI); TO = cerebellar tonsils; VER = vermis.

• **Arachnoidal layer:** Cerebello-medullary cistern.
• **Cranial nerves:** Spinal roots of the accessory nerve (XI).
• **Arteries:** Posterior inferior cerebellar arteries (PICAs), posterior spinal artery.
• **Veins:** Posterior spinal vein, tonsillar veins, major veins of the cerebellar hemispheres.

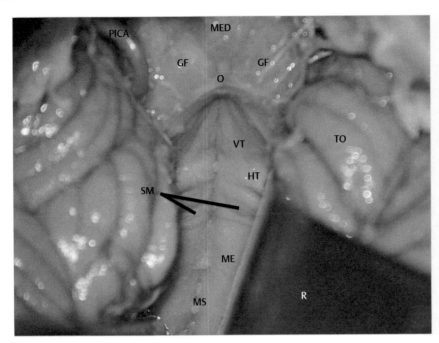

Fig. 25.11 View of the floor of the fourth ventricle after performing a telo-velo-tonsillar approach.
Abbreviations: GF = gracile fasciculus; HT = hypoglossal triangle; ME = medial eminence; MED = medulla oblongata; MS = median sulcus; O = obex; PICA = posterior inferior cerebellar artery; R = retractor; SM = stria medullaris; TO = cerebellar tonsils; VT = vagal triangle.

References

1. Bertalanffy H, Sure U, Petermeyer M, Becker R, Gilsbach JM. Management of aneurysms of the vertebral artery-posterior inferior cerebellar artery complex. Neurol Med Chir (Tokyo) 1998;38(Suppl):93–103

2. König SA, Spetzger U. Surgical strategies for supra- and infratentorially grown occipital meningeomas. J Neurol Surg A Cent Eur Neurosurg 2012;73(2):79–83

26 Retrosigmoid Approach

Marcio S. Rassi, Jean G. de Oliveira, Daniel D. Cavalcanti, and Luis A. B. Borba

26.1 Introduction

The retrosigmoid approach is a lateral approach to the posterior fossa compartment. It is suitable for surgical exposure of the ipsilateral surface of the cerebellar hemisphere, the posterior surface of the petrous bone, as well as the cisternal space defined as cerebellopontine angle (CPA).

Surgical exposure can be further widened caudally toward the magnum foramen and rostrally until the tentorium, which can be cut and opened, providing a transtentorial route to reach the supratentorial space.

The approach is extremely versatile and can be tailored according to the pathology, which must be treated.

The approach is indicated for lesions involving the CPA as well as for microvascular decompression in case of trigeminal neuralgia.

26.2 Indications

- Neoplastic and vascular disorders of the cerebello-pontine angle (CPA).
- Neurovascular decompressions in trigeminal neuralgia.

26.3 Neurophisiological Monitoring

- Somatosensory evoked potentials.
- Facial nerve electromyography.
- Auditory brain stem response.

26.4 Patient Positioning (Fig. 26.1)

- **Position:** Patient is positioned in lateral decubitus; the contralateral arm is positioned below the surgical table with a slight flexion.
- **Head:** The head is positioned neutral, parallel to the ground, fixed on a Mayfield head holder.

- The ipsilateral shoulder is slightly displaced inferiorly, with cushions under contralateral armpit and between the knees.
- The ipsilateral thigh is flexed and prepared for possible fat and fascia harvest.

26.5 Skin Incision (Fig. 26.1)

- **Linear incision**
  - **Landmark:** Mastoid tip.
  - **Starting point:** Incision starts 2 cm behind the external ear at the level of the pinna.
  - **Course:** Incision line runs inferiorly in a straight line.
  - **Ending point:** It ends 1 cm inferior to the mastoid tip.

26.6 Soft Tissue Dissection (Fig. 26.2)

- **Muscles**
  - Incised according to the skin incision.
  - Subperiosteal dissection is carried out laterally, medially, superiorly and inferiorly.

26.6.1 Critical Structures

- Mastoid emissary vein.
- Vertebral artery at the atlanto-occipital joint.

26.7 Craniotomy

- **Burr holes (Fig. 26.3)**
  - **I:** The burr hole is placed on the asterion and performed with a regular cranial perforator or a high-speed drill.
- **Craniotomy landmarks (Fig. 26.4)**
  - **Posteriorly:** Craniotomy runs about 3 cm posterior to the burr hole.
  - **Inferiorly:** It runs 4 cm inferiorly, turning anteriorly, just parallel to the burr hole.

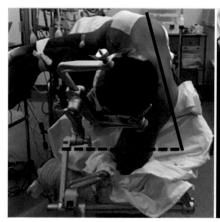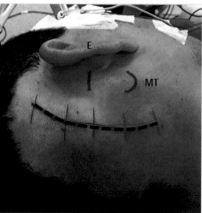

Fig. 26.1 Patient positioning and skin incision.
Abbreviations: E = ear; MT = mastoid tip.

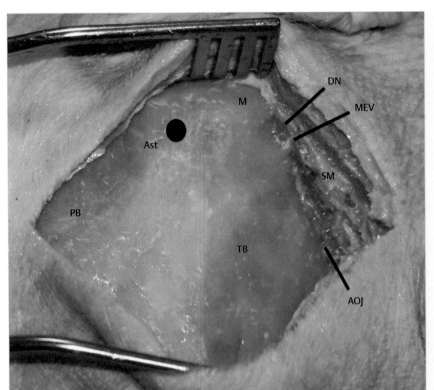

Fig. 26.2 Soft tissue dissection and bone exposure.
Abbreviations: AOJ = atlanto-occipital joint; Ast = asterion; DN = digastric notch; M = mastoid; MEV = mastoid emissary vein; PB = parietal bone; SM = sternocleidomastoid muscle; TB = temporal bone.

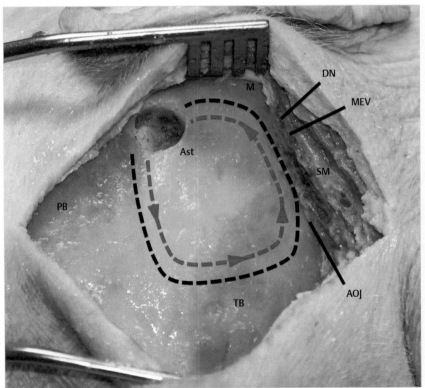

Fig. 26.3 Craniotomy. Burr hole and osteotomy.
Abbreviations: AOJ = atlanto-occipital joint; Ast = asterion; DN = digastric notch; M = mastoid; MEV = mastoid emissary vein; PB = parietal bone; SM = sternocleidomastoid muscle; TB = temporal bone.

○ **Anteriorly:** The remaining anterior cut is performed with the drill.

○ The sigmoid and transverse sinuses have to be exposed by using the drill.

26.7.1 Critical Structures

• Sigmoid and transverse sinus.

26.7.2 Variants

• **Extended transmastoid retrosigmoid approach**
  ○ Indicated for lesions extending medial to the trigeminal nerve (V) but limited at the infratentorial compartment.
  ○ Conventional suboccipital craniotomy is followed by partial mastoidectomy and skeletonization of the total length of the sigmoid sinus.

○ Dura mater is opened along the sigmoid and transverse sinuses, which are reflected anteriorly and superiorly, respectively.

26.8 Dural Opening (Fig. 26.4)

• C-shaped fashion.
• Incision runs just posteriorly to the sigmoid sinus and inferiorly to the transverse sinus.

26.8.1 Critical Structures

• Sigmoid and transverse sinus.
• Dural emissary veins.

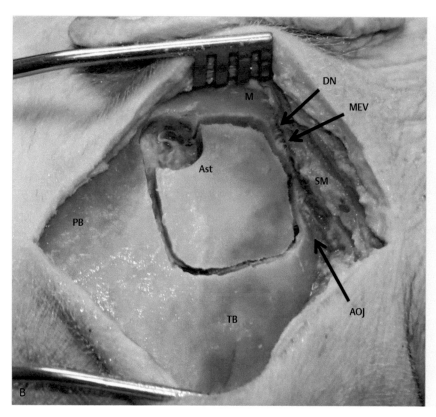

Fig. 26.4 Craniotomy.
Abbreviations: AOJ = atlanto-occipital joint; Ast = asterion; DN = digastric notch; M = mastoid; MEV = mastoid emissary vein; PB = parietal bone; SM = sternocleidomastoid muscle; TB = temporal bone.

26.9 Intradural Exposure (Figs. 26.5–26.7)

- **Parenchymal structures:** Petrosal cerebellar surface, flocculus, choroid plexus and brain stem.
- **Arachnoidal layer:** Lateral cerebellomedullary cistern.
- **Cranial nerves:** Trigeminal (V), abducens (VI), facial (VII), vestibulocochlear (VIII), glossopharyngeal (IX), vagus (X) and accessory (XI) nerves.
- **Arteries:** Superior cerebellar artery (SCA) and anterior inferior cerebellar artery (AICA).
- **Veins:** Petrosal vein.

26.10 Pearls

- Bleeding from emissary veins can be controlled with hemostatic agents and bone wax.
- Packing of large amounts of bone wax must be avoided, due the risk of sinus thrombosis.
- Sinus bleeding can be controlled with a patch of muscle or suture, depending on the extension of the tearing.
- Placing sutures on the anterior margin of the dural opening and slightly reflecting it, could offer additional exposure.
- Starting the intradural procedure, by opening the cerebellomedullary cistern, to release some cerebrospinal fluid, usually provides a good cerebellar relaxation.

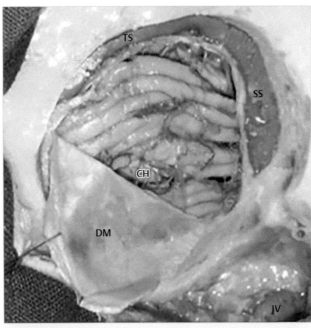

Fig. 26.6 Dural opening.
Abbreviations: CH = cerebellar hemisphere; DM = dura mater; JV = jugular vein; SS = sigmoid sinus; TS = transverse sinus.

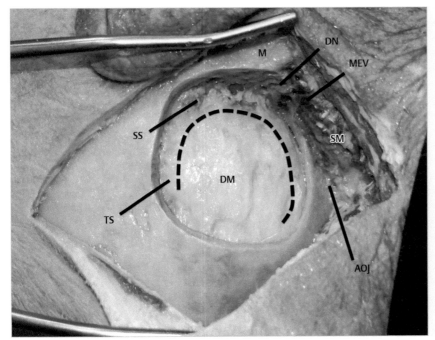

Fig. 26.5 Exposure of the dura mater and venous sinuses.
Abbreviations: AOJ = atlanto-occipital joint; DM = dura mater; DN = digastric notch; M = mastoid; MEV = mastoid emissary vein; SM = sternocleidomastoid muscle; SS = sigmoid sinus; TS = transverse sinus.

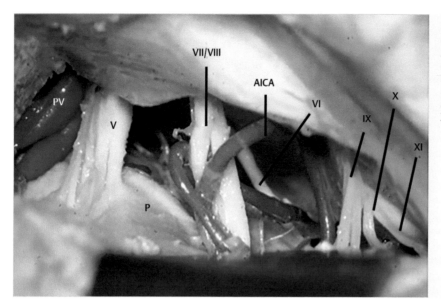

Fig. 26.7 Intradural exposure of the cerebello-pontine angle.
Abbreviations: AICA = anterior inferior cerebellar artery; IX = glossopharyngeal nerve; P = pons; PV = petrosal vein; V = trigeminal nerve; VI = abducens nerve; VII/VIII = facial and vestibule-cochlear nerves complex; X = vagus nerve; XI = accessory nerve.

References

1. Abolfotoh M, Dunn IF, Al-Mefty O. Transmastoid retrosigmoid approach to the cerebellopontine angle: surgical technique. Neurosurgery 2013;73(1, Suppl Operative): ons16–ons23, discussion ons23

2. Al-Mefty O. The retrosigmoid approach to meningiomas of the cerebellopontine angle. In: Al-Mefty O, ed. Operative Atlas of Meningiomas. Philadelphia, PA : Lippincott-Raven; 1988:323–330

3. Matsushima T. The cerebellopontine angle: basic structures and the "rules of three". In: Matsushima T, ed. Microsurgical anatomy and surgery of the posterior cranial fossa. Tokyo: Springer; 2006:101–107

4. Samii M, Gerganov VM. Suboccipital lateral approaches (retrosigmoid). In: Cappabianca P, Califano L, Iaconetta G, eds. Cranial, Craniofacial and Skull Base Surgery. Milan: Springer; 2010:143–150

27 Endoscopic Retrosigmoid Approach

Kerry A. Vaughan and John Y. K. Lee

27.1 Indications

- Microvascular decompression for cranial nerve pathology including
  - Trigeminal neuralgia.
  - Hemifacial spasm.
  - Glossopharyngeal neuralgia.
  - Geniculate neuralgia.
- Cerebellopontine angle tumors.
- Brainstem tumors and vascular malformations.

27.2 Patient Positioning (Figs. 27.1, 27.2)

- **Position:** The patient is positioned in full lateral position with the head fixed in a Mayfield skull clamp.
- **Body:** The body is aligned horizontally and fully lateral, with the patient lying on contralateral side. Pillows or other padding devices should be used liberally to support the body (namely between the knees and ankles, and along the torso anteriorly and posteriorly) before securing the patient to the operating room table.
- **Head:** The head is rotated no more than 30° toward the floor and contralateral side, slightly flexed forward and translated posteriorly such that the chin is slightly tucked ("Military chin tuck").
- Axillary roll is placed under the contralateral axilla.

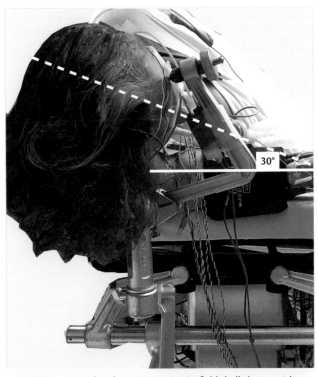

Fig. 27.1 Patient head positioning in Mayfield skull clamp, with no more than a 30° turn to the contralateral side.

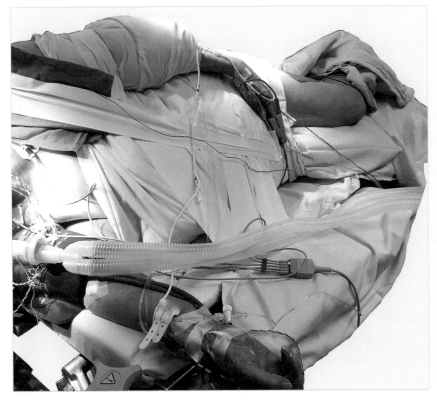

Fig. 27.2 Patient body in fully lateral position with ipsilateral arm tucked and contralateral arm extended anteriorly in front of body.

- Contralateral upper extremity is extended out anteriorly away from the body.
- Ipsilateral arm folded is positioned across the body reaching anteriorly, with appropriate supportive cushioning.
- Ipsilateral shoulder is pulled down and secured with padding and tape to maximize the distance between the head and shoulder.
- **The mastoid process** should be the highest point in the surgical field.

27.3 Endoscopic Pneumatic Arm Setup (Fig. 27.3)

- Mitaka (Storz, Tuttlingen, Germany) bed mount is attached to the side of the anesthesiologist.
- The first joint (most distal) of Mitaka pneumatic arm is extended just over the linear incision to gauge distance from incision.
- During endoscope visualization, the Mitaka should be curved cephalad or caudal in order to reach appropriate depth.
- Double check should be performed that all joints are tightened.
- 100 psi output pressure should be kept for nitrogen hose.
- The pneumatic arm should be raised in vertical direction to drape in sterile fashion.

27.4 Skin Incision (Fig. 27.4)

- **Retrosigmoid linear incision**
  - **Starting point:** The starting point corresponds to the retroauricular area, immediately inferior to the junction of the transverse and sigmoid sinuses and approximately 1 cm behind the patient's hairline.
  - **Run:** Incision line designs a linear path from the starting point, posterior and inferior, toward the posterior inferior border of the mastoid.

- Length of incision should be approximately 4 cm, which is often adequate in patients with average occipito-cervical musculature; a longer incision may be required in those with more muscle bulk.
- **Ending point:** Incision line ends in the retroauricular area, posterior and inferior to the starting point, and posterior and inferior to the cephalad end of the digastric groove.
- **Retrosigmoid sinusoidal incision (useful for larger tumors such as acoustic neuroma)**
  - **Starting point:** The starting point corresponds to the retroauricular area, approximately 3 cm posterior to the superior edge of the pinna and helix, or just behind the patient's hairline.
  - **Run:** Incision line is S-shaped and curves inferiorly at first, then curves posteriorly along the mastoid process and past the tip of the process and away from the ear.
  - **Ending point:** Incision line ends approximately 2 cm behind the mastoid tip along the anterior margin of the sternocleidomastoid muscle.

27.4.1 Critical Structures

- Occipital artery.
- Lesser occipital nerve.
- Greater auricular nerve.

27.5 Soft Tissue Dissection

- **Myofascial level**
  - Myofascial level is incised and dissected deep to skin incision.
- **Muscles**
  - The sternocleidomastoid muscle is detached and reflected anteriorly and inferiorly.

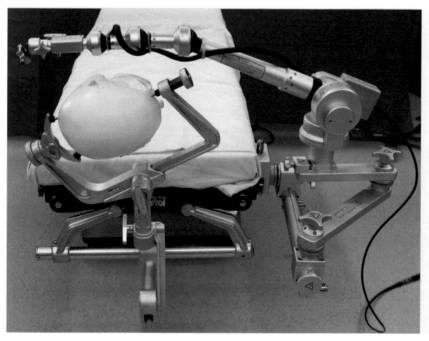

Fig. 27.3 Superior lateral view showing the lowered pneumatic arm, overlying incision site.

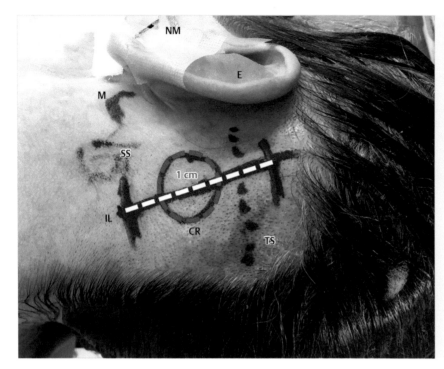

Fig. 27.4 Retrosigmoid incision with external landmarks and planned craniotomy. The mastoid tip is palpated externally and traced. The transverse sinus can be approximately identified by a straight line between zygoma and inion. The white dashed line shows the planned incision, and the red arrow points to the planned circular craniotomy, posterior and inferior to the transverse and sigmoid sinuses.
Abbreviations: CR = craniotomy; E = ear; IL = incision line; M = mastoid; NM = neuro-monitoring; SS = sigmoid sinus; TS = transverse sinus.

○ Posterior belly of the digastric muscle is detached at the digastric groove and reflected anteriorly and inferiorly.
○ The splenius capitis and longissimus capitis muscles are also detached and reflected inferiorly for access.
• **Bone exposure**
○ Subperiosteal dissection of the mastoid region of the temporal bone and mastoid process is performed anteriorly toward the posterior border of the external auditory meatus, taking care not to enter in the meatus.
○ The dissection should be carried out posteriorly toward the parieto-mastoid and occipito-mastoid sutures and inferiorly toward the tip of the mastoid process.

27.5.1 Critical Structures

• External auditory meatus

27.6 Craniectomy (Fig. 27.4)

27.6.1 Retrosigmoid craniotomy landmarks

• **Burr hole**
○ **I:** Only one burr hole is placed, posteriorly and inferiorly to the junction of the transverse and sigmoid sinuses.
• **Craniotomy landmarks**
○ **Anteriorly:** The anterior limit corresponds to the sigmoid sinus.
○ **Posteriorly:** Approximately 2-2.5 cm posterior from the sigmoid sinus.

○ **Superiorly:** The superior limit corresponds to the transverse sinus.
○ **Inferiorly:** Craniotomy should extend approximately 2-2.5 cm inferior to the transverse sinus.

27.6.2 Variants

• The craniotomy might be extended inferiorly toward the tip of the mastoid process, if the approach is intended for a lower cranial nerve pathology (VII to XII cranial nerves).

27.6.3 Critical Structures

• Osseous communicating sinuses and diploic bone.
• Mastoid air cells.

27.7 Dural Opening

• Dura is opened in a C-shaped fashion.
• Diameter of the dural opening measures 1 cm for microvascular decompression and 3 cm diameter for tumors.
• Edges of dural opening are based on the sigmoid sinus.
• The C-shaped flap is reflected anteriorly toward sigmoid sinus.

27.7.1 Critical Structures

• Transverse venous sinus.
• Sigmoid venous sinus.
• Petrosal vein (Dandy's vein).

27.8 Intradural Exposure (Figs. 27.5–27.13)

- **Parenchymal structures:** Antero-lateral aspect of cerebellar surface facing the petrous dura.
- **Arachnoidal layer:** Arachnoid leaflets bridging the anterior cerebellar surface and the petrous dura, the arachnoid covering of the lower cranial nerve bundle (IX to XI cranial nerves).

- **Cranial nerves:** Trigeminal nerve, facial/vestibulocochlear nerve complex, lower cranial nerves complex (glossopharyngeal/vagus/accessory).
- **Arteries:** Superior cerebellar artery (SCA), anterior inferior cerebellar artery (AICA), posterior inferior cerebellar artery (PICA), vertebral artery (VA).
- **Veins:** Dural bridging veins, petrosal vein (Dandy's vein).

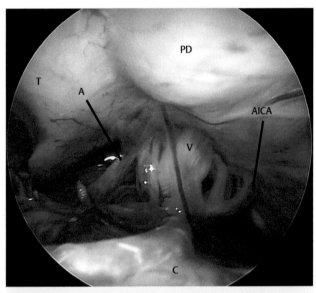

Fig. 27.5 Approach for **right-sided** trigeminal neuralgia, with arachnoid dissection around trigeminal nerve and surrounding vessels. Abbreviations: A = arachnoid; AICA = anterior inferior cerebellar artery; C = cerebellum; PD = petrous dura; T = tentorium; V = fifth cranial nerve.

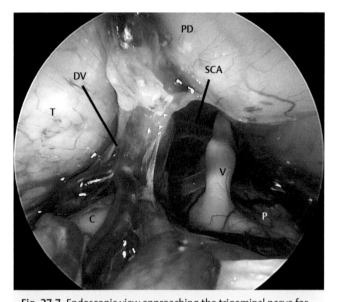

Fig. 27.7 Endoscopic view approaching the trigeminal nerve for **right-sided** trigeminal neuralgia, with clear compression of the nerve by the superior cerebellar artery.
Abbreviations: C = cerebellum; DV = Dandy's vein; P = pons; PD = petrous dura; SCA = superior cerebellar artery; T = tentorium; V = fifth cranial nerve.

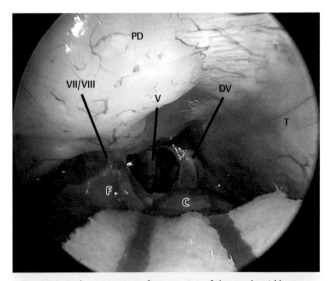

Fig. 27.6 Endoscopic view after opening of the arachnoid layers overlying the trigeminal nerve for **left-sided** trigeminal neuralgia, along with the facial and vestibulocochlear complex (VII/VIII), and the Dandy's vein.
Abbreviations: C = cerebellum; DV = Dandy's vein; F = flocculus; PD = petrous dura; T = tentorium; V = fifth cranial nerve; VII/VIII = facial and vestibulocochlear complex.

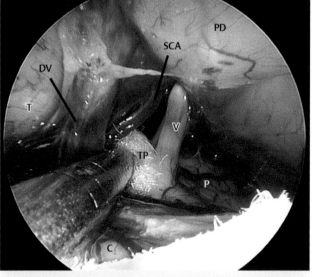

Fig. 27.8 Separation of the superior cerebellar artery from the trigeminal nerve to relieve compression (**right-side**), with insertion of rolled Teflon pad.
Abbreviations: C = cerebellum; DV = Dandy's vein; P = pons; PD = petrous dura; SCA = superior cerebellar artery; T = tentorium; TP = Teflon pad; V = fifth cranial nerve.

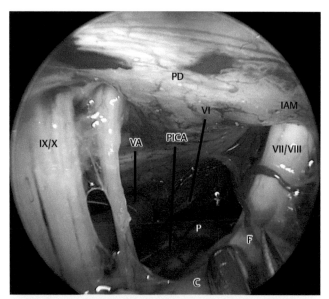

Fig. 27.9 Endoscopic view with 0-degree scope of approach for **left-sided** hemifacial spasm, with the facial and vestibulocochlear complex visible (VII/VIII), vertebral artery, abducens nerve, and the posterior inferior cerebellar artery compressing the root entry zone of the facial nerve. The glossopharyngeal and vagus complex can be seen inferiorly (IX/X).
Abbreviations: C = cerebellum; F = flocculus; IAM = internal acoustic meatus; IX/X = glossopharyngeal and vagus complex; P = pons; PD = petrous dura; PICA = posterior inferior cerebellar artery; VA = vertebral artery; VI = sixth cranial nerve; VII/VIII = facial and vestibulocochlear complex.

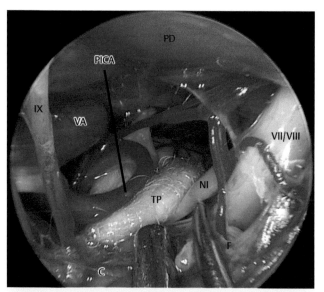

Fig. 27.11 View of posterior inferior cerebellar artery compressing the root entry zone of the facial nerve, seen with a 30-degree endoscope directed medially. Rolled Teflon pads have been inserted to decompress the facial nerve from the PICA loop seen inferior to it, and the nervus intermedius (can be seen separately from the rest of the facial and vestibulocochlear nerve complex).
Abbreviations: C = cerebellum; F = flocculus; IX = glossopharyngeal nerve; NI = nervus intermedius; PD = petrous dura; PICA = posterior inferior cerebellar artery; TP = Teflon pad; VA = vertebral artery; VII/VIII = facial and vestibulocochlear complex.

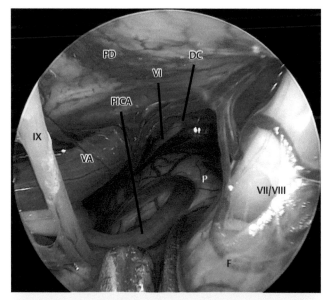

Fig. 27.10 View of posterior inferior cerebellar artery compressing the root entry zone of the facial and vestibulocochlear nerve complex (VII/VIII), seen with a 30-degree endoscope directed medially. Also visible are the superior portion of the glossopharyngeal and vagus nerves (IX/X), and deep to the complex are the vertebral artery and the abducens nerve entering Dorello's canal.
Abbreviations: DC = Dorello's canal; F = flocculus; IX = glossopharyngeal nerve; P = pons; PD = petrous dura; PICA = posterior inferior cerebellar artery; VA = vertebral artery; VI = sixth cranial nerve; VII/VIII = facial and vestibulocochlear complex.

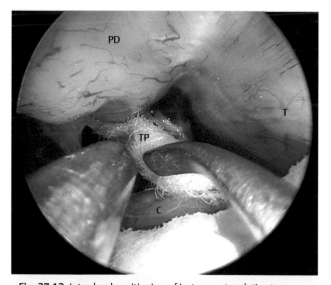

Fig. 27.12 Intradural positioning of instruments relative to endoscope, at the two lower angles of an equilateral triangle, or approximately 8 o'clock and 4 o'clock.
Abbreviations: C = cerebellum; PD = petrous dura; T = tentorium; TP = Teflon pad.

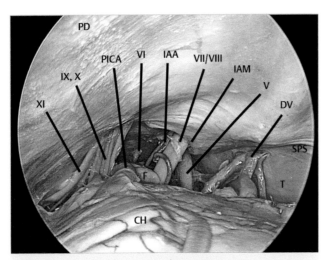

Fig. 27.13 Intradural anatomy in the cadaver.
Abbreviations: CH = cerebellar hemisphere; DV = Dandy's vein; F = flocculus; IAA = internal auditory artery; IAM = internal acoustic meatus; IX = glossopharyngeal nerve; PD = petrous dura; PICA = posterior inferior cerebellar artery; SPS = superior petrosal sinus; T = tentorium; V = trigeminal nerve; VI = abducens nerve; VII/VIII = facial and vestibulocochlear complex; X = vagus nerve; XI = accessory nerve.

27.9 Endoscope Intradural Positioning (Fig. 27.12)

- The position of the endoscope (2.7 mm outer diameter) should be kept at the apex of an imaginary equilateral triangle.
- Endoscope should be parallel to the petrous face/ petrous bone.
- Instruments (teardrop suction, bipolar, microscissors) are introduced at the opposite points of the imaginary equilateral

triangle at 4 o'clock and 8 o'clock, under the endoscope, just parallel to the cerebellum.

References

1. Bohman L-E, Pierce J, Stephen JH, Sandhu S, Lee JYK. Fully endoscopic microvascular decompression for trigeminal neuralgia: technique review and early outcomes. Neurosurg Focus 2014;37(4):E18 10.3171/2014.7.FOCUS14318

2. da Silva OT, de Almeida CC, Iglesio RF, de Navarro JM, Teixeira MJ, Duarte KP. Surgical variation of microvascular decompression for trigeminal neuralgia: A technical note and anatomical study. Surg Neurol Int 2016;7(Suppl 21):S571–S576

3. Jarrahy R, Eby JB, Cha ST, Shahinian HK. Fully endoscopic vascular decompression of the trigeminal nerve. Minim Invasive Neurosurg 2002;45(1):32–35

4. Kabil MS, Eby JB, Shahinian HK. Endoscopic vascular decompression versus microvascular decompression of the trigeminal nerve. Minim Invasive Neurosurg 2005; 48(4):207–212

5. Lang S-S, Chen HI, Lee JYK. Endoscopic microvascular decompression: a stepwise operative technique. ORL J Otorhinolaryngol Relat Spec 2012;74(6):293–298

6. Piazza M, Lee JYK. Endoscopic and Microscopic Microvascular Decompression. Neurosurg Clin N Am 2016; 27(3):305–313

7. Rhoton AL Jr. The cerebellopontine angle and posterior fossa cranial nerves by the retrosigmoid approach. Neurosurgery 2000;47(3, Suppl):S93–S129

8. Rhoton AL Jr. Microsurgical anatomy of the posterior fossa cranial nerves. Clin Neurosurg 1979;26:398–462

9. Takemura Y, Inoue T, Morishita T, Rhoton AL Jr. Comparison of microscopic and endoscopic approaches to the cerebellopontine angle. World Neurosurg 2014;82(3-4):427–441

28 Far Lateral Approach and Principles of Vertebral Artery Mobilization

João Paulo Almeida, Mateus Reghin Neto, and Evandro de Oliveira

28.1 Introduction

The far lateral approach is a lateral approach, which provides access to the postero-lateral aspect of the posterior cranial fossa. It is suitable to treat intra- and extra-axial lesions located at the antero-lateral aspect of the craniocervical junction.

One of the most technically demanding steps of the approach is the mobilization of the vertebral artery, to optimize the surgical exposure.

28.2 Indications

- Lesions located at the anterior and lateral aspect of the craniocervical junction:
  - Vertebral artery (VA), vertebro-basilar junction and posterior inferior cerebellar artery (PICA) aneurysms.
  - Tumors located at the anterior part of the foramen magnum and upper cervical spine.
  - Tumors located at the lower third portion of the clivus and posterior aspect of the foramen jugular.

28.3 Patient Positioning

- **Semi-sitting position (See Chapter 24)**
  - Initially in the supine position, the patient's head is fixed to the Mayfield or Sugita head holder with three or four pins placed bilaterally over the superior temporal lines.
  - The patient's body is gradually brought to a semi-sitting position such that the knees are level with the heart. The head holder adaptor is attached to the table between the hips and the knees and arched back as necessary to accommodate patient's body habitus, connecting to the Mayfield head holder.
  - From a neutral position, the head is carefully flexed toward the chest. This maneuver improves the exposure of the craniovertebral junction at the atlas (C1)-occipital condyle articulation and facilitates the dissection of muscles of the suboccipital region.
  - During flexion of the head the distance between the chin and chest should not be smaller than 2 cm, in order to avoid obstruction of the venous return by the internal jugular veins.

28.4 Skin Incision

- **Horseshoe cutaneous incision (Fig. 28.1)**
  - **Starting point:** The incision begins in the midline, approximately 3 cm below the inion.
  - **Course:** Incision runs straight upward until 2 cm above the external occipital protuberance, then it turns laterally, above the superior nuchal line, toward the asterion. Finally, it turns downward and laterally over the posterior border of the sternocleidomastoid muscle. Abundant irrigation of operative field with physiological solution is imperative at

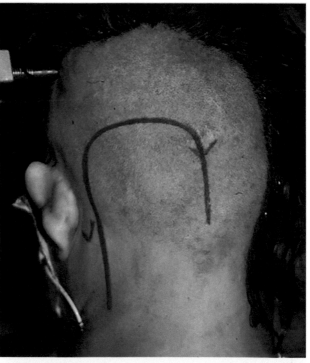

Fig. 28.1 Skin incision

all times during the procedure in order to avoid gaseous embolization.
  - **Ending point:** It ends approximately 5 cm below the mastoid apex, where the transverse process of the atlas can be palpated through the skin.

28.4.1 Critical Structures

- Occipital artery.
- Greater and lesser occipital nerves.

28.5 Soft Tissues Dissection

- **Muscles dissection**
  - After inferomedial retraction of the scalp flap toward the midline, the most superficial layer of muscles, formed by the sternocleidomastoid and splenius capitis muscles (laterally), and trapezius and semispinalis capitis muscles (medially) are exposed **(Fig. 28.2).**
  - The sternocleidomastoid muscle is divided below its insertion, with preservation of its upper attachment for closure. Lateral retraction of that muscle exposes the superior portion of the splenius capitis muscle.
  - The trapezius and splenius capitis muscles are detached, while preserving an upper cuff of their attachment for

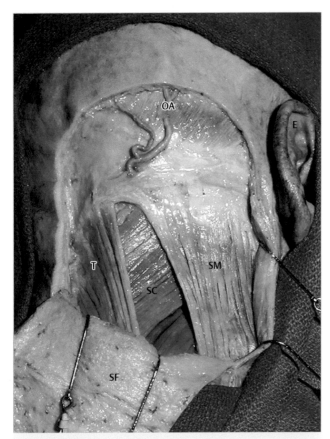

Fig. 28.2 Exposure of the superficial muscle layer.
Abbreviations: E = ear; OA = occipital artery; SC = splenius capitis; SF = skin flap; SM = sternocleidomastoid muscle; T = trapezius

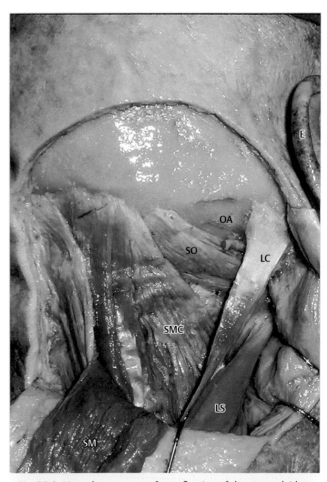

Fig. 28.3 Muscular exposure after reflection of the sternocleidomastoid and trapezius muscles.
Abbreviations: E = ear; LC = longissimus capitis muscle; LS = levator scapulae muscle; OA = occipital artery; SM = sternocleidomastoid muscle; SMC = semispinalis capitis muscle; SO = superior oblique muscle.

closure. After medial and inferior reflection of these muscles, the longissimus capitis, semispinalis and levator scapulae muscles are exposed **(Fig. 28.3).**

○ The longissimus capitis is reflected downward exposing the semispinalis capitis, superior and inferior oblique muscles, and the transverse process of the atlas.

○ Medial reflection of the semispinalis capitis muscles is done in order to expose the suboccipital triangle **(Fig. 28.4).**

○ The suboccipital triangle is defined above and medially by the rectus capitis posterior major, above and laterally by the superior oblique muscle and below and laterally by the inferior oblique muscle **(Fig. 28.4).** These muscles are reflected medially to expose the contents of the suboccipital triangle.

○ In summary, with exception of the sternocleidomastoid, medial retraction of the muscles rather than lateral and inferior reflection is recommended. This maneuver avoids the presence of a muscular bulk between the surgeon and the dura mater, reducing the depth of the exposure.

• **Exposure of the vertebral artery** (Fig. 28. 5)

○ The vertebral artery (VA), venous plexus of the vertebral artery and first cervical (C1) nerve root run in the suboccipital triangle.

○ Adequate exposure of the VA at the suboccipital triangle demands partial obliteration and dissection of the vertebral artery venous plexus.

○ The artery is usually found after dissection of the superior border of the posterior arch of atlas. C1 nerve usually runs on the lower surface of the artery, between the VA and the posterior arch of C1.

○ Careful dissection of the venous plexus until exposure of entrance of the VA into the intradural space is recommended.

• **Mobilization of the vertebral artery**

○ After dissection of the suboccipital triangle and exposure of the extradural extra-foraminal segment of the VA (V3 segment) mobilization of this vessel may be performed.

○ Removal of half of the posterior arch of C1 and the posterior root of its transverse foramen allows for downward and medial mobilization of the VA, which improves the exposure of the occipital condyle **(Fig. 28.6).**

○ Opening of the dura surrounding the VA at the entrance of the intradural space and cut of the first dentate ligament allow further mobilization of the VA.

28.5.1 Critical Structures

• Vertebral artery
• First (C1) and second (C2) cervical nerves

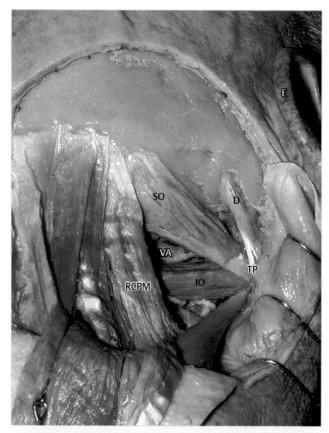

Fig. 28.4 The suboccipital triangle is observed after reflection of the longissimus capitis muscle.
Abbreviations: D = digastric muscle; E = ear; IO = inferior oblique muscle; RCPM = rectus capitis posterior major muscle; SO = superior oblique muscle; TP = transverse process of C1; VA = vertebral artery inside the suboccipital triangle.

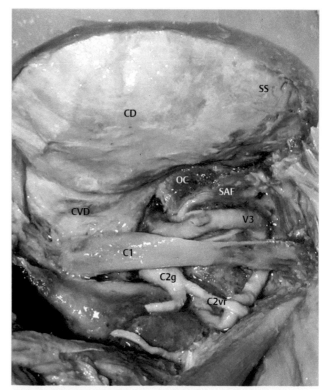

Fig. 28.5 Exposure of the V3 segment of the vertebral artery. Abbreviations: C1 = posterior arch of C1; C2g = C2 ganglion; C2vr = ventral ramus of C2; CD = dura over the suboccipital surface of the cerebellum; CVD = dura over the upper cervical spine; OC = occipital condyle; SAF = superior articular facet of C1; SS = sigmoid sinus; V3 = V3 segment of the vertebral artery.

28.6 Craniotomy

28.6.1 Lateral Suboccipital Craniotomy

- **Limits**
  - **Superiorly:** Transverse sinus.
  - **Laterally:** Sigmoid sinus.
  - **Medially:** External occipital crest.
  - **Inferiorly:** Foramen magnum.
- **Burr holes**
  - **I:** The first burr hole is placed at the asterion (at the junction of the parieto-mastoid, occipito-mastoid, and lambdoid sutures).
  - **II:** The second one is made superiorly and paramedian (below the superior nuchal line).
  - **III:** The third is inferior paramedian (above the foramen magnum).

28.6.2 Removal of the Occipital Condyle

- The occipital condyles project downward along the lateral edge of the anterior half of the foramen magnum.

- The hypoglossal canal crosses the occipital condyle and runs forward and laterally at a 45°angle with the sagittal plane. Its intracranial end is located at the junction of the posterior and middle third of the occipital condyle, while its extracranial end is placed above the junction of anterior and middle third of the condyle.
- The hypoglossal canal is surrounded by cortical bone. It contains the hypoglossal nerve, the meningeal branch of the ascending pharyngeal artery and the venous plexus of the hypoglossal canal (**Fig. 28.6**).
- By drilling the posterior third of the occipital condyle, one sequentially encounters the superficial layer of cortical bone, cancellous bone and the deep layer of cortical bone, which surrounds the hypoglossal canal.
- After exposing the hypoglossal canal, the jugular tubercle may be removed to improve the surgical exposure. It is located above the hypoglossal canal and medially to the lower half of the intracranial end of the jugular foramen.
- Removal of the jugular process, which forms the posterior margin of the jugular foramen, may be performed for extension of the lateral exposure or opening of the jugular foramen from behind. The junction of the sigmoid sinus, jugular bulb and internal jugular vein is exposed after removal of the jugular process.
- Once the bone removal is complete, the bony ridge is covered with rectangular cotton blocks followed by blue drapes, in order to delimitate the surgical field for the intradural phase and minimize light reflection from the surgical microscope.

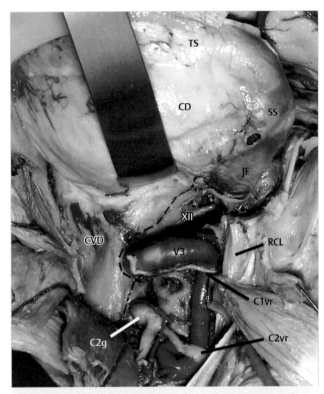

Fig. 28.6 Surgical exposure after removal of the posterior arch of C1 and drilling of the occipital condyle and jugular process. Abbreviations: C1vr = ventral ramus of C1; C2g = C2 ganglion; C2vr = ventral ramus of C2; CD = dura over the suboccipital surface of the cerebellum; CVD = dura over the upper cervical spine; JF = posterior aspect of the jugular foramen; RCL = rectus capitis lateralis muscle; SS = sigmoid sinus; TS = transverse sinus; V3 = vertebral artery; XII = hypoglossal canal.

28.6.3 Critical Structures

- Hypoglossal canal and nerve.
- Jugular tubercle.
- Posterior condylar emissary vein: Communication between the sigmoid sinus and the vertebral venous plexus. It runs in the condylar canal, located posterior to the occipital condyle, and does not communicate with the hypoglossal canal.

28.7 Dural Opening

- The dural incision begins behind the sigmoid sinus and extends behind the VA in the upper cervical region.
- The upper extension of the dural opening depends on how much of the cerebellopontine angle has to be exposed.
- Large lesions may benefit of wide dural openings. In those cases, the dural cut is done close to the medial wall of the sigmoid sinus and inferior wall of the transverse sinus, in a C-shaped fashion, and runs downward to the upper cervical region, behind the entry point of the VA in the intradural space.
- Drilling of the occipital condyle and jugular process improves the lateral retraction of the dura. It allows the dural flap to be flat while reflected laterally toward the sigmoid sinus. The superior edge of the flap is retracted toward the transverse sinus, the medial edge to the occipital bone, and the inferior edge to the occipital bone.

- The dural flap should be tightly held with nylon 4.0 sutures in order to maximize the exposure of the surgical field.

28.7.1 Critical Structures

- Sigmoid and transverse sinus.
- Marginal sinus (encircles the foramen magnum).
- Posterior meningeal artery (branch of the VA).
- Posterior spinal artery.

28.8 Intradural Exposure (Fig. 28.7)

28.8.1 Cisterns

- Cisterna magna.
- Lateral medullary cistern.
- Cerebellopontine cistern.

28.8.2 Parenchymal exposure

- Suboccipital surface of the cerebellum and tonsils.
- Upper cervical spine.
- Cervico-medullary junction.

28.8.3 Dentate ligament

At the craniocervical junction the dentate ligament is located between the VA and ventral roots of C1 anteriorly and the posterior spinal artery and spinal accessory nerve posteriorly.
- Sectioning of the upper two dentate ligaments increases access to the anterior portion of the upper spinal cord.

28.8.4 Cranial nerves

- IX, X, XI cranial nerves in the jugular foramen.
- XII cranial nerve in the hypoglossal canal.
- VII, VIII cranial nerve in the cerebellopontine angle.
- Between the cranial nerves, two windows are available for further dissection:
  ○ The space between the IX cranial nerve and the complex of X and XI nerves.
  ○ The space between the IX cranial nerve and the VII/VIII nerves complex.

28.8.5 Arteries

- Vertebral artery: Anterior to the first dentate ligament at the craniocervical junction.
- Posterior inferior cerebellar artery (PICA): Observed at the lateral medullary cistern.
- Anterior inferior cerebellar artery (AICA): Observed at the cerebellopontine cistern.
- Posterior spinal artery: Posterior to the first dentate ligament at the craniocervical junction.

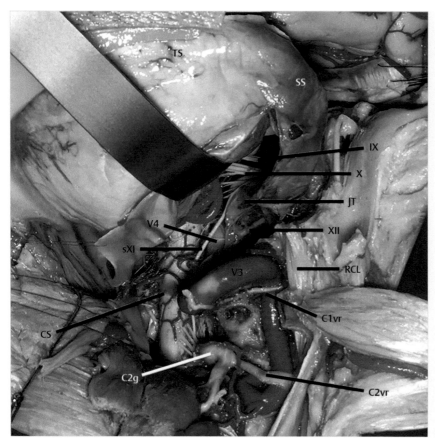

Fig. 28.7 Intradural exposure. Abbreviations: C1vr = ventral ramus of C1; C2g = C2 ganglion; C2vr = ventral ramus of C2; CS = upper cervical spinal cord; IX = IX nerve; JT = jugular tubercle; RCL = rectus capitis lateralis muscle; SS = sigmoid sinus; sXI = spinal accessory nerve; TS = transverse sinus; V3 = V3 segment of the vertebral artery; V4 = intradural segment (V4) of the vertebral artery; X = X nerve; XII = hypoglossal canal.

References

1. Dória-Netto HL, Campos Filho JM, Reghin-Neto M, Rothon AL Jr, Oliveira Ed. The far-lateral craniotomy: tips and tricks. Arq Neuropsiquiatr 2014;72(9):699–705

2. Rhoton AL Jr, Peace D. Microsurgical anatomy of the region of the foramen magnum. Surg Neurol 1985;24(3):293–352

3. Oliveira EO, Wen HT, Tedeschi H, et al. Far lateral transcondylar for lesions of foramen magnum. Tech Neurosurg 2003;9(2):93–105

4. Wen HT, Rhoton AL Jr, Katsuta T, de Oliveira E. Microsurgical anatomy of the transcondylar, supracondylar, and paracondylar extensions of the far-lateral approach. J Neurosurg 1997;87(4):555–585

29 Trans-Frontal-Sinus Subcranial Approach

Nicola Boari, Filippo Gagliardi, Alfio Spina, and Pietro Mortini

29.1 Introduction

The trans-frontal-sinus subcranial approach is well suited for the treatment of tumors of the median anterior skull base. This technique provides early devascularization of the tumor by division of the ethmoidal arteries, direct tumor access from the base, atraumatic frontal lobes decompression, broad exposure of sphenoid and ethmoidal sinuses. It also provides good visual exposure for the dissection of the optic nerves and anterior cerebral arteries, and affords access to a pedicled pericranial flap for dural reconstruction.

29.2 Indications

- Olfactory grove and planum sphenoidale meningiomas.
- Tuberculum sellae and diaphragma sellae meningiomas.
- Giant pituitary adenomas.
- Clival chordomas.
- Esthesioneuroblastomas.
- Malignancy of the anterior skull base - sinonasal tumors.

29.3 Patient Positioning

- **Position:** The patient is positioned supine with the head fixed to a horseshoe head holder.
- **Body:** The body is placed in neutral position with the trunk elevated 30° to increase venous backflow and the legs elevated at the level of the heart.

- **Head:** The head is in neutral position, elevated 15° and extended 20° with the vertex kept downward.
- **Anti-decubitus devices**: Rolls are placed under the knees.
- **The zygoma** has to be the highest point in the surgical field.

29.4 Skin Incision

- Coronal incision (See Chapters 6 and 7)
  - **Starting point:** Incision starts 1 cm anterior and above the tragus.
  - **Run:** Incision line should stay behind the hairline.
  - **Ending point:** It ends 1 cm anterior and above the tragus of the contralateral side.

29.4.1 Critical Structures

- Superficial temporal artery.
- Facial nerve.

29.5 Soft Tissues Dissection (Fig. 29.1)

- **Myofascial level**
  - A subgaleal dissection posterior to the coronal plane of the incision may be performed to maximize the length of the pericranial flap.
  - The pericranial flap is then gently elevated from the cranial vault from posterior to anterior.

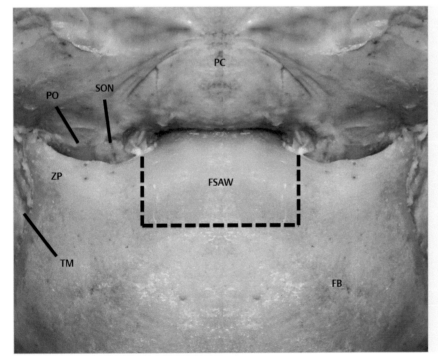

Fig. 29.1 Frontonasal osteotomy. The osteotomy of the anterior wall of the frontal sinus is performed using an oscillating saw (*dotted lines*).
Abbreviations: FB = frontal bone; FSAW = frontal sinus anterior wall; PC = pericranium; PO = periorbit; SON = supraorbital nerve; TM = temporal muscle; ZP = zygomatic process.

- **Muscles**
  - Temporal fascia and muscle are not detached from the temporal fossa.
- **Bone exposure**
  - The scalp is raised forward to expose the supraorbital ridge bilaterally and the nasal process of the frontal bone up to the fronto-naso-maxillary suture in the midline.
  - The periorbit is detached from the superior and medial wall of the orbit on both sides.
- **Supraorbital nerve and artery**
  - They can be freed from the supraorbital notch bilaterally to avoid traction on the orbital contents.

29.5.1 Critical Structures

- Supraorbital nerve and artery.
- Periorbit.
- Lacrimal gland.

29.6 Osteotomy (Fig. 29.2)

An osteotomy of the anterior wall of the frontal sinus, including the upper medial aspect of the superior orbital rims is performed with a reciprocating saw.

- **Cuts**
  - **I:** The first cut is made at the nasofrontal suture on the axial plane down the medial orbital wall and along the nasomaxillary grooves just anterior to the lacrimal crest.
  - **II and III:** Two symmetric cuts are made medial to the supraorbital notch vertically on the sagittal plane.
  - **IV:** A horizontal cut is made on the axial plane across the frontal bones, connecting the previous two, at a level corresponding to the superior limit of the frontal sinus.

29.7 Anterior Skull Base Exposure

- The anterior wall of the sinus is lifted after fracturing the frontal intersinus septa with a chisel.
- Intersinus septa are removed with a rongeur. The mucosa lining the anterior and posterior walls of the sinus is resected **(Fig. 29.3)**.
- Posterior sinus wall is thinned using a diamond drill and piecemeal removed using a Kerrison punch.
- Frontal dura is dissected from the apex and lateral surfaces of the crista galli, which is detached from the ethmoidal cribriform plate, and removed.
- Dissection in a subperiorbital plane along the medial wall of the orbit is performed to identify the anterior and posterior ethmoidal arteries, which are coagulated and divided bilaterally **(Fig. 29.4)**.
- The falx with the origin of the superior sagittal sinus are coagulated and cut.
- Bone from the medial orbital walls is removed and the ethmoid can be drilled to obtain access to the nasal and sphenoethmoidal cavities and to the upper clivus.
- Drilling of the planum sphenoidalis up to the tuberculum sellae can be accomplished **(Fig. 29.5)**.
- The medial optic canals can be unroofed bilaterally to perform an extradural optic nerves and chiasm decompression.

29.7.1 Critical Structures

- Anterior and posterior ethmoidal arteries.
- Internal carotid arteries (ICAs) (C4 and C5 segments).
- Optic nerves and chiasm.

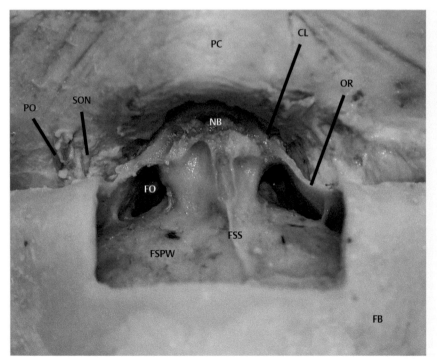

Fig. 29.2 By removing the bony wall and the sinus mucosa the posterior wall of the sinus comes into view.
Abbreviations: CL = canthal ligament; FB = frontal bone; FO = frontal ostium; FSPW = frontal sinus posterior wall; FSS = frontal sinus septum; NB = nasal bone; OR = orbital roof; PC = pericranium; PO = periorbit; SON = supraorbital nerve.

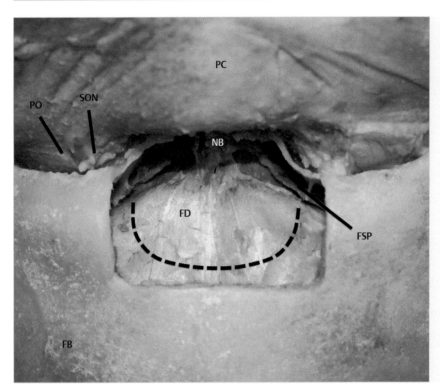

Fig. 29.3 After drilling the posterior sinus wall the frontal dura is exposed. Abbreviations: FB = frontal bone; FD = frontal dura; FSP = frontal sinus pneumatization; NB = nasal bone; PC = pericranium; PO = periorbit; SON = supraorbital nerve; dotted line depicts the following dural opening.

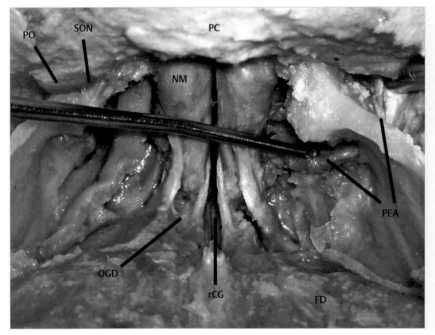

Fig. 29.4 Crista galli is detached from the frontal dura and from nasal mucosa and the anterior and posterior ethmoidal arteries are skeletonized and divided. Olfactory grooves dura is cut with the olfactory filaments. Abbreviations: FD = frontal dura; NM = nasal mucosa; OGD = olfactory groove dura; PC = pericranium; PEA = posterior ethmoidal artery; PO = periorbit; rCG = resected crista galli; SON = supraorbital nerve.

29.8 Dural Opening (Fig. 29.6)

• The dura is divided circumferentially around the olfactory groove.

29.8.1 Critical Structures

• Optic nerves and chiasm.

29.9 Intradural Exposure (Fig. 29.7)

• **Parenchymal structures:** Basal frontal lobes.
• **Arachnoidal layer:** Chiasmatic cistern.
• **Cranial nerves:** Optic and olphactory nerves.
• **Arteries:** Anterior communicating artery (ACoA), anterior cerebral artery (A1 and A2 segments), Heubner's arteries.
• **Veins:** Anterior aspect of the superior sagittal sinus.

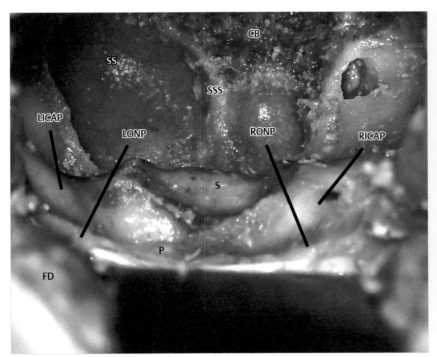

Fig. 29.5 After performing the ethmoidectomy and opening of the sphenoid sinus, the sellar floor, carotid, and optic protuberances come into view.
Abbreviations: CB = clival bone; FD = frontal dura; LICAP = left internal carotid artery prominence; LONP = left optic nerve prominence; P = planum; RICAP = right internal carotid artery prominence; RONP = right optic nerve prominence; S = sella; SS = sphenoid sinus; SSS = sphenoid sinus septum.

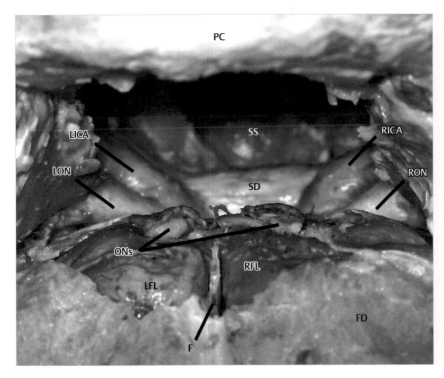

Fig. 29.6 Frontal dura is divided circumferentially exposing the olfactory bulbs and tracts and the frontal lobes.
Abbreviations: F = falx; FD = frontal dura; LFL = left frontal lobe; LICA = left internal carotid artery; LON = left optic nerve; ONs = olfactory nerves; PC = pericranium; RFL = right frontal lobe; RICA = right internal carotid artery; RON = right optic nerve; SD = sellar dura; SS = sphenoid sinus.

29.10 Reconstruction

- Dural defect is repaired by using a free pericranium patch sutured to the dural edges with a 6/0 prolene under microscopic magnification.
- The suture is sealed with fibrin glue.
- A wide pedicled frontal pericranial flap is harvested and then reflected along the anterior skull base. The flap is fixed with fibrin glue.
- Abdominal fat can be positioned to fill the dead space inside the pedicle pericranial flap.

- The anterior wall of the frontal sinus is repositioned and fixed with micro titanium screws and plates.
- A lumbar drain can be positioned if a watertight closure could not be obtained.

29.11 Pearls

- For small frontal sinuses, bone flap has to be extended beyond the limits of the sinus, including the external layer of the frontal vault, which is cut tangentially.

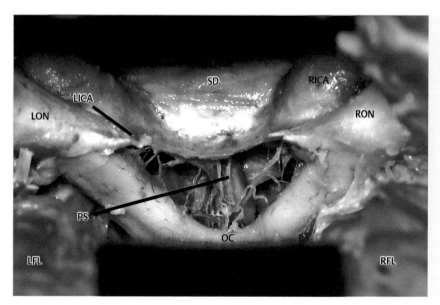

Fig. 29.7 By slight retraction of the frontal lobes, optic nerves, chiasm, and pituitary stalk come into view.
Abbreviations: LFL = left frontal lobe; LICA = left internal carotid artery; LON = left optic nerve; OC = optic chiasm; PS = pituitary stalk; RFL = right frontal lobe; RICA = right internal carotid artery; RON = right optic nerve; SD = sellar dura.

- Identification, coagulation and section of anterior and posterior ethmoidal arteries is crucial in obtaining an early devascularization of the tumor.
- Extensive drilling of the ethmoidal bone allows for an early tumor debulking from below, without any retraction on the frontal lobes; the tumor tends to collapse downward, pushed down by the re-expansion of the edematous frontal lobes.
- Dissection and removal of the posterior pole of the tumor has to be done very carefully in order to identify and preserve the anterior cerebral arteries (ACAs) with the anterior communicating artery (ACoA), that are usually covered by tumor.
- Meticulous multilayer dural reconstruction is crucial in order to avoid cerebrospinal fluid (CSF) leak through the nose.

References

1. Boari N, Gagliardi F, Roberti F, Barzaghi LR, Caputy AJ, Mortini P. The trans-frontal-sinus subcranial approach for removal of large olfactory groove meningiomas: surgical technique and comparison to other approaches. J Neurol Surg A Cent Eur Neurosurg 2013;74(3):152–161
2. Gagliardi F, Boari N, Mortini P. Reconstruction techniques in skull base surgery. J Craniofac Surg 2011;22(3):1015–1020
3. Hallacq P, Moreau JJ, Fischer G, Béziat JL. Trans-sinusal frontal approach for olfactory groove meningiomas. Skull Base 2001;11(1):35–46
4. Raveh J, Turk JB, Lädrach K, et al. Extended anterior subcranial approach for skull base tumors: long-term results. J Neurosurg 1995;82 (6):1002–1010

30 Transbasal and Extended Subfrontal Bilateral Approach

Harminder Singh, Mehdi Zeinalizadeh, Harley Brito da Silva, and Laligam N. Sekhar

30.1 Indications

- The transbasal approach is a transcranial extradural anterior approach to the midline anterior skull base, sellar region-suprasellar region, and clivus.
- It is considered the workhorse for removing a variety of benign and malignant tumors of the anterior skull base.
- Anterior skull base pathology extending intradurally can also be resected via this approach.
- Pathology: Chordomas, chondrosarcomas, meningiomas, craniopharyngiomas, sino-nasal malignancies with cranial extension.

30.2 Patient Positioning (Fig. 30.1)

- **Pre-positioning**: A spinal drain or a frontal ventriculostomy is inserted for brain relaxation.
- **Position**: The patient is positioned supine with the head fixed in a Mayfield head holder.
- **Head:** The head is translated up and slightly extended to allow the frontal lobes to fall away from the skull base.
- **The glabella** must be the highest point in the surgical field.

30.3 Skin Incision (Fig. 30.2)

- **Bifrontal curvilinear incision**
  - **Starting point:** Incision starts at the level of the zygoma.
  - **Course:** It runs behind the hairline, preferably 2 cm posterior to the proposed edge of the craniotomy, so that the skin incision does not overlie the bony opening.
  - **Ending point:** It ends at the contralateral zygoma.
- **Variations**
  - Bow shaped incision (yellow dotted line–**Fig. 30.2**)
  - Zig-zag incision (red dotted line–**Fig. 30.2**)

30.4 Soft Tissue Dissection

- **Myofascial level** (**Fig. 30.3**)
  - The scalp flap along with the pericranium is reflected inferiorly over the face.
  - The temporal fascia is sharply incised, and further dissection is carried inferiorly in an interfascial or subfascial plane to protect the branches of the facial nerve.

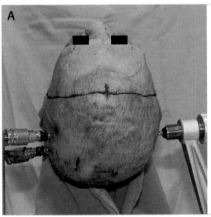
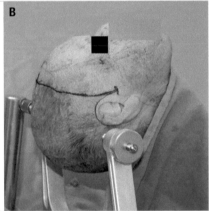

Fig. 30.1 **(A,B)** Patient head positioning in a Mayfield head-holder.

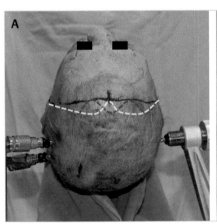
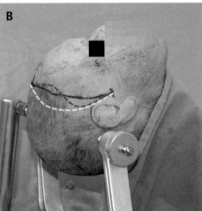

Fig. 30.2 **(A,B)** Variations in incision planning. Curvilinear incision (*black solid line*), bow-shaped incision (*yellow dotted line*), zig-zag incision (*red dotted line*).

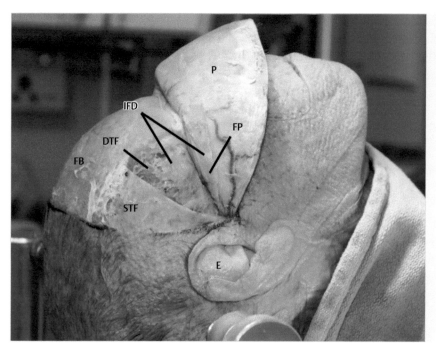

Fig. 30.3 Myofascial soft tissue dissection, with preservation of the branches of the facial nerve.
Abbreviations: DTF = deep temporal fascia; E = ear; FB = frontal bone; FP = fat pad; IFD = inter-fascial dissection; P = pericranium; STF = superficial temporal fascia.

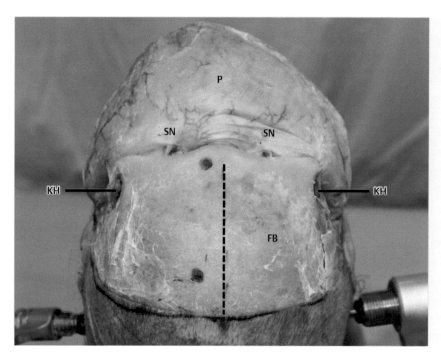

Fig. 30.4 Dissection of the supraorbital nerves, and craniotomy planning.
Abbreviations: FB = frontal bone; KH = keyhole; P = pericranium; SN = supraorbital nerve.

○ The branches of the facial nerve travel through the superficial fat pad, which lies in the plane between the superficial temporal fascia and the scalp.

○ The superficial temporal fascia and fat pad are reflected inferiorly together with the scalp.

○ The orbital rims are exposed bilaterally, and the supraorbital nerves are mobilized out of the supraorbital notches and reflected inferiorly with the scalp (**Fig. 30.4**).

○ The temporal muscle and fascia over the keyhole is sharply incised and pushed inferiorly to create space for placement of a burr hole.

30.4.1 Critical Structures

• Facial nerve branches.
• Supraorbital nerves.

30.5 Craniotomy

30.5.1 Bifrontal Craniotomy

• **Burr holes** (**Fig. 30.4**)
  ○ One over each keyhole.

○ One over the frontal sinus, slightly superior to the orbital rim and medial to the superior sagittal sinus (dotted line).

○ One anterior to the coronal suture in a parasagittal location.

• **Craniotomy**

○ A unifrontal craniotomy flap is turned using a craniotome (**Fig. 30.5**).

○ The dura over the superior sagittal sinus is stripped from the overlying bone using a Penfield under direct tangential view (**Fig. 30.5**).

○ The craniotomy is extended to the contralateral keyhole for a bi-frontal craniotomy (**Fig. 30.6**).

○ The edge of the craniotomy is kept at least 2 cm in front of

the skin incision to facilitate wound healing and reduce the incidence of infection.

• **Orbitofrontal osteotomy**

○ With spinal fluid drainage, the dura mater of the anterior fossa is dissected from the anterior cranial base bilaterally.

○ Similarly, the periorbit is dissected from the roof of the orbit.

○ Osteotomy cuts are made with a reciprocating saw near the nasofrontal suture to the crista galli, and through the roof of the orbits and laterally to the orbital rims (**Figs. 30.7,30.8**).

○ An alternate smaller orbitofrontal osteotomy cut is shown with red dotted lines (**Fig. 30.7**).

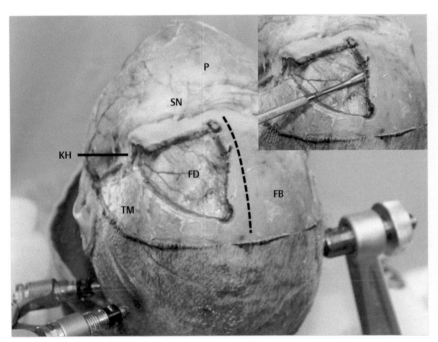

Fig. 30.5 Unifrontal craniotomy, with stripping of the superior sagittal sinus under tangential view (insert).
Abbreviations: FB = frontal bone; FD = frontal dura; KH = keyhole; P = pericranium; SN = supraorbital nerve; TM = temporal muscle.

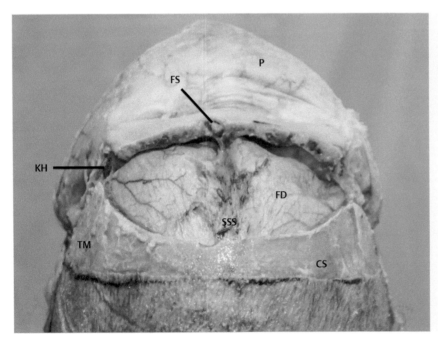

Fig. 30.6 Bifrontal craniotomy.
Abbreviations: CS = coronal suture; FD = frontal dura; FS = frontal sinus; KH = keyhole; P = pericranium; SSS = superior sagittal sinus; TM = temporal muscle.

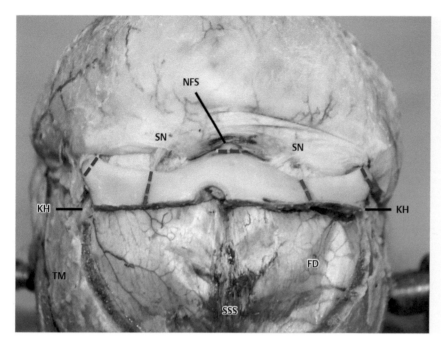

Fig. 30.7 Orbitofrontal osteotomy cuts (*blue dotted lines*). Alternate smaller orbitofrontal osteotomy cuts are shown with red dotted lines.
Abbreviations: FD = frontal dura; KH = keyhole; NFS = nasofrontal suture; SN = supraorbital nerve; SSS = superior sagittal sinus; TM = temporal muscle.

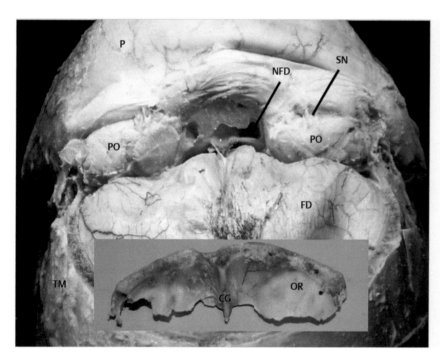

Fig. 30.8 Removal of the naso-orbital bar (insert).
Abbreviations: CG = crista galli; FD = frontal dura; NFD = nasofrontal duct; OR = orbital roof; P = pericranium; PO = periorbit; SN = supraorbital nerve; TM = temporal muscle.

30.5.2 Dural Opening

- Dura is opened on both sides of the superior sagittal sinus and draped over the periorbit (**Fig. 30.9**).
- The superior sagittal sinus is tied off using a stitch and divided near the skull base. It can then be reflected superiorly (**Fig. 30.10**).

Critical Structures

- Superior sagittal sinus.

30.6 Intradural/Extradural Exposure (Figs. 30.11, 30.15)

- **Parenchymal structures:** Bilateral frontal lobes, pituitary stalk.
- **Arachnoidal layer:** Optic-carotid cistern, lamina terminalis.
- **Cranial nerves:** Optic nerve, third cranial nerve.
- **Arteries:** Carotid, ophthalmic, hypophyseal, A1 segment of the anterior cerebral artery (ACA), anterior communicating artery (AcoA), M1 segment of the middle cerebral artery (MCA).
- **Veins:** Cavernous sinus, intercavernous sinus.

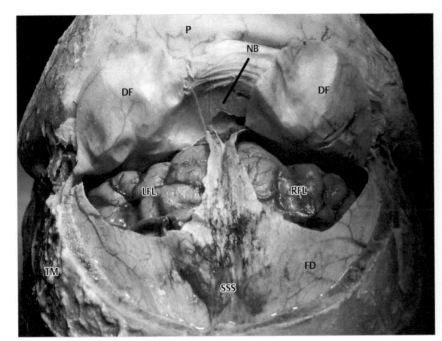

Fig. 30.9 Dural opening.
Abbreviations: DF = dural flap; FD = frontal dura; LFL = left frontal lobe; NB = nasal bones; P = pericranium; RFL = right frontal lobe; SSS = superior sagittal sinus; TM = temporal muscle.

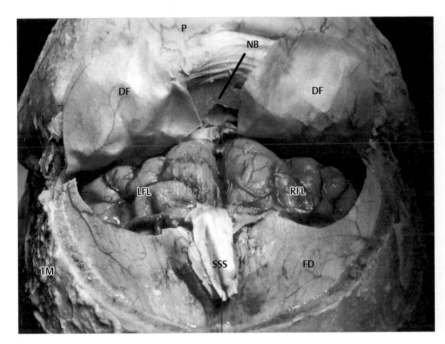

Fig. 30.10 The superior sagittal sinus is tied, cut, and reflected superiorly.
Abbreviations: DF = dural flap; FD = frontal dura; LFL = left frontal lobe; NB = nasal bones; P = pericranium; RFL = right frontal lobe; SSS = superior sagittal sinus; TM = temporal muscle.

30.7 Variations

- In an attempt to save olfaction, a dural sleeve can be cut around the olfactory nerves (**Figs. 30.11,30.13**).
- Once the bony osteotomy surrounding the dural sleeve is performed, the nasal septum and olfactory mucosa are divided and retracted up with the frontal dura. This preserves olfaction in many but not all patients.
- If the tumor invades into the cribriform plate, the osteotomy cut can be extended to the back of the cribriform plate, into the ethmoid (**Fig. 30.12**). Olfaction is thus sacrificed.
- **Fig. 30.14** illustrates the craniotomy, osteotomy and ethmoid resection cuts in a sagittal plane.

30.8 Exposure of Cavernous Sinus – Extradural (Figs. 30.15–30.17)

- After performing a sphenoidotomy and ethmoidectomy, the medial wall of the cavernous sinus can be exposed on either side.
- The medial wall of the cavernous sinus can be opened to expose the cavernous carotid siphon.
- The anterior intercavernous sinus can also be exposed. It travels between the folds of the diaphragma sellae and the sellar dural layer.

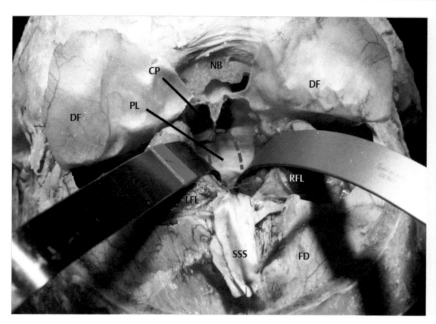

Fig. 30.11 Exposure of the cribriform plate and dura. A dural sleeve can be cut around the olfactory bulbs to preserve olfaction. Abbreviations: CP = cribriform plate; DF = dural flap; FD = frontal dura; LFL = left frontal lobe; NB = nasal bones; PL = planum; RFL = right frontal lobe; SSS = superior sagittal sinus.

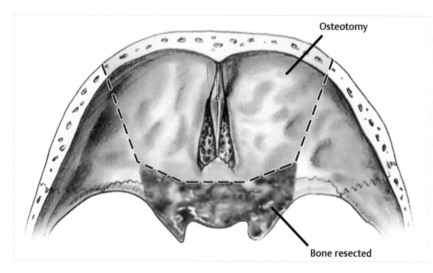

Fig. 30.12 Diagrammatic representation of osteotomy cuts. No olfactory preservation. (Reproduced from Sekhar LN, Fessler RG. Atlas of Neurosurgical Techniques: Brain. 2016. Thieme, New York).

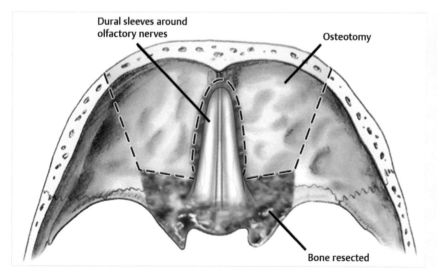

Fig. 30.13 Diagrammatic representation of osteotomy cuts. Potential olfactory preservation. (Reproduced from Sekhar LN, Fessler RG. Atlas of Neurosurgical Techniques: Brain. 2016. Thieme, New York).

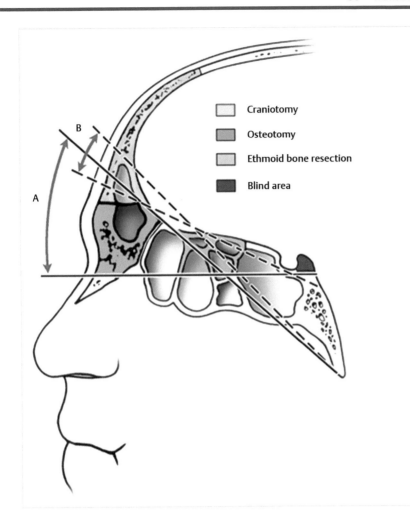

Fig. 30.14 Diagrammatic representation of craniotomy, osteotomy, and ethmoid resection cuts in a sagittal plane. A: extended subfrontal approach; B: craniotomy alone. (Reproduced from Sekhar LN, Fessler RG. Atlas of Neurosurgical Techniques: Brain. 2016. Thieme, New York.)

Craniotomy

Osteotomy

Ethmoid bone resection

Blind area

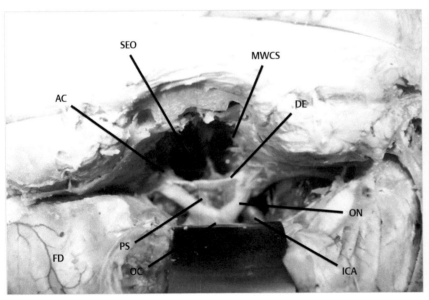

Fig. 30.15 Intradural and extradural exposure of anterior midline skull base. Abbreviations: AC = anterior clinoid; DE = dural edge; FD = frontal dura; ICA = internal carotid artery; MWCS = medial wall of the cavernous sinus; OC = optic chiasm; ON = optic nerve; PS = pituitary stalk; SEO = spheno-ethmoidal opening.

- The diaphragma sellae continues on laterally to become the distal dural ring (DDR), which marks the transition between the clinoid and ophthalmic segments of the internal carotid artery.

30.9 Pearls

- The brain must be very slack when doing this procedure extradurally. The senior author prefers a ventriculostomy over a lumbar drain, in addition to mannitol, furosemide, and hyperventilation.
- In patients older than 60 years, and those with hyperostosis frontalis interna, the dura may be very adherent to the bone, making the peeling of the dura and the superior sagittal sinus difficult.
- Olfactory preservation requires that all of the surrounding bone around the olfactory dural sleeve be carefully removed, and the olfactory mucosa be preserved.
- It has been described as an X-shaped approach: in order to view the contralateral side, one has to look from the ipsilateral orbit, which has been unroofed **(Figs. 30.16,30.17)**.

- Cavernous sinus bleeding can be readily controlled by fibrin glue injection.
- The cavernous internal carotid artery (ICA) is usually exposed readily in the anterior vertical and posterior vertical segments, and then followed into the petrous bone.
- The dura mater can be opened to remove intradural clival tumor; care must be exercised around the basilar artery and its branches, as well as the abducens nerves. Any clival dural defect can be repaired with a fascial graft.
- The dorsum sellae is a blind spot with this approach. However, lesions in this region can be pulled inferiorly, dissected from the dura, and removed.
- Laterally, the approach is limited by the petrous apices.
- Inferiorly, one can reach as low as the atlas (C1), but inferolaterally, the hypoglossal nerves are the limit.
- Reconstruction of the skull base takes place using the vascularized pericranial flap, and free fat graft **(Fig. 30.18)**.
- Enough orbital roof must be included in the osteotomy and preserved, in order to avoid enophthalmos.

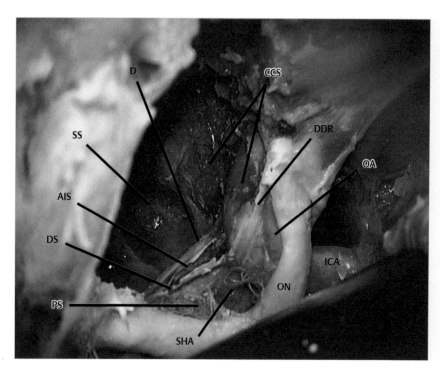

Fig. 30.16 Extradural exposure of the right cavernous sinus, as seen from the contralateral (left) side.
Abbreviations: AIS = anterior intercavernous sinus; CCS = cavernous carotid siphon; D = dura; DDR = distal dural ring; DS = diaphragma sellae; ICA = internal carotid artery; OA = ophthalmic artery; ON = optic nerve; PS = pituitary stalk; SHA = superior hypophiseal artery; SS = sphenoid sinus.

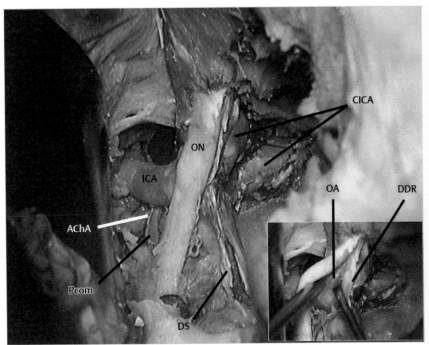

Fig. 30.17 Extradural exposure of the left cavernous sinus, as seen from the contralateral (right) side. Inset: Showing the ophthalmic artery and the distal dural ring. Abbreviations: AChA = anterior choroidal artery; CICA = cavernous carotid artery; DDR = distal dural ring; DS = diaphragma sellae; ICA = internal carotid artery; OA = ophthalmic artery; ON = optic nerve; Pcom = posterior communicating artery.

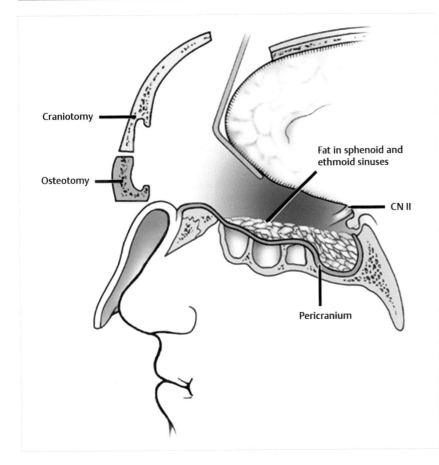

Fig. 30.18 Diagrammatic representation of skull base reconstruction with fat graft and pericranium. (Reproduced from Sekhar LN, Fessler RG. Atlas of Neurosurgical Techniques: Brain. 2016. Thieme, New York).

References

1. Chandler JP, Silva FE. Extended transbasal approach to skull base tumors. Technical nuances and review of the literature. Oncology (Williston Park) 2005;19(7):913–919, discussion 920, 923–925, 929

2. Ramakrishna R, Brito da Silva H, Ferreira M Jr, et al. Chordomas and chondrosarcomas. In: Sekhar LN, Fessler R, eds. Atlas of Neurosurgical Techniques, Brain. 2nd ed. New York, NY: Thieme Medical Publishers;2015

3. Sekhar LN, Nanda A, Sen CN, Snyderman CN, Janecka IP. The extended frontal approach to tumors of the anterior, middle, and posterior skull base. J Neurosurg 1992;76(2):198–206

4. Terasaka S, Day JD, Fukushima T. Extended transbasal approach: anatomy, technique, and indications. Skull Base Surg 1999;9(3):177–184

31 Trauma Flap and Osteo-Dural Decompression Techniques

Michele Bailo, Filippo Gagliardi, Alfio Spina, Cristian Gragnaniello, Anthony J. Caputy, and Pietro Mortini

31.1 Indications

- Acute subdural hematomas.
- Decompressive hemi-craniectomy for trauma or stroke with unilateral hemisphere swelling and midline shift.

31.2 Unilateral Craniectomy

31.2.1 Patient Positioning

- **Position**: Patient is positioned supine.
- **Head**: The head is flexed 10–15°, rotated 45° to the contralateral side (if no contraindications).
- In case of unstable cervical spine: hard collar has to be kept with ipsilateral shoulder roll; alternatively, the patient might be placed in the lateral position to keep neck in neutral position.
- Axillary roll is placed under the contralateral axilla.
- Ipsilateral shoulder is pulled down to maximize the opening between head and shoulder.

31.2.2 Skin Incision

- **Reverse question-mark incision** (**Fig. 31.1**)
  - **Starting point**: Incision starts at the zygomatic arch, < 1 cm anterior to the tragus.
  - **Run**: Incision line runs superiorly and then curves posteriorly at the level of top of the pinna till 4-8 cm behind the pinna, then it is taken superiorly. The incision resembles a "reverse question-mark" shape.
  - **Ending point**: It ends 1-2 cm lateral to the midline, behind the hairline.
  - In case of scalp lacerations, it is advisable to try to incorporate them into the incision. Seek for foreign bodies and excise contused skin edges in elliptical fashion.

Critical Structures

- Branch of the facial nerve to the frontalis muscle.
- Branches of the superficial temporal artery.

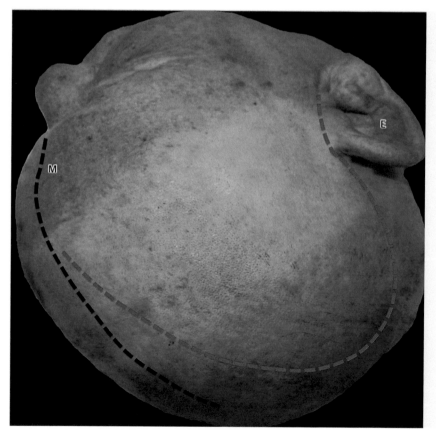

Fig. 31.1 Reverse question-mark skin incision.
Abbreviations: E = ear; M = midline.

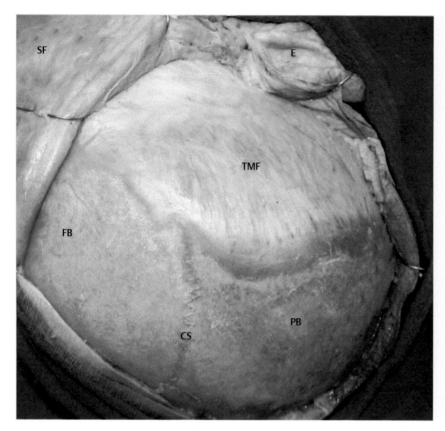

Fig. 31.2 Soft tissue dissection. Abbreviations: CS = coronal suture; E = ear; FB = frontal bone; PB = parietal bone; SF = superficial fascia; TMF = temporal muscle fascia.

31.2.3 Soft Tissues Dissection (Fig. 31.2)

- **Myofascial level**
  - Myofascial level is incised according to skin incision.
- **Muscles**
  - The periosteum and the temporal muscle are divided using monopolar electrocautery.
  - Using periosteal elevator and monopolar electrocautery, the scalp flap is detached along with the temporal muscle and reflected (as a single unit) antero-inferiorly.

Critical Structures

- Branch of the facial nerve to the frontalis muscle

31.2.4 Craniotomy/Craniectomy (Figs. 31.3, 31.4)

- **Burr holes**
  - **I**: The first burr hole is placed at the low temporal area (temporal squama), right above the zygomatic arch.
  - **II**: The second burr hole is made at the keyhole.
  - **III**: The third burr hole might be placed, as preferred, along the planned craniotomy route.
- **Craniotomy landmarks**
  - **Anterior**: Orbital rim.
  - **Lateral**: Zygomatic arch.
  - **Medial**: 1 cm from the midline, sagittal suture.
  - **Posterior**: Lambdoid suture.

Critical Structures

- Parenchymal, pial vessels or dural sinuses injury when elevating depressed fractures.
- Dural sinuses.

31.2.5 Dural Opening (Figs. 31.5, 31.6)

- "Cruciate/stellate" or in a C-shaped fashion.

Critical Structures

- Brain cortex.

31.2.6 Intradural Exposure (Fig. 31.7)

- **Parenchymal structures**: Lateral aspect of frontal, temporal and parietal lobes.
- **Arachnoidal layer**: Sylvian fissure.
- **Arteries**: Middle cerebral artery.
- **Veins**: Superficial Sylvian vein, superior and inferior anastomotic veins, cortical veins of the lateral surface.

31.3 Variants

31.3.1 Bilateral Frontal Craniectomy

- **Indications**: Bilateral brain swelling.
- Schematic representation in **Fig. 31.8**
- Full description in **Chapter 14.**

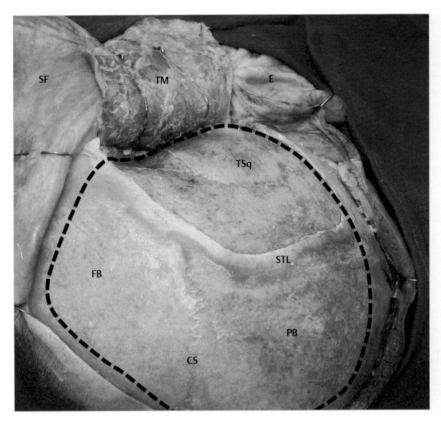

Fig. 31.3 Muscles dissection.
Abbreviations: CS = coronal suture; E = ear;
FB = frontal bone; PB = parietal bone;
SF = superficial fascia; STL = superior
temporal line; TM = temporal muscle;
TSq = temporal squama.

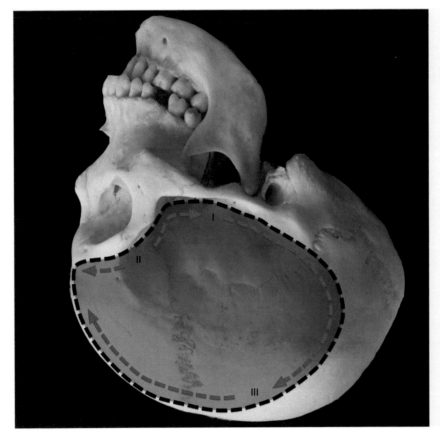

Fig. 31.4 Craniotomy.
Abbreviations: I = first burr holes; II = second
burr hole; III = third burr hole; red dotted
line (craniotomy cuts direction); purple
shape (craniectomy).

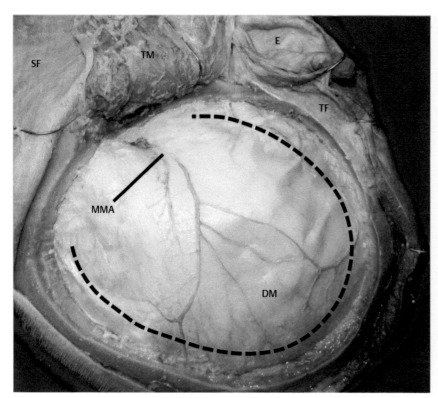

Fig. 31.5 Dural opening.
Abbreviations: DM = dura mater; E = ear;
MMA = middle meningeal artery;
SF = superficial fascia; TF = temporal fascia;
TM = temporal muscle.

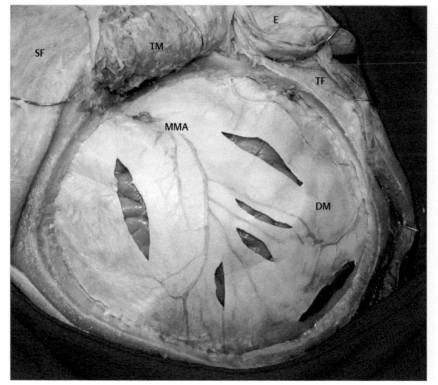

Fig. 31.6 Exploratory openings through the
dura mater.
Abbreviations: DM = dura mater; E = ear;
MMA = middle meningeal artery;
SF = superficial fascia; TF = temporal fascia;
TM = temporal muscle.

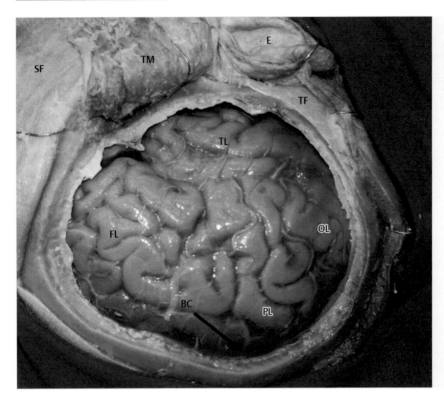

Fig. 31.7 Intradural exposure.
Abbreviations: BC = blood collection in the subdural space; E = ear; FL = frontal lobe; OC = occipital lobe; PL = parietal lobe; SF = superficial fascia; TF = temporal fascia; TL = temporal lobe; TM = temporal muscle.

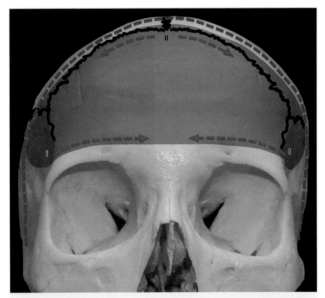

Fig. 31.8 Schematic picture resembling decompressing bifrontal craniectomy.
Abbreviations: I = first burr holes; II = second burr hole; blue dotted line (skin incision); red dotted line (craniotomy cuts direction); purple shape (craniectomy).

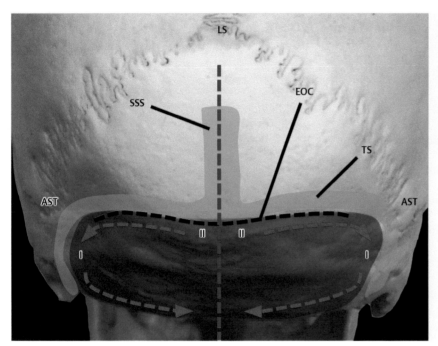

Fig. 31.9 Schematic picture resembling decompressive sub-occipital craniectomy. Abbreviations: AST = asterion; EOC = external occipital crest; LS = lambdoid suture; SSS = superior sagittal sinus; TS = transverse sinus; I = first burr holes; II = second burr holes; blue dotted line (skin incision); red dotted line (craniotomy cuts direction); purple shape (craniectomy).

31.3.2 Posterior Fossa Decompression

- **Indications**: Cerebellar swelling/hematoma.
- Schematic representation in **Fig. 31.9**
- Full description in **Chapter 25.**

References

1. Adewumi D, Colohan A. Decompressive craniectomy: surgical indications, clinical considerations and rationale. INTECH Open Access Publisher;2012

2. Connolly ES, McKhann GM, Huang J. Fundamentals of Operative Techniques in Neurosurgery. New York, NY: Thieme Medical Publishers;2011

3. Greenberg MS. Handbook of Neurosurgery. New York, NY: Thieme Medical Publishers;2010

4. Jandial R, McCormick P, Black PM. Core techniques in operative neurosurgery. Philadelphia, PA: Elsevier Health Sciences;2011

32 Surgical Anatomy of the Petrous Bone

Martina Piloni, Filippo Gagliardi, Cristian Gragnaniello, Anthony J. Caputy, and Pietro Mortini

32.1 Introduction

A comprehensive knowledge of the complex anatomy of the petrous bone and its relationships with surrounding regions (petroclival region, middle and posterior cranial fossa) is the mainstay for lateral skull base surgical approaches directed through the temporal bone. The petrous bone is a pyramid-shaped structure that lies between the sphenoidal and occipital bones, participating to the formation of the skull base.

- **Petrous pyramid includes the following parts:**
  - Base.
  - Apex.
  - Antero-superior surface.
  - Posterior surface.
  - Inferior surface.
  - Superior ridge.
  - Anterior border.
  - Postero-inferior border.
- **Critical anatomical structures of the petrous bone:**
  - Facial canal and nerve.
  - Osseous labyrinth of the inner ear (cochlea, vestibule and semicircular canals).
  - Petrous internal carotid artery.

32.2 Base of the Petrous Bone

- The base of the petrous pyramid continues in the mastoid process, a grossly triangular bony prominence projecting downward and located behind the external auditory canal in the outer surface of the temporal bone
- It gives attachment to the insertions of
  - Sternocleidomastoid muscle.

- Splenius capitis and longissimus capitis muscles.
- Posterior belly of the digastric muscle at the mastoid notch on its medial side.
- The occipital artery courses in a groove medially to the mastoid notch.
- The mastoid process is variably pneumatized.
  - The largest air-filled cell is the mastoid antrum and it communicates through the aditus ad antrum with the posterior part of the tympanic cavity of the middle ear at the epitympanic recess.
  - An important superficial landmark for the mastoid antrum is the suprameatal triangle (MacEwen's triangle), a depression delimited by
    - ❖ The postero-superior border of the external acoustic meatus (Henle's spine).
    - ❖ The supramastoid crest.
    - ❖ A tangential line to the external acoustic meatus joining the two **(Fig. 32.1).**
- The supramastoid crest is a bony ridge corresponding to the level of the middle fossa floor; it represents the inferior extension of the superior temporal line and continues anteriorly as the upper edge of the zygomatic arch.

32.3 Petrous Apex

- The apex of the petrous pyramid is directed antero-medially.
- It is wedged between the body and posterior border of the greater wing of the sphenoid bone and the basilar part of the occipital bone.
- It faces the intracranial end of the carotid canal.

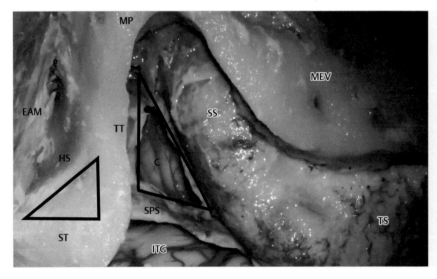

Fig. 32.1 Lateral view of the middle and posterior cranial fossa on the right side. A temporal craniotomy has been performed and drilling of the mastoid process allows to expose the sinodural angle and Trautmann's triangle. Access to the cerebellopontine angle is gained through dural opening in the presigmoid area; a supratentorial dural incision is made on the floor of the temporal fossa while preserving the superior petrosal sinus.
Abbreviations: C = cerebellum; EAM = external acoustic meatus; HS = Henle's spine; ITG = inferior temporal gyrus; MEV = mastoid emissary vein; MP = mastoid process; SPS = superior petrosal sinus; SS = sigmoid sinus; ST = suprameatal triangle; TS = transverse sinus; TT = Trautmann's triangle.

32.4 Antero-Superior Surface of the Petrous Bone

- It forms the posterior part of the floor of the middle cranial fossa.
- In the central part, the bulging of the arcuate eminence overlies the superior semicircular canal.
- Farther laterally, a thin osseous layer, the tegmen tympani, separates the middle cranial fossa from the underlying tympanic cavity.
- The trigeminal impression represents a shallow depression near the apex where the semilunar ganglion sits in Meckel's cave.
- The greater superficial petrosal nerve (GSPN) courses postero-laterally to the trigeminal impression until it reaches the facial hiatus, the opening through which the nerve leaves the geniculate ganglion.
- A smaller canal anterolateral to the facial hiatus occasionally provides passage to the lesser petrosal nerve (LPN).
- The GSPN joins the sympathetic fibers coming from the carotid plexus (deep petrosal nerve) to form the vidian nerve that passes forward in the vidian canal through the root of the pterygoid process.
- The greater and lesser petrosal nerves run parallel beneath the dura of the middle fossa in the spheno-petrosal groove, immediately superior and lateral to the horizontal segment of the petrous internal carotid artery (ICA).
- The anterior surface of the petrous ICA is separated by a thin osseous lamina from the tensor tympani muscle and the Eustachian tube.
- The position of the cochlea below the middle fossa floor can be approximated by the angle between the GSPN and the labyrinthine segment of the facial nerve.
- On the petrous surface, the cochlea corresponds to the lateral apex of Kawase's triangle, which is delimited by the GSPN, the lateral border of the third division of the trigeminal nerve (V3) and a line connecting the facial hiatus to Meckel's cave.
- The cochlea lies medially to the geniculate ganglion, anteriorly to the internal acoustic meatus (IAC) and postero-superiorly to the genu of the petrous internal carotid artery.

32.5 Posterior Surface of the Petrous Bone

- It delimitates the anterior wall of the posterior cranial fossa.
- The internal acoustic meatus is located in the central part and transmits the facial, cochlear and vestibular nerves (**Fig. 32.2**).
- Superolaterally, the subarcuate fossa divides the internal acoustic meatus by the vestibular aqueduct, which connects the vestibule to the endolymphatic sac located beneath the dura.
- The anteromedial part of the jugular foramen is delimited by the lower edge of the posterior surface of the petrous bone, and it receives the venous drainage of the inferior petrosal sinus descending through the petroclival fissure; the postero-lateral border corresponds to the notch on the jugular process of the occipital bone and receives the sigmoid sinus directed at the jugular bulb after coursing down the sulcus grooved on the intracranial surface of the mastoid process.
- One or more emissary veins to the sigmoid sinus perforate the posterior border of the mastoid process.
- Glossopharyngeal, vagus and accessory nerves traverse the jugular foramen through the intrajugular compartment (**Fig. 32.2**).

32.6 Inferior Surface of the Petrous Bone

- It is exocranial and joins the clivus through the interposition of fibrocartilaginous tissue.
- Near the apex, an irregular surface gives attachment to the levator veli palatini and to the cartilaginous portion of the Eustachian tube.
- Behind the external end of the carotid canal, the jugular fossa lodges the superior bulb of the internal jugular vein.
- On the lateral edge of the jugular foramen, the mastoid canaliculus transmits the auricular branch of the vagus nerve.
- The ridge between the carotid canal opening and the jugular foramen presents the cochlear canaliculus, which provides

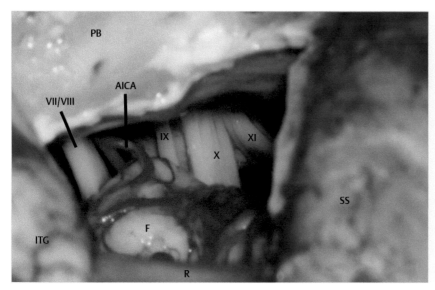

Fig. 32.2 Microsurgical view of the right cerebellopontine angle through the presigmoid area. The petrosal surface of the cerebellum is retracted backward. Abbreviations: AICA = anterior inferior cerebellar artery; F = flocculus; ITG = inferior temporal gyrus; PB = petrous bone; SS = sigmoid sinus; R = retractor; VII/VIII = facial and vestibulocochlear complex; IX = glossopharyngeal nerve; X = vagus nerve; XI = accessory nerve.

a communication between the perilymphatic and subarachnoid space, and the small foramen for the tympanic branch of the glossopharyngeal nerve.

- On the lateral side of the inferior petrous surface, the stylomastoid foramen is situated between the styloid and mastoid processes and represents the external opening of the facial canal.

32.7 Superior Ridge

- It is grooved by the superior petrosal sinus, which runs into the sulcus where the tentorial margin attaches.

32.8 Anterior Border

- It joins medially the greater wing of the sphenoid bone delimitating the foramen lacerum and laterally the temporal squama at the petro-squamosal suture.

32.9 Postero-Inferior Border

- It is articulated with the occipital bone along the petroclival fissure, where the inferior petrosal sinus courses.

32.10 Facial Canal

- The intratemporal course of the facial nerve can be divided into four segments: intrameatal, labyrinthine, tympanic, and mastoid.
  - The intrameatal part enters the internal acoustic meatus and passes through the anterosuperior compartment of the fundus. At this level, it is separated from the cochlear nerve by the transverse crest, while the Bill's bar (or vertical crest) divides the facial canal from the superior vestibular area (**Fig. 32.3**).
  - The labyrinthine segment runs from the meatal fundus to the genu, where the geniculate ganglion sits; it is related to the cochlea antero-medially and the vestibular labyrinth

postero-laterally. The superior semicircular canal lies parallel a few millimeters behind.
  - At the geniculate ganglion, the facial nerve gives rise to the GSPN and then turns posteriorly and laterally along the medial wall of the tympanic cavity, where it courses between the lateral semicircular canal and the oval window. The deep location of the tympanic segment is overlaid on the surface by Henle's spine (postero-superior margin of the external acoustic meatus) (**Fig. 32.432.5**).
  - At the level of the stapes, the facial nerve turns downward and descends vertically through the mastoid process until it reaches the stylomastoid foramen (**Figs. 32.6,32.7**).

32.11 Bony Labyrinth

- The auditory and vestibular labyrinths consist of hollow cavities within the petrous part of the temporal bone.
- These are surrounded by a dense bony shell, the otic capsule, that can be easily distinguished compared to the pneumatized petrous apex and mastoid process.
- These cavities contain the sensory organs of the inner ear for acoustic and vestibular functions.
- The osseous labyrinth can be divided into three sections: vestibule, cochlea, and three semicircular canals.
- The bony labyrinth is located medial to the tympanic cavity and above the jugular bulb (**Figs. 32.4,32.5**)
- The opening of the internal acoustic meatus on the posterior surface of the petrous bone allows entry to the cochlea antero-medially and the vestibule postero-laterally.

32.12 Petrosal Segment of the Internal Carotid Artery

- The ICA enters its canal in the petrous part of the temporal bone at the outer surface of the skull base, anterior and medial to the jugular foramen.
- It ascends vertically and, at the genu, it turns antero-medially in the horizontal portion directed toward the petrous apex.

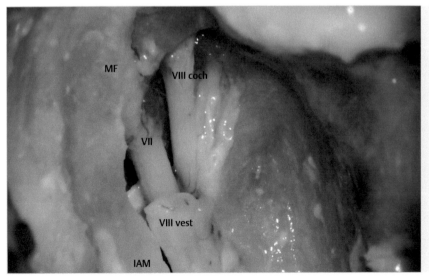

Fig. 32.3 Enlarged view of the nervous bundle of the acoustic-facial complex within the internal acoustic meatus after removal of the posterior wall and dural opening. The vestibular nerve has been sectioned to expose facial and cochlear nerves. Abbreviations: IAM = internal acoustic meatus; MF = meatal fundus; VII = facial nerve; VIII coch = cochlear nerve, VIII vest = vestibular nerve.

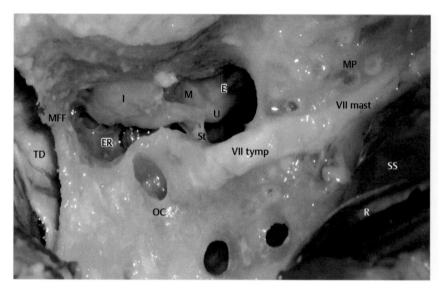

Fig. 32.4 Complete mastoidectomy with exposure of mastoidal and tympanic segments of the facial nerve and the otic capsule. The middle ear cavity is entered through the aditus ad antrum in the epitympanic recess, showing the auditory ossicles.
Abbreviations: E = eardrum; ER = epitympanic recess; I = incus; M = handle of malleus; MFF = middle fossa floor; MP = mastoid process; OC = otic capsule; R = retractor; SS = sigmoid sinus; St = stapes; TD = temporal dura; U = umbo; VII mast = mastoid segment of the facial nerve; VII tymp = tympanic segment of the facial nerve.

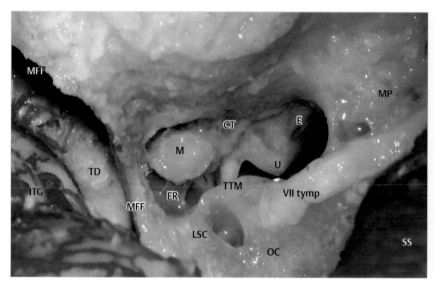

Fig. 32.5 Middle ear cavity (the incus has been removed). The chorda tympani cross the malleus at the level of the neck; the tip of the malleolar handle adheres to the inner surface of the tympanic membrane, while the upper part is the site of attachment of the tendon of the tensor tympani muscle.
Abbreviations: CT = chorda tympani; E = eardrum; ER = epitympanic recess; ITG = inferior temporal gyrus; LSC = lateral semicircular canal; M = head of the malleus; MFF = middle fossa floor; MP = mastoid process; OC = otic capsule; SS = sigmoid sinus; TD = temporal dura; TTM = tendon of the tensor tympani muscle; U = umbo; VII tymp = tympanic segment of the facial nerve.

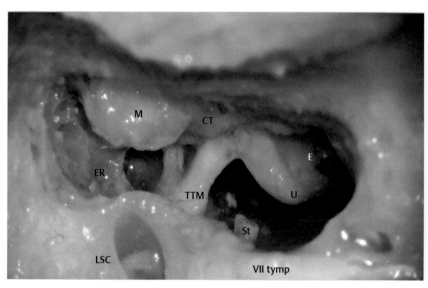

Fig. 32.6 Detailed view of the tympanic cavity (the incus has been removed).
Abbreviations: CT = chorda tympani; E = eardrum; ER = epitympanic recess; LSC = lateral semicircular canal; M = head of the malleus; St = head of the stapes; TTM = tendon of the tensor tympani muscle; U = umbo; VII tymp = tympanic segment of the facial nerve.

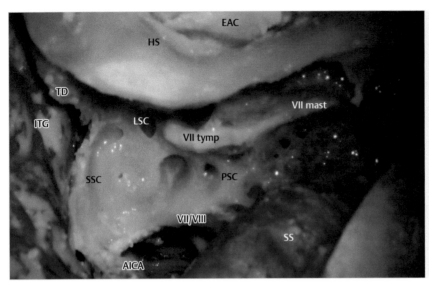

Fig. 32.7 Labyrinthectomy. The deep position of tympanic segment of the facial nerve and lateral semicircular canal is approximated by Henle's spine. The upper end of the posterior semicircular canal merges with the posterior end of the superior semicircular canal in the common crus, which opens in the bony vestibule and is located medially to the tympanic cavity.
Abbreviations: AICA = anterior inferior cerebellar artery; EAC = external acoustic canal; HS = Henle's spine; ITG = inferior temporal gyrus; LSC = lateral semicircular canal; PSC = posterior semicircular canal; SS = sigmoid sinus; SSC = superior semicircular canal; TD = temporal dura; VII mast = mastoid segment of the facial nerve; VII tymp = tympanic segment of the facial nerve; VII/VIII = facial and vestibulocochlear complex.

- The ascending segment of the petrous ICA is separated by a thin osseous layer from the anterior wall of the tympanic cavity. At the genu, the cochlea is situated posterior and superior to the ICA.
- The GSPN courses parallel to the lateral aspect of the horizontal segment of the petrous ICA, posteriorly to the third division of the trigeminal nerve.
- Deeper within the temporal bone, the tensor tympani muscle and the osseous portion of Eustachian tube lie along the anterior surface of the horizontal segment.
- The intracranial end of the petrosal carotid artery can be recognized as it passes above the foramen lacerum, a bone defect obliterated by thick fibrocartilaginous tissue, to continue toward the cavernous sinus at the lateral surface of the sphenoid body.
- The main collateral branches arising from the petrous ICA are the vidian and the caroticotympanic arteries. The first one passes antero-inferiorly through the foramen lacerum and crosses the pterygoid canal; the latter one reaches the tympanic cavity.

32.13 Surgical Considerations

The surgical corridors running through the superior and posterior surfaces of the petrous pyramid provide a panoramic view of middle cranial fossa, cerebellopontine angle (CPA), and petroclival region.

32.13.1 Antero-Superior Surface of the Petrous Bone

- The bony surfaces of temporal fossa, mastoid process and posterior fossa are exposed after elevation of the skin flap; the temporal muscle in retracted antero-inferiorly, while sternocleidomastoid muscle insertion on the mastoid process is detached and retracted postero-inferiorly.
- The asterion is a fundamental craniometric point at the lateral view of the skull. It is defined by the junction of the lambdoid, occipitomastoid, and parietomastoid sutures and corresponds to the meeting point of the transverse and sigmoid sinuses.
- The floor of the middle cranial fossa is exposed performing a temporal craniotomy.

- The temporal lobe is carefully retracted and dura mater is elevated, exposing the middle meningeal artery as it enters the cranial cavity through the foramen spinosum of the sphenoid bone.
- Antero-medially to the foramen spinosum, the mandibular nerve (V3) enters the foramen ovale.
- A further posterior extradural exposure of the superior aspect of the petrous bone allows identity of the GSPN, which can be followed backward to its exit through the hiatus fallopii, and the arcuate eminence harboring the superior semicircular canal.
- The middle portion of the angle delimitated by the GSPN and the arcuate eminence helps to identify the deep position of the internal acoustic canal.
- The geniculate ganglion and the petrous segment of the internal carotid artery may not be covered by the bone of the floor of the middle cranial fossa.
- Bone removal at the level of the tegmen tympani opens the roof of the tympanic cavity and exposes the head of the incus in the epitympanic recess (**Figs. 32.4–32.6**).
- The posterior fossa can be reached by splitting the tentorium behind the point where the trochlear nerve pierces the free tentorial edge.
- An anterior petrosectomy provides a wider exposure of the lateral side of the clival region by additional bone removing between the porus acusticus and trigeminal roots entrance in Meckel's cave.

32.13.2 Base and Posterior Surface of the Petrous Bone

- The suboccipital extension of the temporal craniotomy and a complete mastoidectomy allow exposure of the supra- and infratentorial compartments.
- The anatomical limits of the mastoid drilling are the mastoid tip inferiorly, the asterion posteriorly, and Henle's spine anteriorly.
- The transverse-sigmoid junction is skeletonized in correspondence of the asterion and the sigmoid sinus is followed down to the roof of the jugular bulb (**Fig. 32.1**).
- The sinodural angle (Citelli's angle) is used as a landmark for the position of the superior petrosal sinus draining in the sigmoid sinus (**Fig. 32.1**).

- The mastoid air-cells behind the posterior wall of the external acoustic canal are resected until the mastoid antrum is
identified.
- Medially to the antrum, the compact bone that encloses
the otic capsule can be easily recognized and the mastoid
segment of the facial nerve can be followed toward the stylomastoid foramen, where it exits (**Figs. 32.5,32.7**).
- The digastric ridge represents an important landmark for the
initial extracranial course of the facial nerve.
- In the presigmoid area, the dura mater of the posterior fossa
is exposed as described by the Trautmann's triangle; this triangular dural patch gives access to the pontocerebellar angle
and is bounded anteriorly by the posterior semicircular canal
of the vestibular labyrinth, posteriorly by Citelli's sinodural

angle and superior petrosal sinus, and inferiorly by the jugular bulb (**Figs. 32.1,32.2**).
- Drilling of the petrous bone can continue performing a
translabyrinthine or transcochlear approach, depending on
lesion location or whether a wider surgical access is required.
- The labyrinthectomy consists in the removal of the posteri-
or and lateral semicircular canals and vestibule to gain the
exposure of the internal acoustic meatus and fundus (**Figs.
32.3,32.8.32.10**).
- The lateral semicircular canal is medial to the epitympanic
recess of the middle ear cavity and marks the tympanic segment of the facial nerve.
- The extension of the drilling antero-medially to the fundus of
the internal meatus through the cochlea defines the transco-

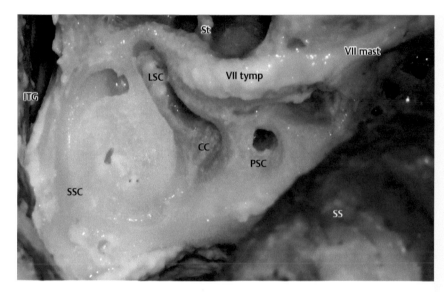

Fig. 32.8 Enlarged view of the bony labyrinth and of the course of facial nerve. The tympanic segment of the facial nerve courses between the lateral semicircular canal and the stapes in the oval window. The facial nerve eventually turns downward as the mastoid segment toward the stylomastoid foramen. The superior semicircular canal bulges upward in the floor of the middle cranial fossa corresponding to the superior surface of the petrous bone. The lateral semicircular canal is located postero-medially to the epitympanic area, and the posterior semicircular canal is situated laterally to the posterior wall of the internal acoustic meatus. Abbreviations: CC = common crus; ITG = inferior temporal gyrus; LSC = lateral semicircular canal; PSC = posterior semicircular canal; SS = sigmoid sinus; SSC = superior semicircular canal; St = stapes; VII mast = mastoid segment of the facial nerve; VII tymp = tympanic segment of the facial nerve.

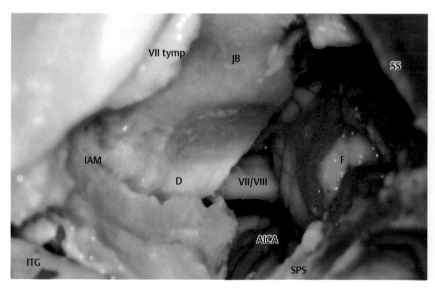

Fig. 32.9 Removal by drilling of the petrous bone through the vestibular labyrinth and exposure of the dura mater lining the posterior wall of the internal acoustic meatus.
Abbreviations: AICA = anterior inferior cerebellar artery; D = dura mater; F = flocculus; IAM = internal acoustic meatus; ITG = inferior temporal gyrus; JB = jugular bulb seen through the bone; SPS = superior petrosal sinus; SS = sigmoid sinus; VII/VIII = facial and vestibulocochlear complex; VII tymp = tympanic segment of the facial nerve.

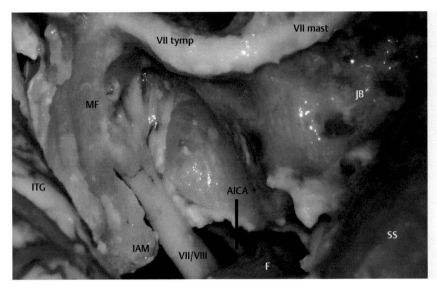

Fig. 32.10 Dural opening within the internal acoustic canal.
Abbreviations: AICA = anterior inferior cerebellar artery; F = flocculus; IAM = internal acoustic meatus; ITG = inferior temporal gyrus; JB = jugular bulb seen through the bone; MF = meatal fundus; SS = sigmoid sinus; VII/VIII = facial and vestibulocochlear complex; VII mast = mastoid segment of the facial nerve; VII tymp = tympanic segment of the facial nerve.

chlear approach and allows widening the exposure of the petroclival region.

References

1. Alonso F, Dekker SE, Wright J, et al. The retrolabyrinthine presigmoid approach to the anterior cerebellopontine region: expanding the limits of Trautmann triangle. World Neurosurg 2017;104:180–185

2. Rhoton AL. The Temporal Bone and Transtemporal Approaches. Cranial anatomy and surgical approaches.Neurosurgery. Rhoton's anatomy. Part 3. 2003:643–697

3. Troude L Jr, Carissimi M Jr, Lavieille JP, Roche PH. How I do it: the combined petrosectomy. Acta Neurochir (Wien) 2016;158(4):711–715

4. Luo Z, Zhao P, Yang K, Liu Y, Zhang Y, Liu H. The microsurgical anatomy of the modified presigmoid trans-partial bony labyrinth approach. J Craniofac Surg 2015;26(5):1619–1623

Part IV
Transpetrosal Approaches

IV

33 Anterior Petrosectomy

Mohammad Abolfotoh and Khaled El-Bahy

33.1 Introduction

Anterior petrosectomy, which means drilling the apex, is the surgical approach that is defined by the removal of the petrous part of temporal bone to facilitate the exposure of the posterior cranial fossa primarily through any of the middle cranial fossa approaches. It may be done after removal of the zygomatic arch, following either a pterional (fronto-temporal), zygomatic, cranio-orbito-zygomatic approach, or through temporal and subtemporal approaches (**see Chapters 15, 17, 19, 20, 21 respectively**); however, these approaches require significant temporal lobe retraction and give limited access to lower brainstem.

33.2 Patient Positioning (Fig. 33.1)

- **Position:** The patient is positioned supine.
- **Body:** The trunk is elevated 20° from horizontal.
- **Head:** The head is extended and rotated 30° to the contralateral side, then fixed to three point Mayfield fixator. The head should not be over-extended or over-turned to avoid stretching the neck and losing the corridor to the petrous apex.

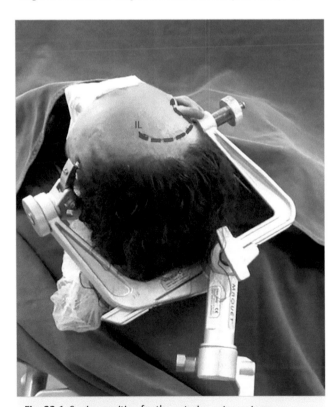

Fig. 33.1 Supine position for the anterior petrosectomy approach. The chest is elevated, the head is rotated to the other side and fixed by 3 pins head clamp.
Abbreviations: IL = incision line.

- The ipsilateral shoulder should be elevated on a roll to avoid stretch of neck veins.
- The aim is to keep the zygoma at the highest point in the patient head and almost horizontal, and middle fossa floor should be almost vertical.

33.3 Skin Incision (Figs. 33.1, 33.2)

Skin incision depends on the craniotomy.
- **Curvilinear skin incision for zygomatic, cranio-orbito-zygomatic, and pterional approaches**.
  - **Starting point:** Incision starts 5 mm just in front of the tragus. Care should be taken to avoid injuring facial nerve branches and the tragus. The way to extend this point down (not routinely needed) is to extend it very superficially in the skin in front of the ear lobule then up to turn around the mandibular angle then down again in the transverse crease of the neck.
  - **Course:** Incision runs upward just behind the hairline.
  - **Ending point:** Incision line ends on the midline behind the hairline; it could be extended beyond the midline to facilitate retraction of the skin flap to the anterior cranial base (if needed).
- **Variants:** Other skin incisions such a straight temporal skin incision for temporal craniotomy or inverted U-shaped incision around ear pinna for subtemporal approach.

33.3.1 Critical Structures

- Superficial temporal artery should be preserved to avoid wound bleeding during surgery, also for better blood supply to the flap *(and may be the muscle)*, and for external-internal carotid (EC-IC) bypass (**see Chapter 48**).

33.4 Soft Tissues Dissection

Soft tissue dissection techniques are already described in **Chapters 15 and 17.**

33.5 Craniotomy/Middle Fossa (Zygomatic) Approach (Fig. 33.2)

- **Zygomatic osteotomy**
  - Zygomatic arch is freed from the deep fascia at its upper edge and kept attached to the masseter muscle at its lower edge. Alternatively, it can be completely freed from muscle insertions and removed.
  - Two V-shaped osteotomies are done on the zygoma. The anterior cut should be placed just behind the malar eminence, while the posterior cut is made just in front of the posterior root of the zygoma. The osteotomy has to be shaped as a "V," in order facilitate further reconstruction.

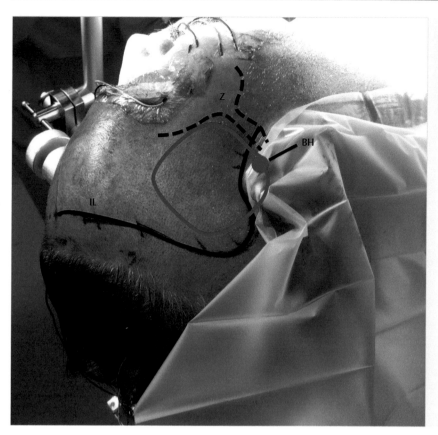

Fig. 33.2 Zygomatic arch (*black dots*), temporal craniotomy (*blue line*), the main burr hole (*blue dot*), at the posterior temporal bone, above the posterior root of the zygomatic arch.
Abbreviations: BH = burr hole; IL = incision line; Z = zygoma.

○ At this point the temporal muscle together with the zygomatic arch can be retracted downward through the zygomatic arch defect.

○ Zygomatic osteotomy gives excellent exposure flush to the middle cranial base and avoids the need for temporal lobe retraction.

• **Temporal craniotomy**
  ○ Single burr hole:
    - The main burr hole in this approach is a posterior basal temporal burr hole.
    - It is placed just above the root of the zygoma.
    - A second burr hole might be placed at the keyhole if frontal or orbital extension is needed (cranio-orbito-zygomatic extension).
  ○ **Cut:** The temporal craniotomy might be performed by a craniotome (cranio-zygomatic approach). It is tailored according to the pathology.
  ○ As mentioned above, the zygoma might be removed separately, or kept attached to the masseter muscle or the cranial flap.

33.6 Middle Fossa Dissection

33.6.1 Identification of the Greater Superficial Petrosal Nerve (GSPN)

• The middle meningeal artery has to be identified on the dural surface at foramen spinosum. Once identified, the artery has to be obliterated and coagulated (**Fig. 33.3**).
  ○ **TIP:** Leaving a few millimeters stump of the artery at the foramen spinosum enables the surgeon to use it as a landmark for surgical orientation.

• The mandibular nerve (V3) might be identified anteriorly and medially to the foramen spinosum, at its entrance into the foramen ovale.

• Close to V3 the greater superficial petrosal nerve (GSPN) might be found. It has to be highlighted that GSPN runs in a shallow bony groove, and that it is accompanied by the lesser petrosal nerve and a blood vessel (the petrosal branch of the middle meningeal artery). Many surgeons find this very tiny blood vessel helpful as a marker of the GSPN (**Fig. 33.4**).
  ○ **TIP:** In this region of the middle fossa floor fibrous bundles of dura are usually encountered, which might be easily mistaken as the GSPN (**Fig. 33.5**).

• The GSPN must be followed backward toward the facial hiatus. In 16% of cases the genu of the facial nerve is protruding from the facial hiatus.
  ○ **TIP:** The separation of the dura at the middle fossa floor in this area should start from posterior to anterior to avoid damaging the nerve.

• Traction on GSPN should be avoided as it might cause facial nerve palsy.

• GSPN division is not recommended as in most cases there is no need for that; nerve division might cause eye dryness, because of the damage on preganglionic parasympathetic fibers to the pterygopalatine ganglion. Moreover, nerve preservation is important, given the GSPN is considered a landmark for the horizontal part of the internal carotid artery (ICA) and the petrous apex.

33.6.2 Identification of the ICA

• One of the most important reasons to identify and preserve the GSPN is to identify the petrous carotid artery. The horizontal part of the petrous ICA runs in the bony petrous canal,

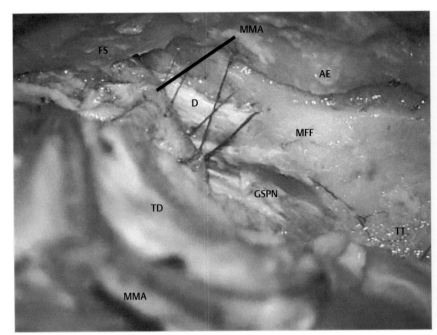

Fig. 33.3 Microscopic middle fossa dissection and anterior petrosectomy. Extradural image showing the middle meningeal artery branches running above the temporal dura, toward foramen spinosum. Abbreviations: AE = arcuate eminence; D = dural fold; FS = foramen spinosum; GSPN = greater superficial petrosal nerve; MFF = middle fossa floor; MMA = middle meningeal artery; TD = temporal dura; TT = tegmen tympani.

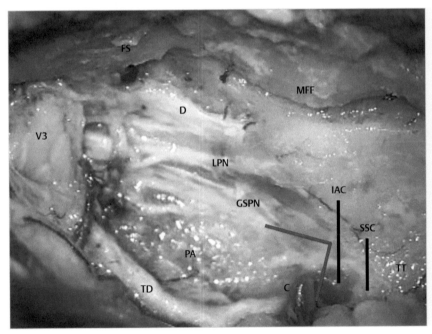

Fig. 33.4 Middle fossa view after cutting the artery and dissecting the middle fossa dura. The superior semicircular canal is located under the arcuate eminence right behind the IAC. Note the cochlear angle (red lines) is found between the greater superficial petrosal nerve and the fundus of the internal auditory meatus.
Abbreviations: C = cochlea; D = dural fold; FS = foramen spinosum; GSPN = greater superficial petrosal nerve; IAC = internal acoustic canal; LPN = lesser petrosal nerve; MFF = middle fossa floor; PA = petrous apex; SSC = superior semicircular canal; TD = temporal dura; TT = tegmen tympani; V3 = third trigeminal branch.

which is located roughly parallel and just below the nerve in the foramen lacerum (**Fig. 33.6**).

○ **TIP:** It must always be kept in mind that the GSPN and the sympathetic plexus surrounding the ICA (deep petrosal nerve) do join each other, giving rise to the vidian nerve.

- The way to find the horizontal petrous ICA is to identify its distal end, underneath the petro-lingual ligament, where the artery exits the petrous canal.
- A gentle elevation of V3 might help to find the ICA, which can be followed backward into the petrous canal.
- In 40% of cases the roof of the petrous canal is dehiscent under the GSPN; in these cases, the identification of ICA is easier, although more risky.
- Opening the roof of the petrous canal with right-angled micro-dissectors and curettes is a crucial step to improve

vascular control during cavernous sinus surgery, however it's not routinely done for this approach.

- After the identification of the GSPN and the ICA, the petrous apex can be drilled, if needed, at Kawase's triangle.

33.6.3 Identification of the Petrous Apex Part to Be Drilled (Figs. 33.4, 33.5)

- The petrous apex is the part of the petrous bone extending from the internal auditory canal (IAC) to the petroclival suture. The tip of the petrous apex is hidden under the trigeminal ganglion, and, in most cases, the anterior limit for the drilling corresponds to the trigeminal impression just supero-lateral to the suture.

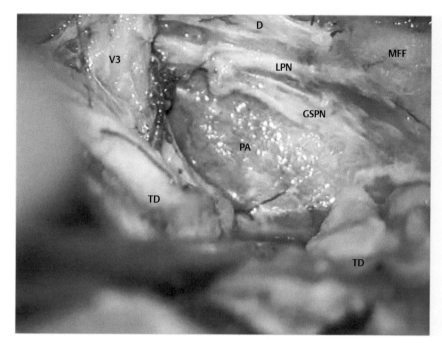

Fig. 33.5 Landmarks of the petrous apex (Kawase's triangle). Abbreviations: D = dural fold; GSPN = greater superficial petrosal nerve; LPN = lesser petrosal nerve; MFF = middle fossa floor; PA = petrous apex; TD = temporal dura; V3 = third trigeminal branch.

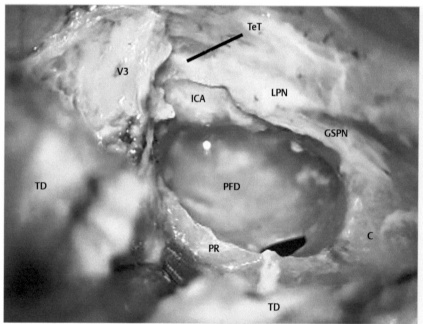

Fig. 33.6 The petrous apex is drilled out with the preservation of the cochlea, and the petrous ridge. Note that the petrous ICA runs parallel and below the GSPN. Two more structures are parallel to the ICA, the tensor tympani above and the Eustachian tube below (not shown). The posterior fossa dura is the medial limit for drilling, and IAC is the posterior limit for drilling. Abbreviations: C = cochlea; GSPN = greater superficial petrosal nerve; ICA = internal carotid artery; LPN = lesser petrosal nerve; PFD = posterior fossa dura; PR = petrous ridge; TD = temporal dura; TeT = tensor tympani; V3 = third trigeminal branch.

- To widen the surgical window, the trigeminal nerve root can be gently elevated. This maneuver enables one to extend the drilling antero-medially, all the way to the clival edge. While performing anterior petrosectomy, care should be taken to avoid the injury of the abducens nerve at the Dorello's canal.
  - TIP: If it is necessary to drill the trigeminal impression, drilling should be directed downward and backward as much as possible, to reduce the risk of damage of the abducens nerve.
    - The abducens nerve runs through the upper end of the superior petrosal sinus and enters the Dorello's canal under the Gruber's (petro-sphenoidal) ligament. The nerve can be found behind and parallel to the first branch of the trigeminal nerve (V1).
    - The posterior limit of drilling is the IAC and the cochlea, to preserve the auditory function.
    - The lateral limit of drilling corresponds to the carotid canal with the GSPN above it.

33.6.4 Identification of the Internal Carotid Artery and Cochlea (Figs. 33.4–33.6)

- Intra-operative navigation might be used to precisely identify the IAC, the cochlea, and the petrous canal; however, it is mandatory for a surgeon to know how to identify the anatomical structures underlying the superior surface of the petrous bone.
- The first impression encountered on the superior surface of petrous bone is the trigeminal impression, which is easy to be identified, because it is underneath the pre-ganglionic trigeminal roots.
- Postero-lateral to the trigeminal impression the trigeminal prominence is encountered, which is the bone to be drilled during the approach.
- By moving further laterally on the upper surface of the petrous bone the meatal impression is encountered just

above the IAC, representing the posterior limit of the bone drilling.

- Lateral to the meatal impression the superior semicircular canal eminence (arcuate eminence) is found.
- If the meatal impression is not evident from above, it can be identified as the bisector of the 120° angle made by the GSPN and the superior semicircular canal eminence.
- The cochlea is found in the area between the facial nerve and the GSPN, the space between the IAC and the GSPN (the cochlear angle). The bone of the cochlea is a hard and compact bone, different from the trabecular bone of the petrous apex. By using the diamond drill the change in consistency of the bone can be appreciated. Some authors refer to the limit of drilling in the angle between the IAC and the GSPN as the cochlear line. Drilling beyond this line puts the cochlea on the risk of damage.

- ○ **TIP:** Drilling area of Kawase's triangle is defined medially by the GSPN and petrous segment of the ICA, anteriorly by V3 and posteriorly by the arcuate eminence. Once the drilling has been completed, the posterior fossa dura covering the cerebellar surface and bounded above by the superior petrosal sinus, and below by the inferior petrosal sinus, is exposed.

33.7 Dural Opening (Figs. 33.7–33.9)

- As previously described, middle fossa dissection is exclusively extradural.
- After drilling the posterior fossa dura comes into view in the depth of the surgical field.

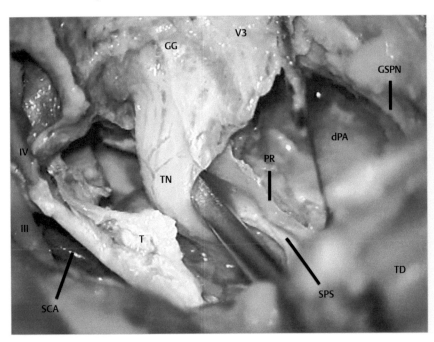

Fig. 33.7 The extended Kawase's approach; the trigeminal nerve roots can be elevated and the drilling might be extended all the way to the petroclival region by drilling out the trigeminal impression.
Abbreviations: dPA = drilled petrous apex; GG = Gasserian ganglion; GSPN = greater superficial petrosal nerve; III = third cranial nerve; IV = fourth cranial nerve; PR = petrous ridge; SCA = superior cerebellar artery; SPS = superior petrosal sinus; T = tentorium; TD = temporal dura; TN = trigeminal nerve; V3 = third trigeminal branch.

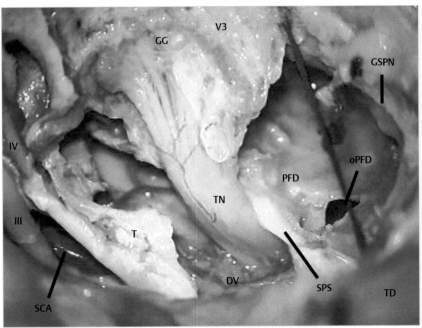

Fig. 33.8 Complete drilling of the petrous ridge exposing the superior petrosal sinus.
Abbreviations: DV = Dandy's vein; GG = Gasserian ganglion; GSPN = greater superficial petrosal nerve; III = third cranial nerve; IV = fourth cranial nerve; oPFD = opened posterior fossa dura; PFD = posterior fossa dura; SCA = superior cerebellar artery; SPS = superior petrosal sinus; T = tentorium; TD = temporal dura; TN = trigeminal nerve; V3 = third trigeminal branch.

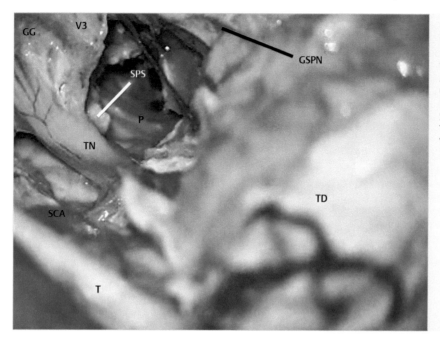

Fig. 33.9 Final exposure of the posterior fossa and lateral part of the upper brain stem after cutting the petrosal sinus and opening the posterior fossa dura.
Abbreviations: GG = Gasserian ganglion; GSPN = greater superficial petrosal nerve; P = pons; SCA = superior cerebellar artery; SPS = superior petrosal sinus; T = tentorium; TD = temporal dura; TN = trigeminal nerve; V3 = third trigeminal branch.

- The superior petrosal sinus runs in the petrous ridge and should be divided and opened in order to open the fossa dura.
  - **TIP:** It is crucial to see the tip of surgical instrument during the sectioning of the posterior petrosal sinus in order to avoid sectioning the trochlear nerve, while crossing the tentorial edge.

References

1.   al-Mefty O, Anand VK. Zygomatic approach to skull-base lesions. J Neurosurg 1990;73(5):668–673.

2.   Kawase T, Toya S, Shiobara R, Mine T. Transpetrosal approach for aneurysms of the lower basilar artery. J Neurosurg 1985;63(6):857–861.

3.   Rhoton AL. Anterior and middle cranial base. Cranial anatomy and surgical approaches. Neurosurgery 2003: 301–330.

34 Presigmoid Retrolabyrinthine Approach

Lucas Troude, Silvestre De La Rosa, Anthony Melot, and Pierre-Hugues Roche

34.1 Introduction

The principle of the retrolabyrinthine approach (RLA) is to achieve an enlarged mastoidectomy, while sparing the neuro-otologic structures. The RLA has been originally described by otological groups for the treatment of refractory Meniere's disease but indications have been gradually extended to the neurosurgical field for various cerebellopontine angle (CPA) tumors or vascular disease.

The RLA is a demanding technique because it requires an excellent knowledge of the petrous bone anatomy and of its main variations. We present herein the technique, limitations and indications of the RLA.

34.2 Indications

In the neurosurgical field, the indications have substantially decreased over years.
- Presigmoid broad based meningeal tumors.
- Tumors infiltrating the transverse and sigmoid sinuses, which require extensive surgery (aggressive/recurrent meningiomas).
- Endolymphatic sac tumors.
- Some surgeons are still operating vestibular schwannomas using the approach in order to preserve hearing.

- Exceptional cases of dural arteriovenous fistulas are treated through a RLA in case of failed endovascular treatment. This approach can extensively disconnect the totality of arterial dural feeders.
- Intra-axial brain diseases like cerebellar or pontine cavernomas.
- In our hands, this approach is mostly used as a first step of combined approaches. We routinely propose the RLA associated with an anterior petrosectomy, the so-called "combined petrosectomy" to resect large petroclival meningiomas. We also combine the RLA with a high cervical dissection for large jugulo-tympanic paragangliomas.

34.3 Surgical Anatomy (Figs. 34.1, 34.2)

- The petrous pyramid makes the junction between the middle and the posterior fossa.
- The base of the pyramid corresponds to its outer surface, which main part is occupied by the cortical bone that covers the mastoid process (MP).
- The external contours of MP grossly describe a triangle delineated by three points, the mastoid tip at the bottom, the posterior zygomatic point at the anterosuperior corner and the asterion at the postero-superior corner.

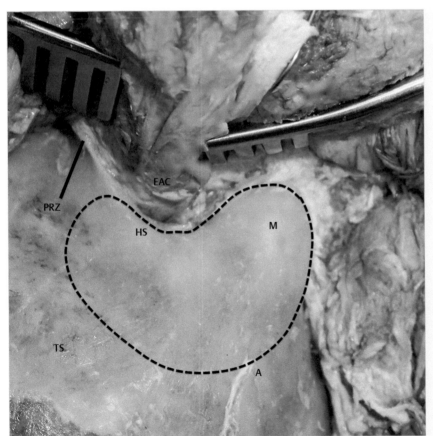

Fig. 34.1 Bone exposure after soft tissues dissection.
Abbreviations: A = asterion; EAC = external auditory canal; HS = spine of Henle; M = mastoid; PRZ = posterior root of the zygoma; TS = temporal squama.

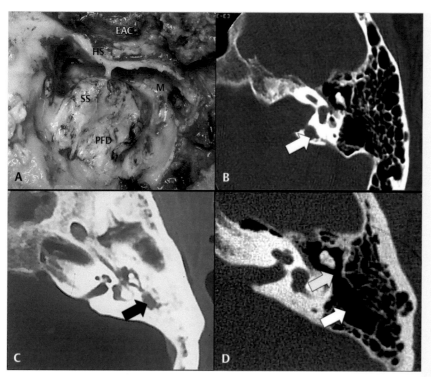

Fig. 34.2 Anatomy and variations of the mastoid air cells and venous sinuses. **(A)** The first step of the approach, superficial drilling and skeletonization of sigmoid sinus have been achieved on the right temporal bone. One can appreciate the forward course of the sigmoid sinus at the close vicinity of the posterior margin of the bony external auditory canal. **(B)** Bone window CT scan of the left petrous bone. The *white arrow* indicates a high jugular bulb position at the same level than the posterior margin of the internal auditory canal. **(C)** Bone window CT scan of the left petrous bone. The pneumatization of the mastoid air cells is dramatically poor and only the mastoid antrum can be seen (*black arrow*). **(D)** Bone window CT scan of the left petrous bone. The pneumatization of the mastoid air cells is huge and will facilitate the drilling process and the identification of the compact bony shell that covers the SCCs. The *white arrow* indicates the mastoid antrum while the *yellow arrow* shows the aditus ad antrum, which is the corridor that makes communication between the middle ear and the antrum.
Abbreviations: EAC = external auditory canal; HS = spine of Henle; M = mastoid; PFD = posterior fossa dura; SS = sigmoid sinus.

- The first step of the surgery is conducted through this triangle with gradual exposure of the posterior surface of the petrous bone and presigmoid dura.
- The drilling of the mastoid will give access to the mastoid antrum that is always identified regardless the degree of pneumatization of the petrous bone. Medially to the antrum, the external contour of the posterior labyrinth is seen.
- The 3 semicircular canals (SCC) display a constant orientation in between them with a 90° angulation to each other. The average diameter of each canal is around 8 mm. The canals are covered by a shell of compact bone with a density that is usually very distinct from the compact bone, different from the cancellous bone of the mastoid air cells.
- Two important landmarks are exposed at the level of the posterior labyrinth. The first one is the loop of the lateral SCC that covers the second portion of the intra-petrous facial nerve that runs into the Fallopian canal. The second is the junction of the posterior SCC to the superior SCC, named the common crus.
- The dura that covers the posterior surface of the petrous bone is framed by venous sinuses (superior and inferior petrosal sinuses, sigmoid sinus), which have variable size and diameter. The petrous ridge is a groove where runs the superior petrosal sinus. This sinus corresponds to the upper limit of the drilling depth. The superior petrosal sinus and tentorium collect part of the venous drainage of the temporal lobe through temporo-basal veins and the vein of Labbé. The optimal knowledge of the individual tailored pattern of drainage is worthwhile before deciding to expose and divide a sinus or tentorium if needed during the approach.

34.4 Variations in Surgical Anatomy

- Several variations of the key structures need to be mentioned (**Fig. 34.2**). These variations should be identified before starting the surgery while checking the preoperative images.

Their diagnosis may influence the operative technique and be responsible for potential complications if overlooked.
- In many cases, the course of the sigmoid sinus is located anteriorly; this anterior location is defined by a distance between the anterior border of the sinus and the posterior wall of the external auditory canal of less than 15 mm (**Fig. 34.2A**).
- The roof of the jugular bulb may be highly seated and reach the level of the posterior SCC or even higher at the level of the posterior wall of the IAC in rare cases (**Fig. 34.2B**); this configuration may hamper the drilling process.
- Another variation involves the degree of aeration of the petrous bone. Indeed, pneumatization may change from very compact petrous bone (**Fig. 34.2C**), where the air cells are almost absent excepting the constant antrum, to the highly aerated petrous bone that makes the approach easier and faster (**Fig. 34.2D**).

34.5 Patient Positioning

- **Position:** The patient is positioned supine with the head fixed in a Mayfield 3-pin holder.
- **Head**: The head is rotated 80° toward the opposite side. Care is taken not to occlude the contralateral jugular vein by excessive rotation.
- The surgeon stands behind the head and the pinna.
- The **facial nerve monitoring** is compulsory.
- **Neuronavigation** may be helpful to find the mastoid antrum and the SCCs in case of very compact mastoid.

34.6 Skin Incision

- **Peri-Auricular skin incision (See Chapter 7)**
  - **Starting point:** Incision starts at preauricular temporal region superiorly.

○ **Course:** It runs 1 cm away from the external circumference of the pinna.
○ **Ending point:** It ends at the level of the mastoid tip inferiorly.

34.7 Soft Tissue Dissection

- **Myofascial Level**
  ○ The skin incision spans the galea and the underlying pericranium.
- **Muscles**
  ○ The muscles and deep fascia are elevated from the bone with a monopolar section, and retracted anteriorly.
  ○ The sternocleidomastoid muscle is detached from the mastoid and mobilized downward.
- **Bone Exposure**
  ○ The base of the petrous pyramid is now clearly exposed with an anterior limit that corresponds to the posterior wall of the external auditory canal, that is marked by the spine of Henle (**Fig. 34.1**).

34.8 Critical Structures

○ Occipital artery, which needs to be ligated.
○ Emissary vein (bone wax hemostasis).
○ The skin of the external auditory canal in case of incision proceeding excessively in front of the spine of Henle.

34.9 Craniectomy (Figs. 34.3–34.9)

- The surgeon is equipped with a 6 to 8 mm cutting burr and will gradually shave the mastoid under copious irrigation. The drill is held like a pen and oriented tangentially to the structures that must be shaved.

- During this step, the key point is to skeletonize the sigmoid sinus and its junction with the SPS, which is named sinodural angle (or angle of Citelli) (**Fig. 34.3**). It is strongly recommended to leave a thin shell of compact bone over the sinuses to avoid any tear. This shell will be subsequently elevated with a sharp dissector.
- Depending on the course of the sigmoid sinus the opening of the angle may be a matter of variation. For instance, in case where the sigmoid sinus (SS) is anteriorly displaced as shown in **Fig. 34.2**, the angle is very narrow which hampers the access to the mastoid cells. In order to increase his working space, the surgeon will extend the drilling process behind the SS and above the superior petrosal sinus (SPS) (floor of the temporal fossa); proceeding in this way, the sinus will be mobilized downward and the angle will become wider.
- The opening of the mastoid antrum that is located at the postero-superior corner behind the external auditory canal (EAC) allows the identification of the posterior labyrinth (**Figs. 34.4, 34.5**). The surgeon keeps drilling with a diamond burr under microscope and continuous irrigation.
- The semicircular canals are covered by a shell of compact yellowish bone which texture is in sharp contrast with the loosely aerated bone around.
  ○ The lateral SCC is seen first and care is taken to avoid any drilling under its surface due to the close vicinity of the second portion of the facial nerve.
  ○ The posterior SCC is then skeletonized. At its posterior border, the notch of the endolymphatic canal is seen under microscope and communicates with a triangular shape thickening of the presigmoid dura that correspond to the endolymphatic sac.
  ○ The last canal to be exposed is the superior SCC lying in the depth and connected posteriorly to the lateral SCC by the common crus. The surgeon should avoid any excessive anterior drilling at the level of the ampulla of the superior and lateral SCCs because the facial nerve runs (junction first and second portion) very nearby.

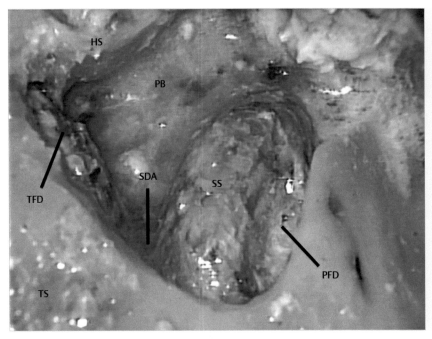

Fig. 34.3 Different steps of a retrolabyrinthine approach conducted under microscope on the right side of an injected cadaver specimen. Superficial step of the drilling. Skeletonization of the sigmoid sinus with exposure of the dura of the temporal fossa that allows the identification of the sinodural angle.
Abbreviations: HS = spine of Henle; PB = petrous bone; PFD = posterior fossa dura; SDA = sino-dural angle; SS = sigmoid sinus; TFD = temporal fossa dura; TS = temporal squama.

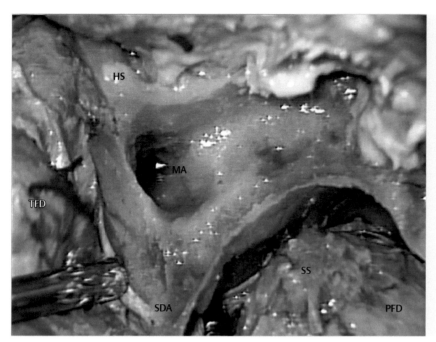

Fig. 34.4 Different steps of a retrolabyrinthine approach conducted under microscope on the right side of an injected cadaver specimen. The gradual drilling in the depth of the mastoid allows more exposure of the presigmoid dura and the one of the temporal fossa, thereby widening the sinodural angle and increasing the corridor of approach. Abbreviations: HS = spine of Henle; MA = mastoid antrum; PFD = posterior fossa dura; SDA = sino-dural angle; SS = sigmoid sinus; TFD = temporal fossa dura.

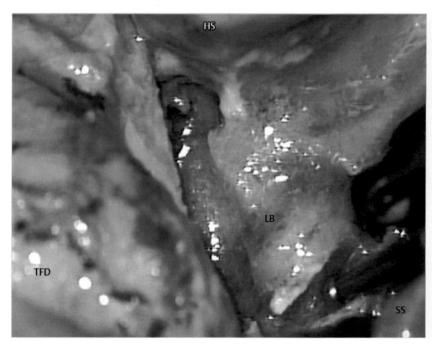

Fig. 34.5 Different steps of a retrolabyrinthine approach conducted under microscope on the right side of an injected cadaver specimen. The drilling has been carried out in the depth as far as the labyrinthine block. The respective position and orientation of the three SCCs can be assessed. Abbreviations: HS = spine of Henle; LB = labyrinthine block; SS = sigmoid sinus; TFD = temporal fossa dura.

- Once the SCCs have been exposed (**Figs. 34.6**, **34.7**), the drilling is conducted inferiorly in the infralabyrinthine area behind the third portion of the facial nerve. While drilling the infralabyrinthine cells, the digastric ridge is encountered inside the mastoid cortex and toward the mastoid tip. This landmark is located just behind the stylomastoid foramen from where the course of the third portion of the facial nerve can be drawn.
- The roof of the jugular bulb is now exposed even though this step may be challenging because the venous wall is extremely thin and fragile (**Figs. 34.8**, **34.9**). Again, it is strongly advised to leave a piece of bone that will protect the vein.

- At the end of the drilling step, the surgeon has achieved a full exposure of the presigmoid dura following the limits described as the Trautmann's triangle (anterior border of the SS, SPS, posterior SCC and third portion of the facial canal).

34.10 Dural Opening

- The dura opening can be carried out in different manners.
- One option is to open it just in front of the SS for the vertical arm and under the SPS for the horizontal arm of the dural flap that will be retracted anteriorly.

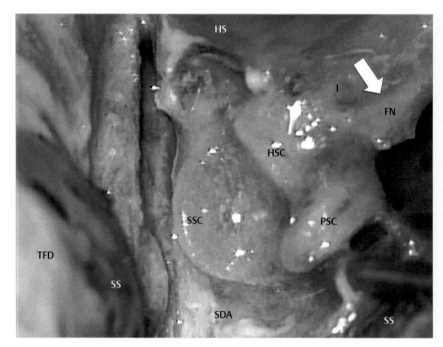

Fig. 34.6 Different steps of a retrolabyrinthine approach conducted under microscope on the right side of an injected cadaver specimen. Close-up view of the SCCs. The drilling has been achieved at the point where the blue line of the posterior SCC is seen under irrigation. More drilling will carry the risk of opening the canal and experience delayed deafness. The *white arrow* indicates the junction between the second and the third portion of the intra-petrous facial nerve. Abbreviations: FN = facial nerve; HS = spine of Henle; HSC = horizontal semicircular canal; I = incus; PSC = posterior semicircular canal; SDA = sino-dural angle; SS = sigmoid sinus; SSC = superior semicircular canal; TFD = temporal fossa dura.

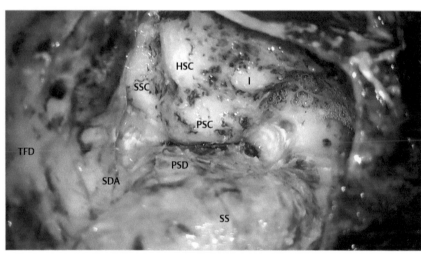

Fig. 34.7 Operative view of the retrolabyrinthine approach on the right side. The temporal fossa and presigmoid dura are shown. The blue color of the sigmoid sinus makes an angle with the temporal fossa named sinodural angle. In the depth, the compact bone that covers the SCCs is clearly seen while the antrum has been opened.
Abbreviations: HSC = horizontal semicircular canal; I = incus; PSC = posterior semicircular canal; PSD = presigmoid dura; SDA = sino-dural angle; SS = sigmoid sinus; SSC = superior semicircular canal; TFD = temporal fossa dura.

34.11 Intradural Exposure

- **Parenchymal structures:** Middle cerebellar peduncle, cerebellar hemisphere, Lushka foramen.
- **Cranial nerves:** From the fifth to the lower cranial nerves.
- **Arteries:** Anterior inferior cerebellar artery (AICA), posterior inferior cerebellar artery (PICA).
- **Veins:** Petrosal vein, subpial pontine venous network.

34.12 Closure

- Once the intradural step has been achieved, the closure is done by re-approaching the dura. At this point the dura cannot be easily closed water-tightly; thus, the usual way is to plug the defect and the mastoid cavity using fat.

- We routinely use stripes of fat that have been harvested from the abdomen. This step requires an additional skin incision and this must be mentioned to the patient before surgery.

- In case of large bony defect the use of titanium mesh that covers the mastoid tip resection may reduce the cosmetic burden.

34.13 How to Prevent Complications

- Careful case selection is the most important point.
- The surgeon carefully checks the preoperative bone window CT of the petrous bone to confirm the amount of pneumatization of the mastoid air cells.
- The surgeon carefully checks the angio-CT or angio-MR to assess the course of the sigmoid sinus and jugular bulb and potential infiltration or occlusion of the sinus.
- During surgery, one important task is to optimize the exposure of the sinodural angle as well as the skeletonization of the common crus. Careful hemostasis will be performed before opening the dura.

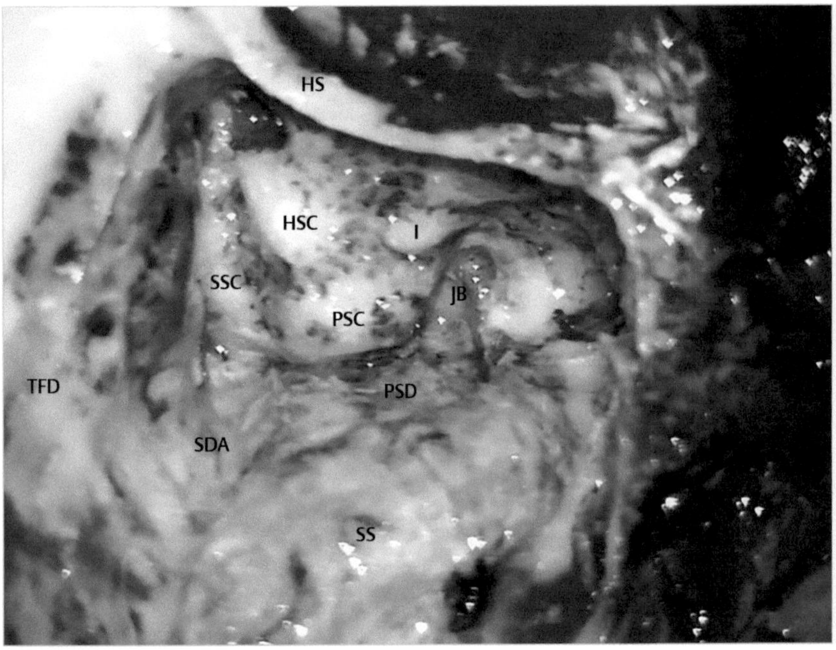

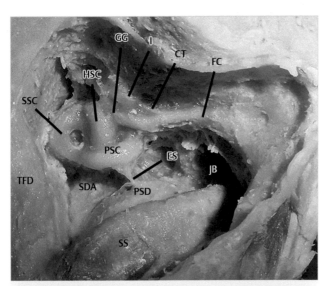

Fig. 34.8 Operative view of the retrolabyrinthine approach on the right side. Final exposure after achieved drilling. The SSCs are fully skeletonized. The whole course of the sigmoid sinus from the sinodural angle to the jugular bulb is exposed.
Abbreviations: HS = spine of Henle; HSC = horizontal semicircular canal; I = incus; JB = jugular bulb; PSC = posterior semicircular canal; PSD = presigmoid dura; SDA = sino-dural angle; SS = sigmoid sinus; SSC = superior semicircular canal; TFD = temporal fossa dura.

Fig. 34.9 Cadaveric view of the retrolabyrinthine approach on the right side. The third portion of the facial nerve and chorda tympani (CT), which usually does not require full exposure is seen as well as the endolymphatic sac (ES).
Abbreviations: CT = chorda tympani; ES = endolymphatic sac; FC = Fallopian canal; GG = geniculate ganglion; HSC = horizontal semicircular canal; I = incus; JB = jugular bulb; PSC = posterior semicircular canal; PSD = presigmoid dura; SDA = sino-dural angle; SS = sigmoid sinus; SSC = superior semicircular canal; TFD = temporal fossa dura.

References

1. Darrouzet V, Martel J, Enée V, Bébéar JP, Guérin J. Vestibular schwannoma surgery outcomes: our multidisciplinary experience in 400 cases over 17 years. Laryngoscope 2004; 114(4):681–688.
2. de Melo JO, Klescoski J, Nunes CF, Cabral GA, Lapenta MA, Landeiro JA. Predicting the presigmoid retrolabyrinthine space using a sigmoid sinus tomography classification: A cadaveric study. Surg Neurol Int 2014;5:131.
3. Roche PH, Moriyama T, Thomassin JM, Pellet W. High jugular bulb in the translabyrinthine approach to the cerebellopontine angle: anatomical considerations and surgical management. Acta Neurochir (Wien) 2006;148(4):415–420.

35 Translabyrinthine and Transcochlear Transpetrosal Approach

Cristian Gragnaniello, Parisa Sabetrasekh, Sam Maghami, Alan Siu, Zachary Litvack, and Ashkan Monfared

35.1 Introduction

Presigmoid approaches decrease the working angle and depth of field as compared to retrosigmoid approaches, and are indicated for extra-axial lesions anterolateral to the brainstem, petroclival lesions, or deep-seated brainstem lesions. Common pathologies in the internal auditory canal (IAC) and cerebellopontine angle (CPA) include vestibular schwannomas, meningiomas, and epidermoids. These approaches can also be combined with a middle fossa craniectomy for lesions extensively involving the temporal bone or spanning both sides of the tentorial incisura.

The translabyrinthine and transcochlear approaches are variations of a posterior transpetrosal approach, which provide access to the IAC and CPA. These approaches are usually used in patients in whom the hearing is already compromised. In the translabyrinthine approach, the labyrinth is removed, sacrificing hearing if present, to provide an anterolateral view of the CPA without cerebellar retraction.

The transcochlear approach, with or without transposition of the facial nerve (placing the VII cranial nerve at increased risk for iatrogenic injury), provides additional access to the mid-clivus, petrous apex, and pre-pontine cistern.

35.2 Indications

- Lesions of the internal auditory canal or cerebellopontine angle.
- Anterior and ventral brainstem lesions in patients with non-serviceable hearing.
- Deep-seated brainstem lesions.
- Petroclival lesions.
- Tumors extending into the cochlea.
- Tumors extending into the temporal bone.
- Tumor remnants from a previous retrosigmoid or middle fossa approach.

35.3 Patient Positioning

Patients may be positioned supine, lateral, or ¾ prone (*aka* park-bench) at the discretion of the surgeon.

Supine position is preferred when possible as it minimizes the risk of pressure ulcers and positional neuropathies, but requires a patient with good cervical range of motion, and can be difficult in obese patients or those with broad shoulders.

If not supine, we prefer ¾ prone to lateral as it drops the shoulder out of the field, increasing the angle of attack toward the tentorium.

35.3.1 Supine

- **Position:** The patient is positioned supine and the head is not pinned (i.e., placed on a foam donut or a cerebellar headrest).

- **Body:** The shoulders and body remain parallel to the floor. The elbows are padded and the arms tucked against the body.
- **Head:** The head is rotated 60° contralateral to the side of the pathology. The auricle of the ear may be folded over the external canal and taped.
- The external ear is the highest point in the surgical field.

35.3.2 Three-Quarters Prone

- **Position:** The patient is positioned three-quarters prone, with the head fixed in a Mayfield head holder.
- **Body:** The body is held in place with a sandbag. An axillary roll is placed about 5 cm below the axilla. The dependent arm is placed in a sling, and the upper arm placed on an armrest. A pillow is placed in between the legs with the top leg flexed 45°. Extensive padding is used on the elbows, hands, hips, knees, ankles, and areola of the breasts to prevent pressure ulcers.
- **Shoulder:** The shoulder is taped downward and away from the ear to minimize hindrance.
- **Head:** The head is rotated 45° contralateral to the side of the pathology.

35.4 Skin Incision (Fig. 35.1)

- **Curvilinear incision**
  - Starting point: The incision starts 3 cm radially, posterior to the post-auricular sulcus.
  - The ending points are just superior to the pinna and inferior to the mastoid tip. A periosteal flap may be elevated separate from the skin incision depending on the soft tissue thickness.

35.4.1 Critical Structures

- The external auditory canal (EAC) is anterior to the spine of Henle.
- Great care should be taken not to lacerate the skin of the external auditory canal while elevating the subperiosteal flap.
- If the skin is transected, the EAC may need to be completely sealed and the contents of the ear canal and middle ear completely removed to prevent cerebrospinal fluid (CSF) fistula formation post-operatively.

35.5 Soft Tissue Dissection

- **Myocutaneous level**
  - A myocutaneous flap is raised just superficial to the deep temporal fascia and the mastoid periosteum (**Fig. 35.2**).
  - Subperiosteal flap is elevated anteriorly and posteriorly after making an incision on the temporal line extending from the root of the zygoma posteriorly and then connected with a separate incision to the mastoid tip (**Fig. 35.3**).

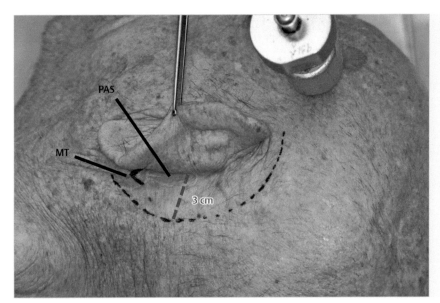

Fig. 35.1 Curvilinear incision with a 3 cm radius posterior to the postauricular sulcus. Abbreviations: MT = mastoid tip; PAS = postauricular sulcus.

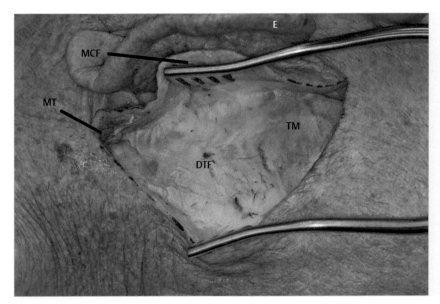

Fig. 35.2 Myocutaneous flap raised to expose the deep temporal fascia. Abbreviations: DTF = deep temporal fascia; E = ear; MCF = myocutaneous flap; MT = mastoid tip; TM = temporal muscle.

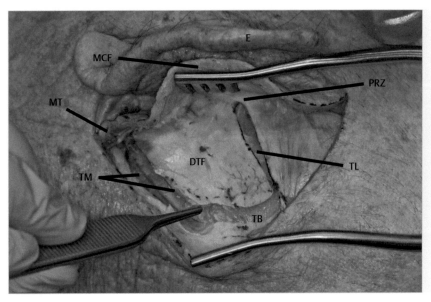

Fig. 35.3 Deep temporal fascia, temporal muscle, and periosteum flap may be elevated separately or all at once as shown here. Incision is made at the posterior root of zygoma on the inferior temporal line and connected with a separate incision to the mastoid tip. Abbreviations: DTF = deep temporal fascia; E = ear; MCF = myocutaneous flap; MT = mastoid tip; PRZ = posterior root of the zygoma; TB = temporal bone; TL = temporal line; TM = temporal muscle.

○ The myocutaneous and periosteal flaps are reflected anteriorly.
- **Bone exposure**
  ○ Spine of Henle.
  ○ Mastoid tip.

35.6 Mastoidectomy/ Labyrinthectomy

- **Mastoidectomy landmarks (Fig. 35.4)**
  ○ MacEwan's Triangle.
    - EAC and Spine of Henle.
    - Mastoid tip.
    - Root of the zygoma.

35.6.1 Critical Structures

- A cortical mastoidectomy will expose the following structures **(Fig. 35.5)**.
  ○ Tegmen or the bone underlying the middle fossa dura.
  ○ Sigmoid sinus and transverse sinus.
  ○ Posterior fossa dura. The junction between the tegmen and the sigmoid sinus is known as sinodural angle. Superior petrosal sinus is located in the junction between middle and posterior fossa dura at the edge of the tentorium.
  ○ Endolymphatic sac is encountered while exposing the dura, and should be sharply divided from the vestibular aqueduct.
  ○ Antrum with incus seen in the fossa incudis.
  ○ Lateral semicircular canal.
  ○ Facial nerve and chorda tympani.
- **Labyrinthectomy landmarks (Figs. 35.6–35.9)**
  ○ Anterior-superior: Antrum and Incus.
  ○ Anterior-inferior: Facial nerve.
  ○ Posterior: Posterior fossa dura.
  ○ Superior: Middle fossa dura.
  ○ Inferior: Retrofacial air cells.

35.6.2 Critical Structures

- Facial Nerve: Intimately associated with the ampulla of the semicircular canals.
- Superior, lateral, posterior semicircular canals.
- Superior petrosal sinus.

- **Cochlectomy landmarks** after removal of the bone of the EAC, tympanic membrane and the ossicles.
  ○ **Anterior:** Petrous internal carotid artery (ICA) and the Eustachian tube.
  ○ **Posterior:** Descending facial nerve.
  ○ **Superior:** Geniculate ganglion and tympanic segment of the facial nerve.
  ○ **Inferior:** Jugular bulb.

35.7 Internal Auditory Canal Dissection (Fig. 35.10)

- Circumferential bony removal 270° by creating superior and inferior troughs over the IAC.

35.7.1 Critical Structures

- Facial nerve and geniculate ganglion.
- Superior and inferior vestibular nerve.
- Cochlear nerve.
- Transverse crest.
- Vertical crest or Bill's bar.

35.8 Dural Opening (Figs. 35.11, 35.12)

- H-shaped incision inferior to the superior petrosal sinus and superior to the horizontal segment of the sigmoid sinus connected posterior to the dura of the porus acusticus.

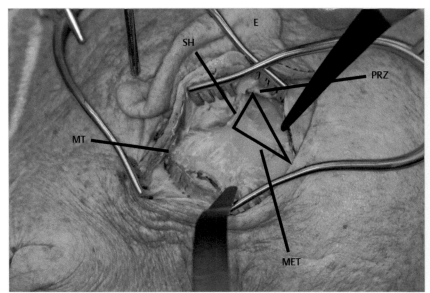

Fig. 35.4 The MacEwan's triangle is a small triangular depression bordered by the spine of Henle (suprameatal spine), posterior root of the zygomatic arch, and the line joining the two borders. The mastoid antrum lies 1 to 2 cm deep to the MacEwan's triangle. Abbreviations: E = ear; MET = MacEwan's triangle; MT = mastoid tip; PRZ = posterior root of the zygoma; SH = spine of Henle.

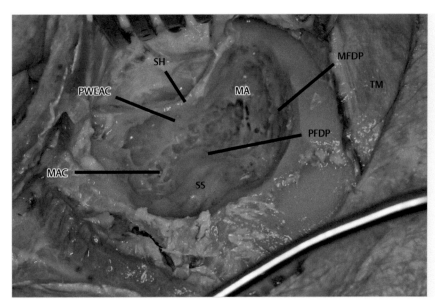

Fig. 35.5 Cortical mastoidectomy with exposure of relevant structures. Abbreviations: MA = mastoid antrum; MAC = mastoid air cells; MFDP = middle fossa dura plate; PFDP = posterior fossa dura plate; PWEAC = posterior wall of the external acoustic canal; SH = spine of Henle; SS = sigmoid sinus; TM = temporal muscle.

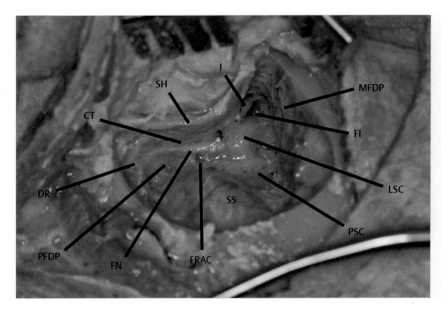

Fig. 35.6 Labyrinthectomy with demonstration of critical structures. Abbreviations: CT = chorda tympani; DR = digastric ridge; FI = fossa incudis; FN = facial nerve; I = incus; LSC = lateral semicircular canal; MFDP = middle fossa dura plate; PFDP = posterior fossa dura plate; PSC = posterior semicircular canal; FRAC = facial recess air cells; SH = spine of Henle; SS = sigmoid sinus.

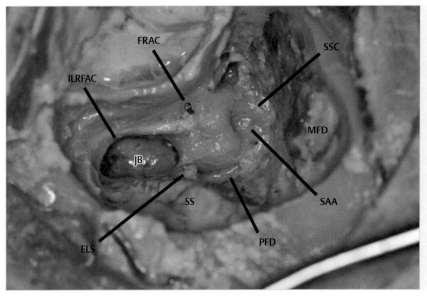

Fig. 35.7 The bones over the middle fossa and posterior fossa plates are removed before labyrinthectomy is performed. Abbreviations: ELS = endolymphatic sac; FRAC = facial recess air cells; ILRFAC = infralabyrinthine retrofacial air cells; JB = jugular bulb; MFD = middle fossa dura; PFD = posterior fossa dura; SAA = subarcuate artery; SS = sigmoid sinus; SSC = superior semicircular canal.

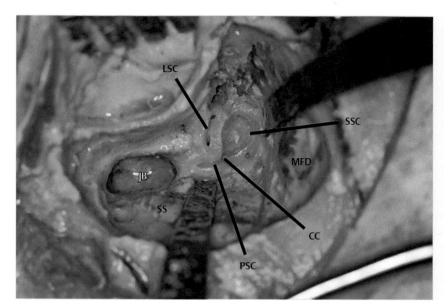

Fig. 35.8 Partial labyrinthectomy has been performed to demonstrate the opening into the balance canals.
Abbreviations: CC = common crus; JB = jugular bulb; LSC = lateral semicircular canal; MFD = middle fossa dura; PSC = posterior semicircular canal; SS = sigmoid sinus; SSC = superior semicircular canal.

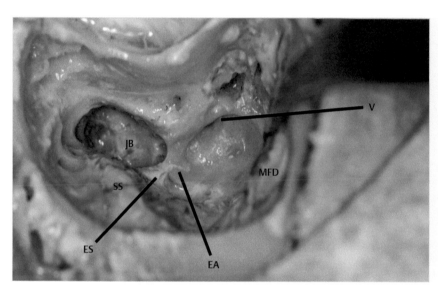

Fig. 35.9 Complete labyrinthectomy.
Abbreviations: EA = endolymphatic aqueduct; ES = endolymphatic sac; JB = jugular bulb; MFD = middle fossa dura; SS = sigmoid sinus; V = vestibule.

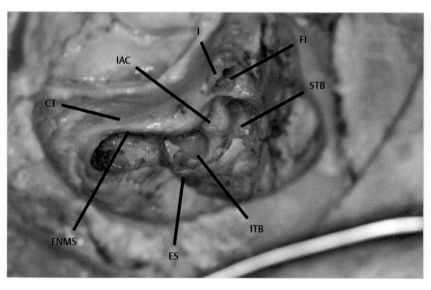

Fig. 35.10 Decompression of the internal auditory canal by creation of superior and inferior troughs of bone over the canal.
Abbreviations: CT = chorda tympani; ES = endolymphatic sac; FI = fossa incudis; FNMS = facial nerve mastoid segment; I = incus; IAC = internal acoustic canal; ITB = inferior trough of bone; STB = superior trough of bone.

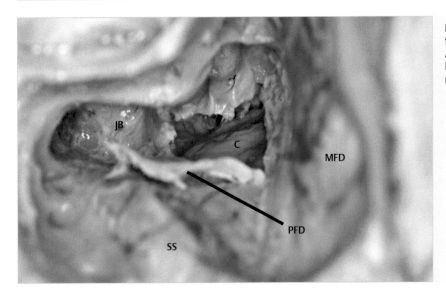

Fig. 35.11 Opening of the posterior fossa dura.
Abbreviations: C = cerebellum; JB = jugular bulb; MFD = middle fossa dura; PFD = posterior fossa dura; SS = sigmoid sinus.

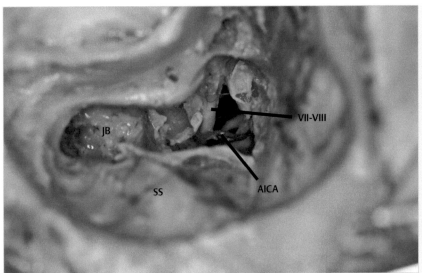

Fig. 35.12 Opening of the dura over the internal auditory canal. Contents of the IAC are facial nerve, vestibulocochlear nerve, and labyrinthine artery (not shown).
Abbreviations: AICA = anterior inferior cerebellar artery; JB = jugular bulb; SS = sigmoid sinus; VII-VIII = facial and vestibule-cochlear nerve.

35.8.1 Critical Structures

- Contents of the IAC including CNVII and VIII as well as labyrinthine artery.
- Superior petrosal sinus.
- Sigmoid sinus and jugular bulb.

35.9 Intradural Exposure (Fig. 35.12)

- **Cranial Nerves:** from the fifth to the ninth cranial nerve.
- **Parenchymal Structures:** cerebellum, anterolateral brainstem, flocculus, choroid plexus.

- **Arteries:** AICA with labyrinthine artery, SCA.
- **Veins:** superior petrosal vein (Dandy's vein).

References

1. Jackler RK, Jackler RK. Atlas of skull base surgery and neurotology, 2nd ed. New York, NY: Thieme Medical Publisher; 2009.

Part V
Endonasal, Transoral, and Transmaxillary Procedures

36 Nasal Surgical Anatomy

Matteo Trimarchi, Salvatore Toma, Francesco Pilolli, and Mario Bussi

36.1 Operative Theater Setup (Fig. 36.1)

- Surgeon typically stands on the right side of the patient (if right-handed).
- Monitor and any intraoperative imaging devices are located facing the first surgeon.

36.2 Patient Positioning

- **Position:** The patient is positioned supine.
- **Body:** The body lines 20° from the horizontal in anti-Trendelenburg position.
- **Head:** The head is flexed 30° and rotated in the direction of the first surgeon.
- Face is draped in order to expose forehead, eyes, nose, and upper lip.

36.3 Endoscopic Instrument Employment (Fig. 36.2)

- The left hand is used to keep the telescope.
- Commercially available telescopes comprise zero-degree and angled view (30°, 45°, 70°, 120°). Zero-degree and 30°telescopes are the minimum equipment required for basic dissections.
- The right hand keeps the surgical instruments: straight and angled forceps, back-biting and down-biting forceps, straight and angled suctions, Cottle periosteal elevator, ostium seeker, sphenoid and frontal punch.
- Powered instruments (drill) can be useful for the sphenoid sinus dissection.

36.4 Exploration of Nasal Fossae

- At the beginning of surgical dissection, the tip of the telescope must be positioned at the nasoseptal angle, retracting the nasal tip cranially.
- The telescope is then directed toward the occipital area in order to progressively visualize
  - Nasal floor.
  - Inferior turbinate.
  - Nasopharynx.
- A 30° telescope is placed in the middle meatus and rotated to identify
  - Uncinate process.
  - Bulla ethmoidalis.
  - Middle turbinate axilla.
  - Frontal recess.

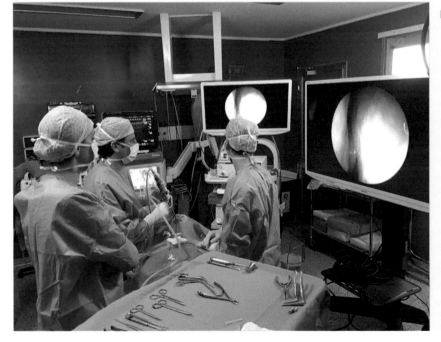

Fig. 36.1 Setup of the operative theatre.

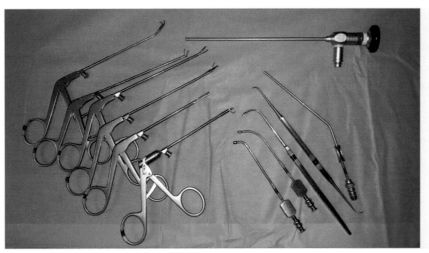

Fig. 36.2 Surgical instruments required for basic nasal endoscopic dissection.

• Zero-degree telescope is useful to identify the sphenoid ostium and the spheno-ethmoidal recess.

36.5 Opening of Maxillary Sinus

• Before starting the surgical dissection, the surgeon must identify fundamental anatomical landmarks such as the inferior turbinate, the head of the middle turbinate and its attachment to the maxillary bone (axilla of the middle turbinate), the nasal septum, and the uncinate process.
• The **uncinate process** is a C-shaped process of the ethmoid bone, which represents a small part of the medial wall of the maxillary sinus posteriorly to the lacrimal bone, and articulates with the axilla of the middle turbinate (**Fig. 36.3**).
• The **maxillary sinus ostium** is found within the concavity designed by the uncinate process, using the ostium seeker. The natural ostium is sloped 45°on the axial plane, and it is perpendicular to the coronal plane.
• The ostium must be enlarged using back-biting and down-biting forceps in order to remove the caudal part of the uncinate process (**Fig. 36.4**), taking care to preserve the cranial part as an important anatomical landmark for the frontal recess. The surgeon should avoid injuries to the lacrimal canal. If needed, the ostium can be enlarged posteriorly, using straight forceps (**Fig. 36.4**).
• Thirty-degree and 45°telescopes allow the exploration of the maxillary sinus including the alveolar as well as infra-orbitary recess, which can be visualized in the roof of the maxillary sinus (**Figs. 36.5, 36.6**).

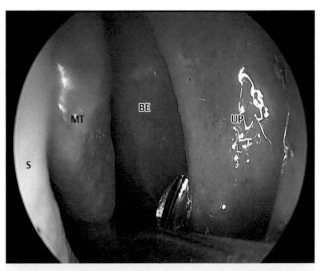

Fig. 36.3 Partial uncinectomy.
Abbreviations: BE = bulla ethmoidalis; MT = middle turbinate; S = septum; UP = uncinate process.

36.6 Opening of the Anterior Ethmoidal Complex

• The pneumatization of the ethmoid labyrinth might present a wide variability, except for the **ethmoidal bulla**, which is constantly represented. It is the most anterior pneumatized cell in the middle meatus, and it is located postero-medially to the uncinate process; its cranial and posterior walls can be either in continuity with the middle turbinate or separated from it by the sovrabullar/retrobullar recess.

- The safe opening of the ethmoidal bulla should be performed starting medially and inferiorly (**Figs. 36.7, 36.8**), keeping in mind that the lateral wall of the bulla corresponds to the lamina papyracea of the orbit, and avoiding injuries to the anterior ethmoidal artery.

36.7 Opening of Posterior Ethmoidal Complex

- The basal lamella of the middle turbinate divides the anterior ethmoidal cells from the posterior ones. Surgeons must identify the midpoint between the nasal septum and the medial wall of the orbit on a horizontal plane, passing through the

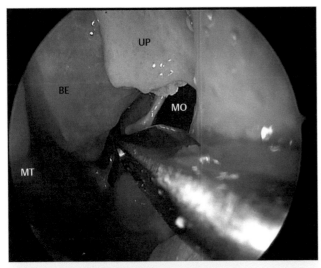

Fig. 36.4 Antrostomy: opening of the maxillary ostium. Abbreviations: BE = bulla ethmoidalis; MO = maxillary ostium; MT = middle turbinate; UP = uncinate process.

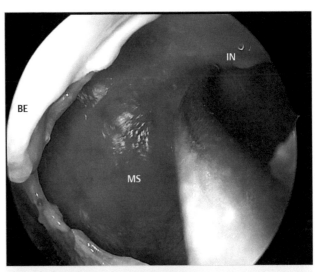

Fig. 36.5 Antrostomy: anatomic landmarks of maxillary sinus. Abbreviations: BE = bulla ethmoidalis; IN = infra-orbital nerve; MS = maxillary sinus.

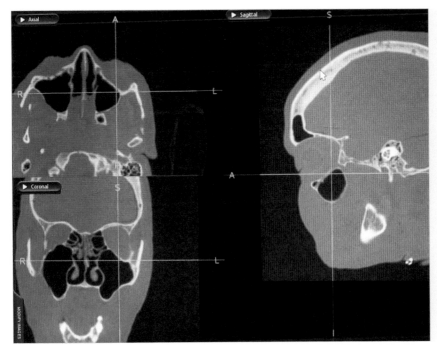

Fig. 36.6 Neuronavigation probe touching the tubercle of the infraorbitary nerve.

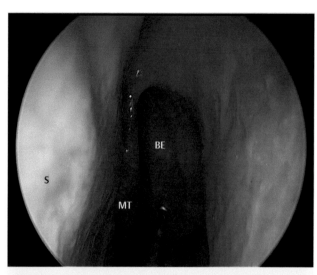

Fig. 36.7 Opening of the ethmoidal bulla. Surgical view. Abbreviations: BE = bulla ethmoidalis; MT = middle turbinate; S = septum.

orbital floor, which represents the safe entry zone to the posterior ethmoidal cells.

• The accurate evaluation of the CT images is important in order to open all pneumatized cells of the ethmoidal complex, taking care not to damage the skull base, the lamina papyracea and the posterior ethmoidal artery (**Fig. 36.9**).

36.8 Opening of Sphenoid Sinus

• The sphenoid ostium (**Figs. 36.10, 36.11**) is located 16-27 mm from the supero-lateral angle of the posterior choana, 2-8 mm from the midline, just medial to the tail of the superior and supreme turbinate.

• The opening of sphenoid sinus can be performed either through the sphenoethmoidal recess, or by performing an ethmoidectomy.

• The ostium might be safely enlarged medially and caudally, where septal branches of the spheno-ethmoidal artery are usually found.

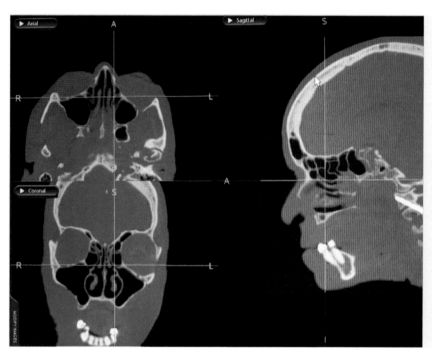

Fig. 36.8 Opening of the ethmoidal bulla. Neuronavigation seeker on the ostium.

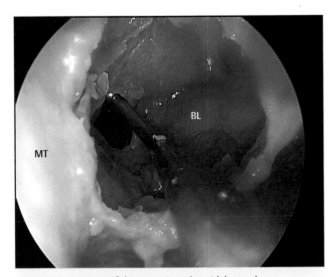

Fig. 36.9 Opening of the posterior ethmoidal complex.
Abbreviations: BL = basal lamella; MT = middle turbinate.

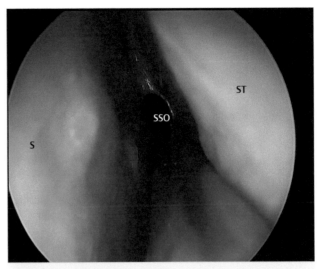

Fig. 36.10 Sphenoid sinus opening.
Abbreviations: S = septum; SSO = sphenoid sinus ostium;
ST = superior turbinate.

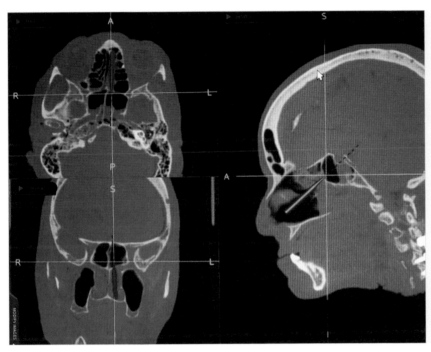

Fig. 36.11 Neuronavigated instrument
demonstrating the physiological ostium of
sphenoid sinus.

- At this point, the entire anterior wall of the sphenoid sinus can be removed.
- The bony septum dividing the sphenoid sinuses can be safely drilled.
- On the posterior and lateral walls, the surgeon can appreciate the carotid protuberances, the clival recess, the medial opticocarotid recesses, the lateral opticocarotid recesses, the optic protuberances, and the sellar floor (**Figs. 36.12, 36.13**).

36.9 Opening of the Frontal Sinus

- The frontal sinus might present a complex and variable drainage, which is usually shaped like an hourglass: the upper portion is the frontal sinus, the lower portion is formed by the frontal recess and the narrowest portion corresponds to the frontal ostium.

- The frontal drainage is surrounded anteriorly either by the *agger nasi* or by the frontal infundibular cells, laterally by the orbital roof, the lamina papyracea and the uncinate process, posteriorly by the suprabullar cells, and medially by the vertical lamella of the middle turbinate.
- The correct access to the frontal recess must be found supero-medially, just adjacent to the vertical lamella of the middle turbinate, and slightly posterior to the uncinate process.
- In a case in which the *agger nasi* is present, the surgeon must remove its posterior and medial walls, to gain access to the frontal sinus.
- CT scan may reveal the presence of frontal cells, which are ethmoidal cells that are encroached into the frontal sinus. If these cells are present, the surgeon has to remove all the bone between them ("uncapping the eggs") (**Figs. 36.14, 36.15**).

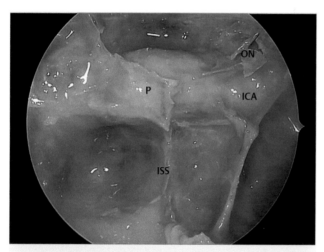

Fig. 36.12 Posterior wall of the sphenoid sinus after removal of the inter-sinusal bone.
Abbreviations: ICA = internal carotid artery; ISS = inter-sinusal I septum; ON = optic nerve; P = pituitary gland.

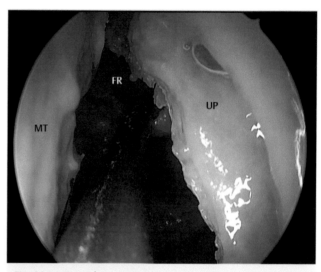

Fig. 36.14 Frontal sinus opening.
Abbreviations: FR = frontal recess; MT = middle turbinate; UP = uncinate process.

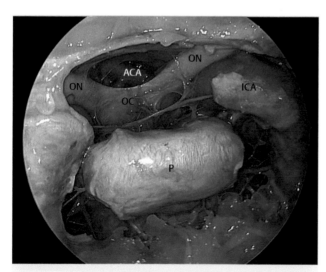

Fig. 36.13 Endoscopic view after removal of all the posterior wall of the sphenoid sinus and opening of the dura mater.
Abbreviations: ACA = anterior cerebral artery; ICA = internal carotid artery; OC = optic chiasm; ON = optic nerve; P = pituitary gland.

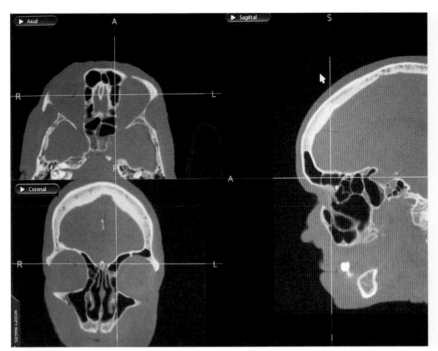

Fig. 36.15 Neuronavigation probe inside the frontal sinus.

References

1. Badia L, Lund VJ, Wei W, Ho WK. Ethnic variation in sinonasal anatomy on CT-scanning. Rhinology 2005;43(3):210–214.

2. Comer BT, Kincaid NW, Smith NJ, Wallace JH, Kountakis SE. Frontal sinus septations predict the presence of supraorbital ethmoid cells. Laryngoscope 2013;123(9):2090–2093.

3. Daniels DL, Mafee MF, Smith MM, et al. The frontal sinus drainage pathway and related structures. AJNR Am J Neuroradiol 2003;24(8):1618–1627.

4. El-Shazly AE, Poirrier AL, Cabay J, Lefebvre PP. Anatomical variations of the lateral nasal wall: The secondary and accessory middle turbinates. Clin Anat 2012;25(3):340–346.

5. Han D, Zhang L, Ge W, Tao J, Xian J, Zhou B. Multiplanar computed tomographic analysis of the frontal recess region in Chinese subjects without frontal sinus disease symptoms. ORL J Otorhinolaryngol Relat Spec 2008;70(2):104–112.

6. Jankowski R. The Evo-Devo Origin of the Nose, Anterior Skull Base and Midface: Springer;2013.

7. Lund VJ, Stammberger H, Fokkens WJ, et alEuropean position paper on the anatomical terminology of the internal nose and paranasal sinuses. 2014;24:1-34.

8. Simmen D, Raghavan U, Briner HR, et al. The surgeon's view of the anterior ethmoid artery. Clin Otolaryngol 2006; 31(3):187–191.

9. Simmen D, Jones NS. Manual of Endoscopic Sinus and Skull Base Surgery: Thieme;2013.

10. Kennedy DW; Anatomic Terminology Group. Paranasal sinuses:anatomic terminology and nomenclature. Ann Otol Rhinol Laryngol Suppl 1995;167:7–16.

11. H, Lund V. Anatomy of the nose and paranasal sinuses. In: Gleeson M, Browning GG, Burton MJ, al e, editors. Scott-Brown's Otorhinolaryngology, Head and Neck Surgery. 2. 7th ed. London: Hodder Arnold;2008:1315-43.

12. Wormald PJ. The agger nasi cell: the key to understanding the anatomy of the frontal recess. Otolaryngology–head and neck surgery : official journal of American Academy of Otolaryngology-. Head Neck Surg 2003;129 (5):497–507.

37 Microscopic Endonasal and Sublabial Approach

Michael Buchfelder and Sven-Martin Schlaffer

37.1 Introduction

The microscopic endonasal and sublabial approach is a midline skull-base approach, which provides direct access to the sellar and parasellar region with a surgical corridor free from major neurovascular structures.

37.2 Indications

- Intra- and suprasellar pituitary adenomas.
- Intra- and suprasellar craniopharyngiomas.
- Any other intrasellar lesions.
- Suprasellar lesions depending on magnitude of sella enlargement.

37.3 Patient Positioning (Fig. 37.1)

- **Position:** Patient is positioned supine with the head on a flat headrest.
- **Body:** The body is positioned straight and flat.
- **Head:** The head is positioned straight, extended 15°.
- Cushion is placed under patient's shoulders.
- The upper lip has to be the highest point in the surgical field.

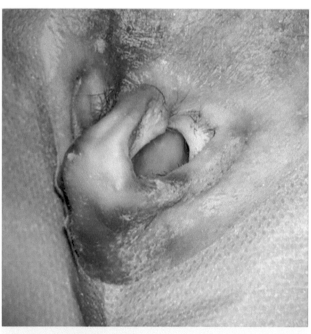

Fig. 37.1 Patient positioning.

37.4 Mucosal Incision for Endonasal Approach (Fig. 37.2)

- The right nostril is exposed (if surgeon is right-handed).
- The base of right nostril is retracted with Langenbeck retractor.
- A straight unilateral incision is performed.
  - **Starting point:** Incision starts 4 mm below the surface of right cartilage.
  - **Course:** It runs straight above nasal cartilage, parallel to nostril.
  - **Ending point:** It ends at the superior medial margin of the right nostril.

37.5 Mucosal Incision for Sublabial Approach (Figs. 37.3–37.5)

- The upper lip is retracted with 2 Langenbeck retractors.
- A straight unilateral incision is performed (**Fig. 37.3**).
  - **Starting point:** Incision starts at the level of medial canines.
  - **Course:** It runs parallel to the plica between gingiva and upper lip (4 mm from plica), crossing the phrenulum.
- The anterior margin of nasal cartilage is exposed (**Fig. 37.4**).
- The mucosa is dissected on a sub-perichondrial plane.
- The self-retaining speculum is inserted (**Fig. 37.5**).

37.6 Soft Tissue Dissection for Endonasal Approach (Figs. 37.6–37.9)

- Mucosa is detached unilaterally from the cartilaginous septum and the submucosal tunnel is created (**Fig. 37.6**).
- Medial nasal mucosa has to be kept intact by careful stepwise dissection.
- A self-retaining speculum is inserted.
- The junction of cartilaginous and bony nasal septum is exposed and dissected (**Fig. 37.7**).
- The mucosa is detached bilaterally from the bony nasal septum (**Figs. 37.7, 37.8**).
- The junction of cartilaginous and bony nasal septum is separated.
- The paraseptal mucosa is detached bilaterally from the bony nasal septum.
- Portions of bony nasal septum are resected (**Fig. 37.8**).
- The self-retaining speculum is inserted (**Fig. 37.9**).

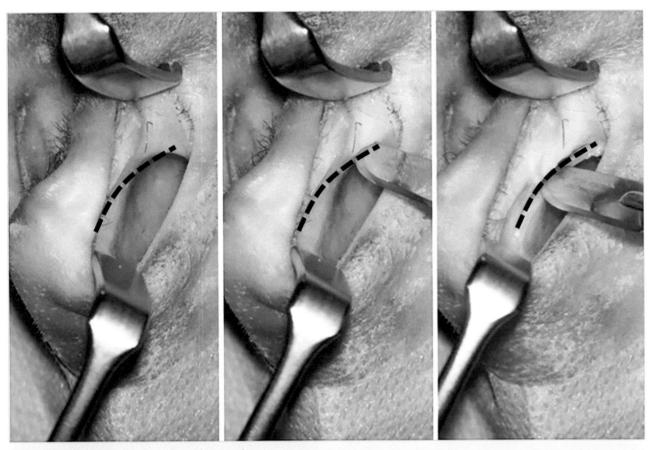

Fig. 37.2 Mucosal incision for endonasal approach.

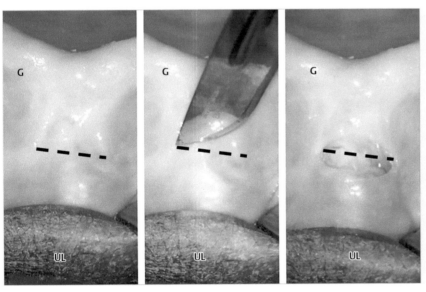

Fig. 37.3 Mucosal incision for sublabial approach.
Abbreviations: G = gingiva; UL = upper lip.

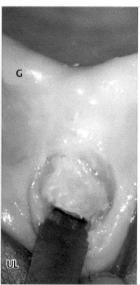
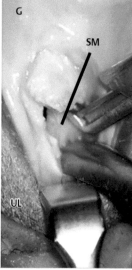
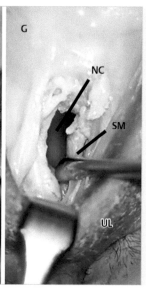

Fig. 37.4 Exposure of anterior margin of nasal cartilage and sub-perichondrial dissection. Abbreviations: G = gingiva; NC = nasal cartilage; SM = septal mucosa; UL = upper lip.

37.6.1 Critical Structures

- Alveolar branches to the frontal teeth.
- Anterior nasal spine.
- Any irregularities in the osseous nasal spine.
- Beware of subluxation of cartilaginous and bony nasal septum.

37.7 Sphenoid Sinus Dissection for Endonasal Approach

37.7.1 Bone Exposure (Figs. 37.10, 37.11)

- Subperiosteal dissection of the anterior surface of the vomer is performed.
- Bilateral exposure of ostium is carried out.
- Sphenoidotomy must be performed with forceps, rongeur, diamond drill.

37.7.2 Resection of Sphenoid Sinus Mucosa (Fig. 37.12)

- The mucosa and mucosal polyps are extracted from the sphenoid sinus.
- Hydrogen peroxide cottonoids are inserted for hemostasis and disinfection.

37.7.3 Resection of Sphenoid Sinus Septa (Fig. 37.13)

- Septa has to be resected, so that a complete view onto the sella floor is provided.

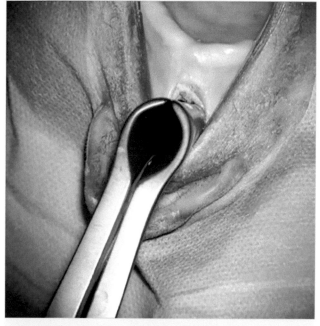

Fig. 37.5 Insertion of the self-retaining speculum.

- Incomplete pneumatization of the sphenoid sinus requires aggressive drilling of clivus so that a sufficient portion of the sellar floor is directly exposed.
- Bleeding from clival bone can be controlled with bone wax.

37.8 Sphenoidotomy Landmarks

Usually, the sphenoidotomy extends from both the anterior ostia until the entire sellar floor can be visualized.

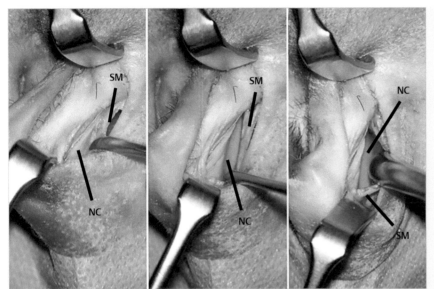

Fig. 37.6 Sub-perichondrial dissection. Abbreviations: NC = nasal cartilage; SM = septal mucosa.

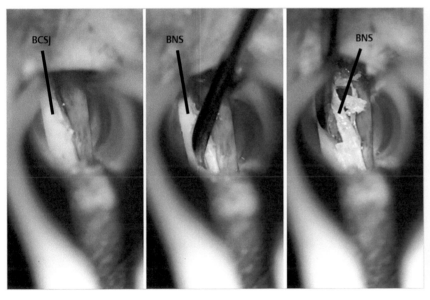

Fig. 37.7 Junction of cartilagenous and bony nasal septum is separated. Abbreviations: BCSJ = bony-cartilage nasal septum junction; BNS = bony nasal septum.

- The entire sellar floor from the planum sphenoidale to the clivus has to be exposed.
- Clival and retro-sellar lesions require more posterior opening.
- Osseous canal of carotid artery is frequently encountered.
- Bone has to be maintained intact around carotid artery.

37.8.1 Exposure of the Sellar Floor

- The sellar floor is resected between both cavernous sinus with rongeur or diamond drill (**Fig. 37.14**).
- Dura has to be kept initially intact (**Fig. 37.15**).

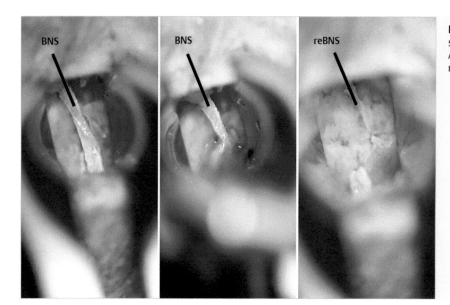

Fig. 37.8 Partial resection of bony nasal septum.
Abbreviations: BNS = bony nasal septum; reBNS = resected bony nasal septum.

- Dural opening may be performed in X-shaped fashion or through a straight incision extended to a dural window (**Fig. 37.16**).
- Edges remain within the course of cavernous sinuses.

37.8.2 Critical Structures

- Cavernous sinuses.
- Internal carotid arteries, particularly in the posterior portion of sphenoid sinus.
- The arachnoid close to the junction with the anterior cranial fossa.

37.9 Intradural Exposure (See Anatomy in Chapters 36 And 39)

- **Parenchymal structures:** Anterior and posterior pituitary gland.
- **Arachnoidal layer:** Optic-chiasmatic cistern.
- **Cranial nerves:** Second, third, fourth, fifth and sixth cranial nerves (only visible with invasive tumors).
- **Arteries**: Internal carotid arteries.
- **Veins:** Cavernous sinuses.

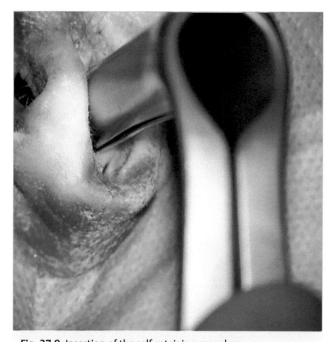

Fig. 37.9 Insertion of the self-retaining speculum.

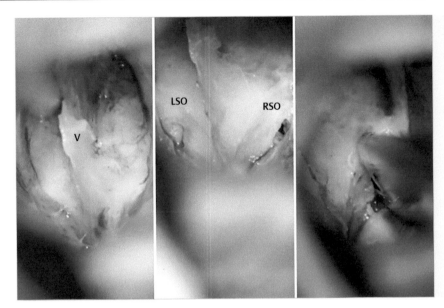

Fig. 37.10 Exposure of the vomer.
Abbreviations: LSO = left sphenoid ostium;
RSO = right sphenoid ostium; V = vomer.

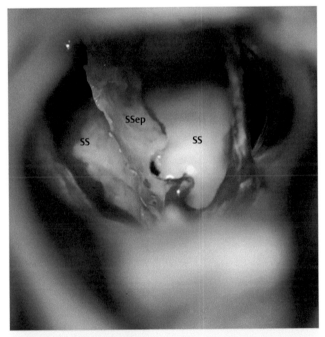

Fig. 37.11 Sphenoidotomy.
Abbreviations: SS = sphenoid sinus; SSep = sphenoid septum.

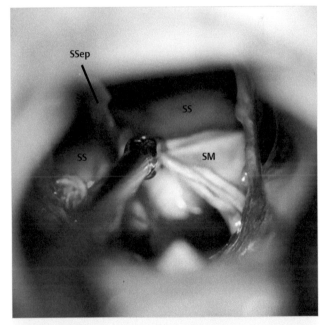

Fig. 37.12 Dissection and resection of mucosa.
Abbreviations: SM = sphenoid mucosa; SS = sphenoid sinus;
SSep = sphenoid septum.

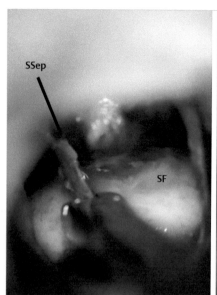

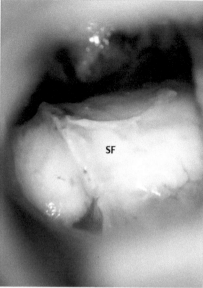

Fig. 37.13 Resection of bony septa. Abbreviations: SF = sellar floor; SSep = sphenoid septum.

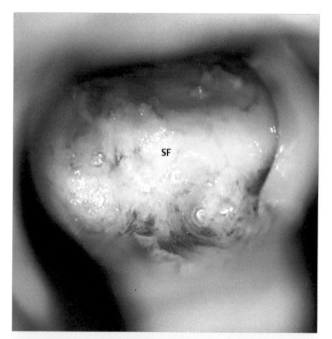

Fig. 37.14 Exposure of the sellar floor. Abbreviations: SF = sellar floor.

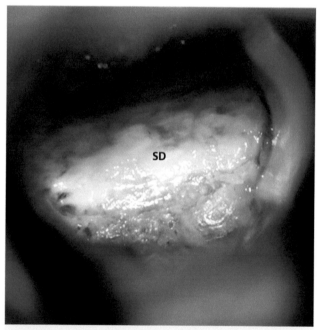

Fig. 37.15 Sellar floor is resected and the dura is exposed. Abbreviations: SD = sellar dura.

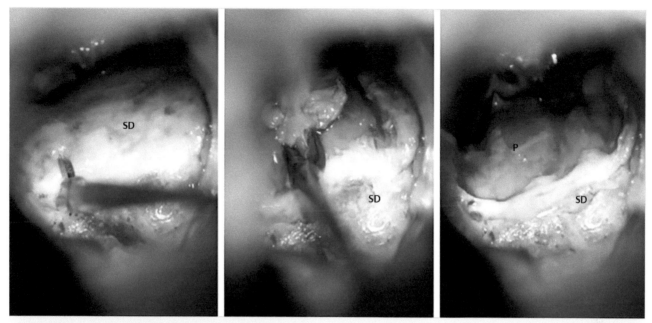

Fig. 37.16 Dural opening and exposure of intrasellar tissue.
Abbreviations: P = pituitary gland; SD = sellar dura.

References

1. Buchfelder M, Fahlbusch R. The "classic" transsphenoidal approach for resection of pituitary tumors. Oper Techn Neurosurg. 2002;5:210–217.
2. Destrieux C, Kakou MK, Velut S, Lefrancq T, Jan M. Microanatomy of the hypophyseal fossa boundaries. J Neurosurg 1998;88(4):743–752.
3. Fatemi N, Dusick JR, de Paiva Neto MA, Kelly DF. The endonasal microscopic approach for pituitary adenomas and other parasellar tumors: a 10-year experience. Neurosurgery 2008;**63**(4, Suppl 2):244–256, discussion 256.
4. Fukushima T, Sano K. Sublabial rhinoseptoplastic technique for transsphenoidal pituitary surgery by a hinged-septum method. Technical note. J Neurosurg 1980;52(6):867–870.
5. Grisoli F, Vincentelli F, Henry JF, et al. Anatomical bases for the transsphenoidal approach to the pituitary gland. Anat Clin 1982;3:207–220.
6. Romano A, Zuccarello M, van Loveren HR, Keller JT. Expanding the boundaries of the transsphenoidal approach: a microanatomic study. Clin Anat 2001;14(1):1–9.

38 Endoscopic Endonasal Transsphenoidal Approach

Kevin Swong, Asterios Tsimpas, Chirag R. Patel, and Anand V. Germanwala

38.1 Patient Positioning

- **Position:** The patient is positioned supine with slight rotation towards operating team.
- **Head:** The head is slightly extended and above the heart with Mayfield pins for intra-arachnoidal lesions.
- The tip of patient's nose should be the highest point in the surgical field.
- Abdomen is usually prepped for potential fat graft.

38.2 Preoperative Settings

- Neurophysiological monitoring (electroencephalogram and somatosensory evoked potentials) is often utilized.
- Image guidance navigation with stereotactic CT and MRI is often used.
- Nasal cavity decongestion with topical vasoconstricting agents (1:1000 Epinephrine, oxymetazoline, or 4% cocaine).

38.3 Skin Incision

- Not applicable.
- Close collaboration with an ENT team is favored.
  - **Option 1:** Single nare technique with or without turbinate resection.
  - **Option 2 (favored):** Bilateral nare technique with or without turbinate resection, which provides a wider viewing angle and area of exposure, more room for skull base instruments, and better haptic feedback.

38.4 Soft Tissue Dissection, Nasal Phase (Figs. 38.1–38.4)

- Depending on the preference of the ENT surgeon, local anesthetic may be injected before or after the patient is draped.
- Additionally, cotton pledgets saturated in a topical vasoconstricting agent placed between the middle turbinate and the nasal septum may aid in decongestion.
- A 0° rigid endoscope is introduced into the nasal cavities; the inferior turbinates and the nasal septum are the first identifiable landmarks.
- The middle turbinates are then moved laterally to allow for increased exposure. If necessary, the middle turbinate can be resected for additional space.
- The sphenoid ostium is identified adjacent to the septum near the inferior edge of the superior turbinate. This is approximately 2 cm above the arch of the choana.

38.4.1 Critical Structures

- Inferior, middle, and superior turbinates.
- Choana, sphenoid ostium.

38.5 Osteotomy, Sphenoid Phase (Fig. 38.4–38.9)

- Care is taken during approach to preserve sphenopalatine arteries in anticipation of possible skull base dural reconstruction with a pedicled vascularized nasoseptal flap.

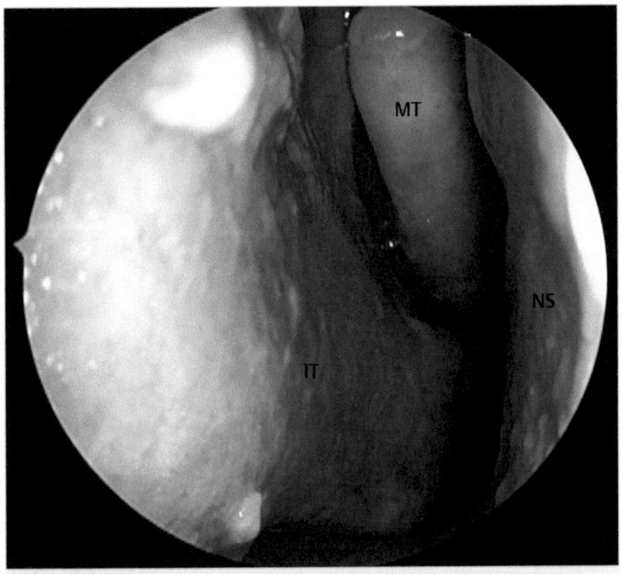

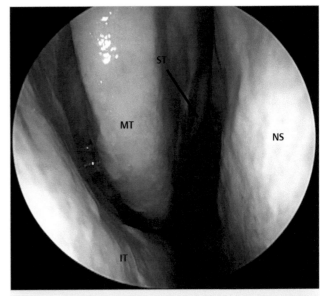

Fig. 38.1 Endoscopic endonasal photo depicting sino-nasal landmarks in the right nasal cavity.
Abbreviations: IT = inferior turbinate; MT = middle turbinate; NS = nasal septum.

Fig. 38.2 Endoscopic endonasal photo depicting sino-nasal landmarks deeper in the right nasal cavity. Identification of the superior turbinate.
Abbreviations: IT = inferior turbinate; MT = middle turbinate; NS = nasal septum; ST = superior turbinate.

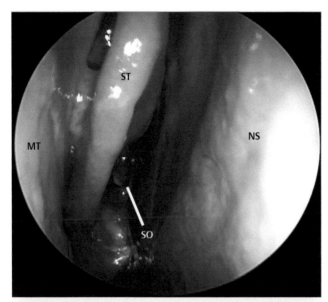

Fig. 38.3 Endoscopic endonasal intraoperative photo depicting location of the right sphenoid ostium. Note that the sphenoid ostium in this specimen is higher than we would typically expect (i.e. closer to the inferior edge of the superior turbinate). Extra caution should be taken during widening of the sphenoid ostium in this situation as it is located much closer to the skull base (i.e. planum sphenoidale).
Abbreviations: MT = middle turbinate; NS = nasal septum; SO = sphenoid ostium; ST = superior turbinate.

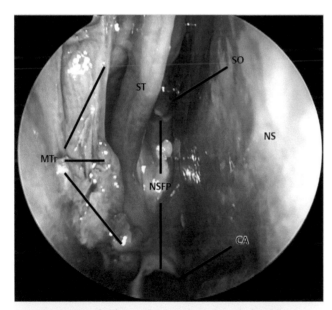

Fig. 38.4 View of right nasal cavity after removal of middle turbinate. Note the location of the vascular pedicle for the nasoseptal flap. Damage to this mucosa should be avoided to preserve the viability of the flap.
Abbreviations: CA = choanal arch; MTr = middle turbinate resected; NS = nasal septum; NSFP = nasoseptal flap peduncle; SO = sphenoid ostium; ST = superior turbinate.

- This neurovascular pedicle runs horizontally across the sphenoid face and extends from the arch of the choana to the level of the natural sphenoid ostium.

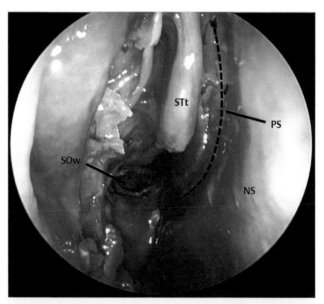

Fig. 38.5 The right sphenoid ostium has been partially widened. A more limited opening has been employed initially in this specimen due to the high position of the natural ostium (thus its proximity to the skull base superiorly) and the need to protect the nasoseptal flap pedicle inferiorly. The posterior septectomy has also been outlined.
Abbreviations: NS = nasal septum; PS = posterior septectomy; SOw = widened sphenoid ostium; STt = trimmed superior turbinate.

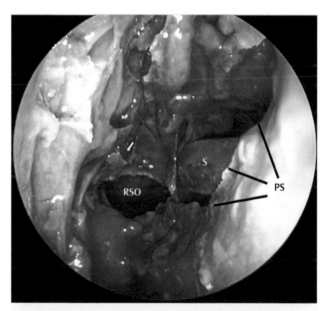

Fig. 38.6 The posterior septectomy has been completed. Instruments passed through the left nasal cavity can now be seen from the right. Also note the sphenoidotomy has been further widened as better visualization has been obtained.
Abbreviations: PS = posterior septectomy; RSO =right sphenoid ostium; S = suction tube in the contralateral nasal fossa.

- The sphenoid ostium is widened first laterally then superiorly on both sides. The superior turbinate can be trimmed as needed to improve visualization and access.
- A small posterior septectomy is then performed to allow binarial access.

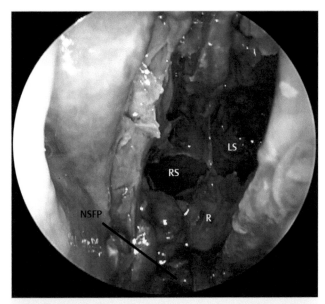

Fig. 38.7 The vascular pedicle is being carefully elevated off the face of the sphenoid to allow widening of the sphenoidotomy inferiorly while protecting the flap pedicle.
Abbreviations: LS = left sphenoid; NSFP = nasoseptal flap peduncle; R = rostrum; RS = right sphenoid.

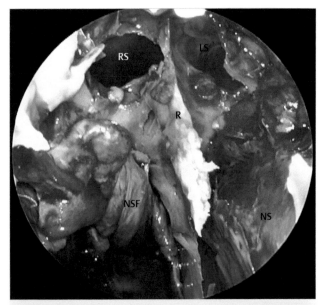

Fig. 38.8 In this view, a right nasoseptal flap has been elevated and tucked into the nasopharynx. The bony nasal septum has been disarticulated from the rostrum, giving us a clear view of the "keel."
Abbreviations: LS = left sphenoid; NS = nasal septum; NSF = nasoseptal flap; R = rostrum; RS = right sphenoid.

- If use of a nasoseptal flap is anticipated for reconstruction, it should be elevated at this point to protect the neurovascular pedicle and the flap mucosa. The flap can be stored in the nasopharynx for safekeeping until needed. Should the flap not be needed, it can be sutured back to the septum at the end of the procedure.
- If use of a nasoseptal flap is not anticipated, the pedicle should still be protected to preserve reconstructive options.

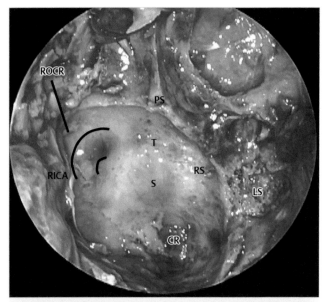

Fig. 38.9 The remainder of the face of the sphenoid and the sphenoid rostrum have been removed. Note the left sphenoid in this specimen is small and under-pneumatized. The clival recess, sella, and right carotid are clearly visible. The optic-carotid recess is not well formed.
Abbreviations: CR = clival recess; LS = left sphenoid; PS = planum sphenoidalis; RICA = right internal carotid artery; ROCR = right optic-carotid recess; RS = right sphenoid; S = sella; T = tuberculum sellae.

The pedicle is elevated inferiorly off the face of the sphenoid to expose the underlying bone. The sphenoidotomy can then be safely widened inferiorly without sacrificing the pedicle.
- The bony nasal septum is detached from sphenoid rostrum, and the rostrum is removed with rongeurs or a drill.
  The anterior wall of the sphenoid sinus is further widened as needed.
- Sphenoid septations are removed, allowing visualization of the bony prominences of the internal carotid artery (ICA), planum, and optic-carotid recess (OCR).

38.5.1 Critical Structures

- OCR: Endonasally visualized pneumatization of optic strut.
- ICA: Cavernous segment.

38.5.2 Pitfalls

- Spheno-ethmoidal air cell (Onodi Cell): posterior ethmoid air cell that lies superior to the sphenoid sinus that may house the ICA or the optic nerve (ON).

38.6 Osteotomy, Sellar Phase (Figs. 38.10–38.13)

- The endoscope may be attached to a holder if desired; however, most surgeons use an assistant to hold the endoscope to allow for continued dynamic manipulation of the field of view.

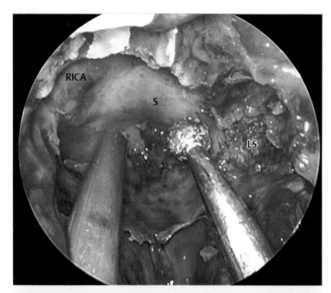

Fig. 38.10 A two-handed binarial technique can now be employed. Here a suction is placed through the right nostril and a drill is passed through the left.
Abbreviations: LS = left sphenoid; RICA = right internal carotid artery; S = sella.

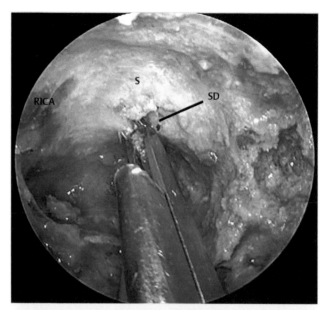

Fig. 38.12 The bone of the sella is thinned and a small bony defect is created to allow further bone removal with Kerrison rongeurs.
Abbreviations: RICA = right internal carotid artery; S = sella; SD = sellar dura.

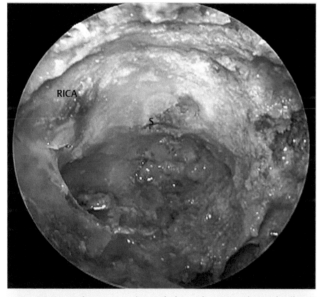

Fig. 38.11 Endoscopic endonasal photo depicting thinned sellar floor after drilling.
Abbreviations: RICA = right internal carotid artery; S = sella.

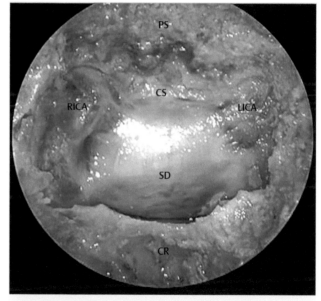

Fig. 38.13 The bone has been removed from the sella, tuberculum, and both carotids.
Abbreviations: CR = clival recess; CS = chiasmatic sulcus; LICA = left internal carotid artery; PS = planum sphenoidalis; RICA = right internal carotid artery; SD = sellar dura.

- The sellar floor is opened using a combination of a high-speed drill and Kerrison rongeurs.
  - Bony work may be less if there is erosion of the bony floor.
  - Footplate of the rongeur should be parallel with the carotid artery.
- Ultrasonic doppler probe and image guidance may be utilized to identify the carotid arteries.

38.7 Dural Opening (Figs. 38.14–38.16)

- Once the bone has been cleared, the dura is opened in a cruciate fashion.

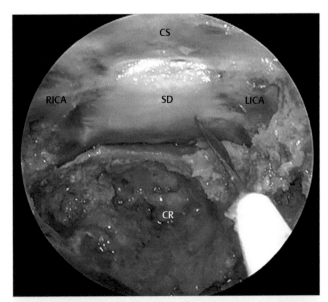

Fig. 38.14 Endoscopic endonasal photo depicting dural opening with a sickle knife blade.
Abbreviations: CR = clival recess; CS = chiasmatic sulcus; LICA = left internal carotid artery; RICA = right internal carotid artery; SD = sellar dura.

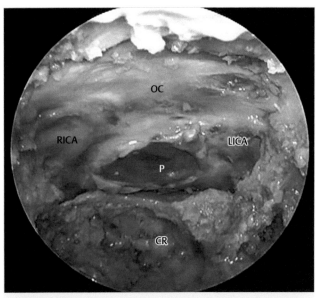

Fig. 38.16 Completed dural opening with underlying gland exposed.
Abbreviations: CR = clival recess; LICA = left internal carotid artery; OC = optic chiasm; P = pituitary gland; RICA = right internal carotid artery.

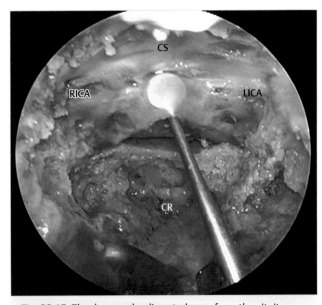

Fig. 38.15 The dura can be dissected away from the pituitary capsule.
Abbreviations: CR = clival recess; CS = chiasmatic sulcus; LICA = left internal carotid artery; RICA = right internal carotid artery.

- Venous bleeding is controlled with gentle pressure, warm irrigation, and hemostatic agents such as Floseal or Gelfoam soaked in thrombin.

38.8 Intradural Exposure (See Anatomy in Chapters 36 And 39)

- Identify tumor capsule if present (and firm) to allow for en-bloc resection.

- ○ If unable to identify plane or tumor is soft, intra-tumoral debulking will be necessary.
- ○ Prefer two suction technique or ultrasonic aspiration for resection under visualization.
- ○ However, at times, curettes can be used to assist in resection more superficially.
- Inferior and lateral aspects of tumor should be approached before the superior aspect to prevent premature downward descent of the diaphragma which may obstruct visualization.
- If there is extension into the medial cavernous sinus, it is helpful to insert the endoscope into the contralateral nostril to improve visualization or consider use of angled endoscopes.
  - ○ A Doppler and image guidance is helpful to identify the carotid arteries.
  - ○ Venous bleeding can be controlled with a combination of hemostatic agents and cotton pledgets.
  - ○ Neurophysiological monitoring of cranial nerves (EMG) may be helpful in this particular case.
- If there is extension into the lateral cavernous sinus, the exposure can be extended by removal of the ethmoidal bullae and medial pterygoid process.
  - ○ The carotid artery is identified with a Doppler probe before the dura is opened.
  - ○ Neurophysiological monitoring of cranial nerves (EMG) may be helpful in this particular case.
- The area of the resection is directly inspected for any residual tumor.
- An angled scope is helpful for seeing around neurovascular structures.

38.8.1 Critical Structures

- Carotid artery.
- Cavernous sinus.
- Diaphragma sellae.

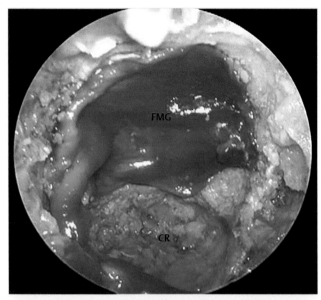

Fig. 38.17 A free mucosal graft was harvested from the previously resected middle turbinate and has been placed over the sellar defect. Note that a rather sizeable graft can be harvested from the middle turbinate. It is important to ensure the periosteal side faces the bone and the mucosal side faces the sinus cavity.
Abbreviations: CR = clival recess; FMG = free mucosal graft.

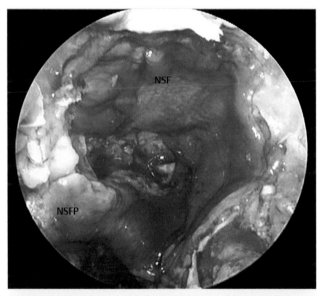

Fig. 38.18 Use of a nasoseptal flap for reconstruction. The flap can be oriented in any position that is favorable as long as the entire perichondrial/periosteal surface is touching denuded bone and the mucosal surface is facing the nasal cavity.
Abbreviations: NSF = nasoseptal flap; NSFP = nasoseptal flap peduncle.

38.9 Reconstruction (Figs. 38.17, 38.18)

- Depends on type of cerebrospinal fluid (CSF) leak.
  - High flow (ventricular) CSF leak.
  - Low flow (cisternal) CSF leak.
  - Pinhole CSF leak.
  - No CSF leak.
- For situations with a pinhole CSF leak or no leak, it is our practice to line the dural defect with an avascular collagen graft and/or a free mucosal graft, and then line the edges with Surgicel.
- A free mucosal graft can be harvested from a previously resected middle turbinate or from the nasal floor.
- For low and high flow leak situations, a vascularized pedicled mucosal flap is favored after repair with an avascular graft.
- It is very rare to utilize a lumbar drain; would consider this, in addition to vascularized reconstruction, in patients with elevated CSF pressure and a high flow leak.

38.10 Postoperative Care

- It is important the close collaboration with ENT for continued follow up.
- Postoperative imaging should be obtained.
- Patients should be monitored for symptoms and signs of CSF leak, infection, and endocrinopathies.

References

1. Cavallo LM, Cappabianca P, Galzio R, Iaconetta G, de Divitiis E, Tschabitscher M. Endoscopic transnasal approach to the cavernous sinus versus transcranial route: anatomic study. Neurosurgery 2005;**56**(2,Suppl):379–389, discussion 379–389.

2. Dallapiazza RF, Jane JA Jr. Outcomes of endoscopic transsphenoidal pituitary surgery. Endocrinol Metab Clin North Am 2015; 44(1):105–115.

3. Elhadi AM, Hardesty DA, Zaidi HA, et al. Evaluation of surgical freedom for microscopic and endoscopic transsphenoidal approaches to the sella. Neurosurgery 2015;11(Suppl 2):69–78, discussion 78–79.

4. Patel MR, Stadler ME, Snyderman CH, et al. How to choose? Endoscopic skull base reconstructive options and limitations. Skull Base 2010;20(6):397–404.

39 Expanded Endoscopic Endonasal Approach

Zachary Litvack, Cristian Gragnaniello, Alan Siu, and Ameet Singh

39.1 Indications

- Craniopharyngioma.
- Tuberculum sellae meningioma.
- Planum sphenoidale meningioma.
- Olfactory groove meningioma.
- Esthesioneuroblastoma.
- Paranasal sinus malignancies.

39.2 Cautions and Contraindications

- Extension of the pathology lateral to the medial edge of the optic canal/orbit.
- Extension of the pathology lateral to the paraclinoid/supra-clinoidal carotid.
- Extension of the pathology ventral to the subfrontal region.
- Caution should be exercised for pathology that circumferentially encases critical structures including the carotid or its major branches, and the optic nerve.
- Caution regarding sinonasal morbidity including atrophic rhinitis, chronic sinusitis, nasal septal perforations, and tooth numbness.

39.3 Room Layout (Fig. 39.1)

- Bed is spun 180° from anesthesia.
- A right-handed surgeon will stand on patient's right side.
- The first assist/co-surgeon can stand at the patient's head to the surgeon's left, or across from the surgeon.

- The scrub nurse stands across from the surgeon at the torso, such that instruments are passed across the sterile field.
- The back table of instruments is arranged as an "L" off the left side of patient's head.
- A Mayo Stand is positioned at patient's head on the side opposite the first assist/co-surgeon.

39.4 Equipment Considerations

- Surgical equipment includes the following:
  - HD Endoscopic Tower, 4 mm × 18 cm rod lenses (0°, 30°, 45°).
  - Ultrasonic aspirator with long (transsphenoidal) bone cutting and tumor ablating attachments.
  - Endonasal bipolar instrumentation.
  - Sinus microdebrider.
  - Neurosurgical microdebrider (NICO Myriad).

39.5 Patient Positioning (Fig. 39.2)

- **Position:** Patient is positioned in semi-recumbent position (supine with bed reflexed) with head held on a cerebellar headrest or in 3-point Mayfield fixation.
- **Body:** The body is placed supine. (**Fig. 39.2**)
  - Shoulders should be kept above the break in the bed prior to removing the headboard to place the cerebellar horseshoe/Mayfield.
  - The bed is reflexed to torso up 20°, and the legs are placed downward 20°.
  - Ipsilateral arm is reverse tucked at the side.
  - Contralateral arm is left accessible on an arm board.
  - Abdomen or thigh is draped out for a possible fat/fascia graft.

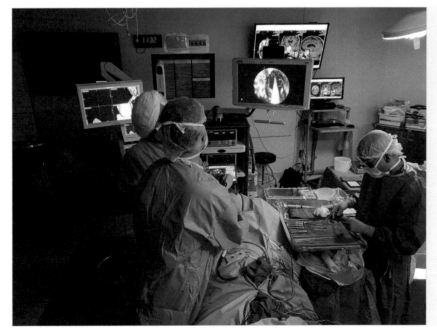

Fig. 39.1 Intraoperative photograph of the room layout demonstrating the position of the patient with the head of the bed 180° from anesthesia and the position of the surgeons and tech as well as the monitors and instrument tables.

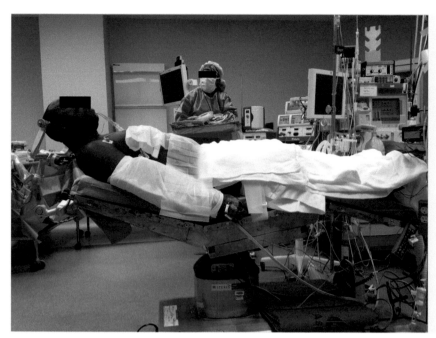

Fig. 39.2 Patient positioning. Patient is placed supine, head in a cerebellar headrest with the torso elevated 20° and the legs lowered 20°. The ipsilateral arm is tucked at the side to increase surgeon's ergonomics. The contralateral arm is kept on an arm board. The abdomen is draped for possible graft harvesting.

- **Head:** (**Fig. 39.3**)
  - The head is flexed 10–15° (bridge of nose approximately parallel to floor), rotated 5° to the right, and tilted 10–15° to the contralateral side.
- **Padding:**
  - Arms are padded with foam or gel pads prior to tucking.
  - Care is taken to ensure hands are supported at the sides, and not hanging free at the wrists. Intravenous (IV) sites are double padded with gauze between the plastic of the IV or stop-cock and the patient's skin.
  - A pillow is placed behind patient's knees. It is combined with the leg-panel of the bed down 20°, which removes pressures from the heels.
  - Heels are padded/wrapped with gel pads.
  - Sacrum is padded with gel or disposable pad.
- The nasal tip is the highest point in the surgical field.

39.6 Skin Incision (Fig. 39.4)

- The only external incisions for this portion are the harvest sites.
- Alternatives include
  - Lower quadrant abdominal.
  - Sub-umbilical.
  - Lateral thigh (fascia lata).

39.7 Endonasal Dissection

- **Nasal passage** (typically completed by an ENT/sinus surgeon)
  - Inferior turbinates are outfractured/reduced.
  - Right middle turbinate is resected. Left turbinate is optionally resected depending on anatomy and type of pathology.
  - Septal flap is harvested according to Hadad-Bassagasteguy and stored in the nasopharynx (**Fig. 39.5**).
  - Superior/posterior septectomy is performed.
  - Bilateral posterior ethmoidectomy, occasional complete ethmoidectomy depending on pathology and anatomy is performed.

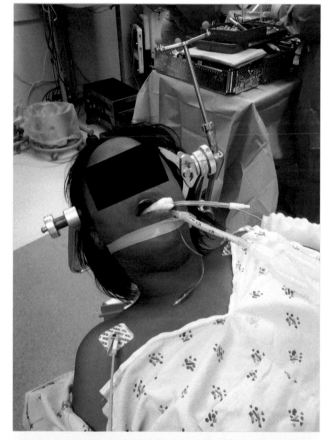

Fig. 39.3 Patient positioning. The head is flexed 10–15°, bringing the bridge of the nose parallel to the floor with a slight 5° rotation to the right and a 10–15° tilt to the opposite side.

  - Wide bilateral sphenoidotomies with removal of horizontal, vertical, or oblique septations are carried out.
  - (Optional) Modified Lothrop approach (for pathology extending up to or ventral to the Crista Galli) (**see Chapter 40).**

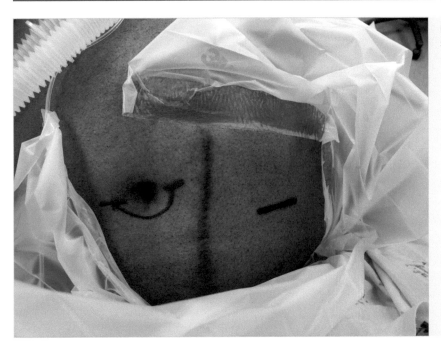

Fig. 39.4 Photograph of the abdomen showing the possible harvesting incision.

- **Bone exposure**
  - ○ Contents of sphenoid from clivus to planum sphenoidale, including carotid prominences, optic-carotid recesses, tuberculum sella, fovea ethmoidalis should be clearly identified. This often requires drilling or ultrasonic bone curettage of intra-sphenoidal septations and ethmoidal septations (**Fig. 39.6**).
  - ○ **Variants**
    - – Removal of endonasal olfactory apparatus via trans-ethmoidal route to reveal the fovea ethmoidalis and cribriform plate for approach to pathology between the planum sphenoidale and the Crista Galli.
    - – Modified Lothrop/Draf III approach to expose the sub-frontal bone for approach to pathology at or ventral to the Crista Galli.

39.7.1 Critical Structures

- Sphenopalatine trunk.
- Septal branch of sphenopalatine artery (must be preserved for flap viability).
- Anterior and posterior ethmoidal arteries.
- Lamina papyracea.
- Olfactory mucosa (typically sacrificed).
- Greater and lesser palatine nerve.

39.8 Craniectomy (Figs. 39.7–39.10)

Craniectomy proceeds in stepwise fashion as follows:
I. Removal of the bone overlying the sella turcica (Fig. 39.7)
  - ○ Exposure from cavernous sinus to cavernous sinus, and tuberculum sella to floor of sella.
  - ○ The inferior extent of exposure may be tailored, but some of the sella must always be exposed to allow for safe resection of the tuberculum sellae.

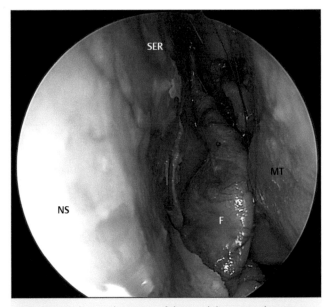

Fig. 39.5 Cadaveric dissection of the nasal dissection showing the nasal flap harvested as per Hadad-Bassagasteguy. The flap is stored in the nasopharynx during surgery.
Abbreviations: F = flap; MT = middle turbinate; NS = nasal septum; SER = spheno-ethmoid recess.

  - ○ This portion of the bony opening may be completed quickly with Kerrison rongeur after a pilot hole is created with a diamond-edge high-speed drill or simply fracturing the sella with a blunt nerve-hook.
II. Removal of the bone of the planum sphenoidale (Fig. 39.8)
  - ○ Exposure from the tuberculum sellae to the posterior ethmoidal artery.
  - ○ Removal may be effected with a diamond edge drill or ultrasonic bone curette, and completed with Kerrison rongeur.
  - ○ The lateral extent of exposure may be tailored, and guided by neuronavigation, but care must be taken

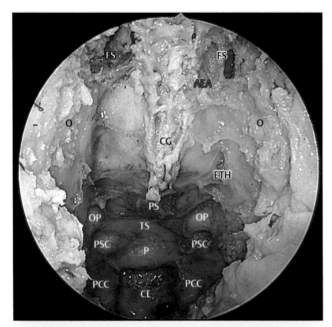

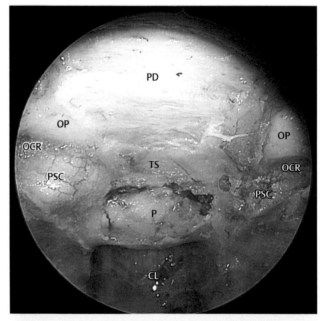

Fig. 39.6 Cadaveric dissection demonstrating contents of sphenoid from clivus to planum sphenoidale, including carotid prominences, optic-carotid recesses, tuberculum sella, fovea ethmoidalis clearly identified. This often requires drilling or ultrasonic bone curettage of intra-sphenoidal septations and ethmoidal septations.
Abbreviations: AEA = anterior ethmoidal artery; CG = crista galli; CL = clivus; ETH = ethmoid; FS = frontal sinus; O = orbit; OP = optic protuberance; P = pituitary gland; PCC = paraclival carotid protuberance; PS = planum sphenoidale; PSC = parasellar segment of the carotid protuberance; TS = tuberculum sellae.

Fig. 39.8 Removal of the bone of the planum sphenoidale. Exposure from the tuberculum sellae to the posterior ethmoidal artery.
Abbreviations: CL = clivus; OCR = lateral optic-carotid recess; OP = optic protuberance; P = pituitary gland; PD = planum dura; PSC = parasellar segment of the carotid protuberance; TS = tuberculum sellae.

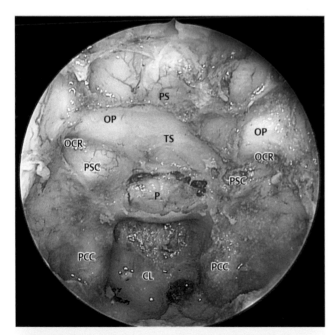

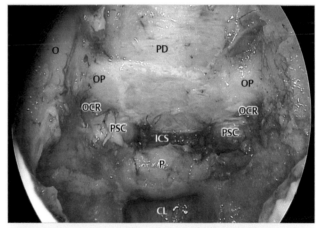

Fig. 39.9 Removal of the limbus sphenoidale and tuberculum sellae. Exposure to the medial edge of optic-carotid recess bilaterally. Removal is most safely effected similar to an anterior clinoidectomy, drilling it out (either with a diamond edge drill or ultrasonic bone curette) to an eggshell and then in-fracturing the cortical bone.
Abbreviations: CL = clivus; ICS = intercavernous sinus; O = orbit; OCR = lateral optic-carotid recess; OP = optic protuberance; P = pituitary gland; PD = planum dura; PSC = parasellar segment of the carotid protuberance.

Fig. 39.7 Removal of the bone overlying the sella turcica. Exposure from cavernous sinus to cavernous sinus, and tuberculum sella to floor of sella. The inferior extent of exposure may be tailored, but some of the sella must always be exposed to allow for safe resection of the tuberculum sellae.
Abbreviations: CL = clivus; OCR = lateral optic-carotid recess; OP = optic protuberance; P = pituitary gland; PCC = paraclival carotid protuberance; PS = planum sphenoidale; PSC = parasellar segment of the carotid protuberance; TS = tuberculum sellae.

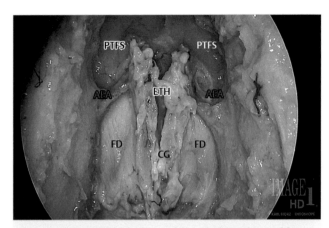

Fig. 39.10 Removal of the bone of the cribriform plate and fovea ethmoidalis. Exposure from posterior to anterior ethmoid or more ventral as pathology requires. The medial edge of the orbit is a hard limit to the lateral extent of exposure for endonasal approaches. The ventral edge of the Crista Galli is a relative ventral limit to the exposure.
Abbreviations: AEA = anterior ethmoidal artery; CG = crista galli; ETH = ethmoid; FD = frontal dura; PTFS = posterior table of the frontal sinus.

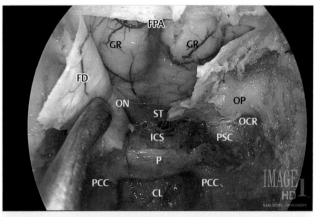

Fig. 39.11 Dural opening: Double I-shaped fashion. Two transverse incisions parallel to the inter-cavernous sinus (above and below). A third transverse incision at the most rostral aspect of exposure (ideally rostral to the pathology to allow definition of normal subarachnoid plane).
Abbreviations: CL = clivus; FD = frontal dura; FPA = frontopolar arteries; GR = gyrus rectus; ICS = intercavernous sinus; OCR = lateral optic-carotid recess; ON = optic nerve; OP = optic protuberance; P = pituitary gland; PCC = paraclival carotid; PSC = parasellar segment of the carotid protuberance; ST = pituitary stalk.

not to inadvertently violate the laminae papyracea. The laminae may be dehiscent depending on the underlying pathology. Dehiscence near the orbital apex may leave the optic nerve exposed in the lateral wall of the sphenoid.

III. Removal of the limbus sphenoidale and tuberculum sellae (Fig. 39.9)
  ○ Exposure to medial edge of optic-carotid recess bilaterally.
  ○ Removal is most safely effected similar to an anterior clinoidectomy, drilling it out (either with a diamond edge drill or ultrasonic bone curette) to an eggshell and then in-fracturing the cortical bone.
  ○ Due to the acute inflections of bone from the sella through tuberculum and limbus to the planum, 90° blunt hooks, micro-curettes and Kerrison rongeurs 1, 1.5, and 2 mm are most useful.
  ○ Care must be taken not to violate the dura of the inter-cavernous sinus, which is densely adherent to the inferior portion of the tuberculum. Sinus bleeding encountered prior to complete removal of the tuberculum may be controlled with either SurgiFlo™ or injecting fibrin glue into the sinus.

IV. (Optional) Removal of the bone of the cribriform plate and fovea ethmoidalis (Fig. 39.10)
  ○ Exposure from posterior to anterior ethmoid or more ventral as pathology requires.
  ○ The medial edge of the orbit is a hard limit to the lateral extent of exposure for endonasal approaches.
  ○ The ventral edge of the Crista Galli is a relative ventral limit to the exposure.
  ○ Extradural removal of the Crista Galli may be effected by dissecting in the subperiosteal dural space and removing it en-block.
  ○ Efforts should be made to skeletonize and cauterize the anterior ethmoidal artery, with sharp controlled transection rather than simply drilling/curetting across it. The artery

can retract into the orbit, and while no arterial bleeding is apparent in the endonasal corridor, entrapment of the orbital contents may ensue due to an intraconal hematoma.

39.8.1 Critical Structures

• Optic nerve (at orbital apex).
• Cavernous and clinoidal carotid artery.
• Medial edge of cavernous sinus.
• Intercavernous sinus.
• Anterior ethmoidal artery.

39.9 Dural Opening (Fig. 39.11)

• Dura is opened in a double I-shaped fashion, as described below:
  ○ Two transverse incisions parallel to the inter-cavernous sinus (above and below).
  ○ A third transverse incision at the most rostral aspect of exposure (ideally rostral to the pathology to allow definition of normal subarachnoid plane).
  ○ A fourth transverse incision (as needed) at the most caudal aspect of the sellar exposure.
• Bipolar cautery across the intercavernous sinus for hemostasis are used (alternatively, small silver clips may be used).
• Mid-sagittal incisions are made transecting the intercavernous sinus and from the rostral transverse incision to the intercavernous sinus.
• Flaps may be reflected laterally or, in case of a meningioma, completely resected.

39.9.1 Critical Structures

• Optic nerve (at orbital apex).
• Medial cavernous sinus.

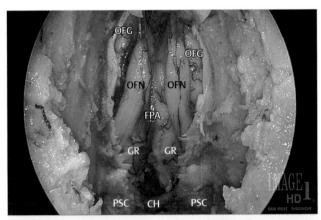

Fig. 39.12 Intradural exposure.
Abbreviations: CH = chiasm; FPA = frontopolar arteries; GR =gyrus rectus; OFG = orbito-frontal gyrus; OFN = olfactory nerve; PSC = parasellar carotid.

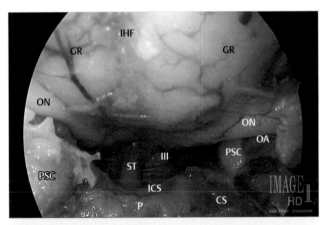

Fig. 39.13 Intradural exposure.
Abbreviations: CS = cavernous sinus; GR =gyrus rectus; ICS = intercavernous sinus; IHF = interhemispheric fissure; III = third cranial nerve; OA = ophthalmic artery; ON = optic nerve; P = pituitary gland; PSC = parasellar carotid; ST = pituitary stalk.

- Carotid siphon (limits extent of lateral opening at the dural ring).
- Ophthalmic artery (often found just above the diaphragm at the lateral extent of the intracranial exposure).
- Intercavernous sinus.
- Olfactory tract and bulb.

39.10 Intradural Exposure (Figs. 39.12–39.14)

- **Parenchymal structures:**
  - Pituitary gland.
  - Infundibulum.
  - Gyri recti.
- **Arachnoidal layer:**
  - Suprasellar cistern arachnoid.
  - Proximal carotid cistern arachnoid.
  - Membrane of Liliequist.
- **Cranial nerves:**
  - Olfactory tracts.
  - Optic nerves and chiasm.

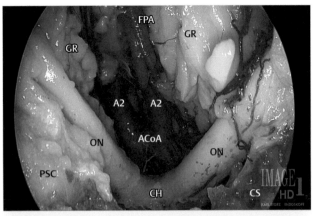

Fig. 39.14 Intradural exposure. Resection of gyri recti has been performed.
Abbreviations: ACoA = anterior communicating artery; A2 = A2 segments of anterior cerebral arteries; CH = chiasm; CS = cavernous sinus; FPA = frontopolar arteries; GR =gyrus rectus; ON = optic nerve; PSC = parasellar carotid.

- **Arteries:**
  - Paraclinoidal carotids.
  - Ophthalmic arteries.
  - Superior hypophyseal artery.
  - Anterior communicating artery.
  - Anterior cerebral arteries (A1, A2 segments).
  - Posterior communicating artery.
  - Fronto-polar arteries.

39.11 Pearls

- Before transitioning from the sinonasal approach to the craniotomy, take a blunt nerve hook or Freer elevator to ensure that the surgeon can reach the skull base as visualized on the endoscope without collision or major restriction. If it is not feasible to outline the planned opening with easy manipulation of the instrument, the surgeon will be limited in their ability to 'reach' what is seen once dura is opened. Expanding the sinonasal exposure with a larger septostomy, expanding the ethmoidectomy and/or turbinate resection will help.
- Care should be taken when using a diamond drill or ultrasonic bone tool at the orbital apex to use copious irrigation as the heat generated by both devices may injure the optic nerve.
- All cuts with knives/scissors should be made from lateral to medial (away from, rather than toward the carotid siphon). Suction is used to help control the extent of the cut in case the knife slips (or collides with the endoscope, which can cause it to jump).
- It is important to have good control of the intercavernous sinus early in the case. It has a tendency to ooze throughout the case, which severely limits your visualization of the suprasellar cistern.
- The pituitary gland and diaphragm sellae (when not disrupted due to pathology) will help to orient the surgeon regardless of pathology. They should always be used as surgeon's "true north."
- Always double confirm location of the carotids with micro-Doppler prior to drilling or making dural incisions in this region. There is a tendency for neuronavigation to have significant errors in this region as it is often at the edge of

the sphere of registration. The combination of Doppler and dead-reckoning based on the sella will always allow the surgeon to identify the carotid as over-reliance on neuronavigation is a recipe for disaster.

• The arachnoid of the suprasellar cistern has to be opened in a vertical fashion in the midline, and then should be swept side-to-side, like a curtain opening on a stage. This minimizes disruption of the infra-chiasmatic perforators from the C4 segment of the carotid, which run from inferolateral to superomedial. Disruption of these perforators can easily cause a chiasmal infarct.

References

1. Bassett E, Farag A, Iloreta A, Farrell C, Evans J, Rosen M, Singh A, Nyquist G. The extended nasoseptal flap for coverage of large cranial base defects. *International Forum of Allergy & Rhinology.* 2016 Nov;6(11)1113–1116.

2. Schwartz TH, Fraser JF, Brown S, Tabaee A, Kacker A, Anand VK. Endoscopic cranial base surgery: classification of operative approaches. Neurosurgery 62:991–1002;discussion 1002-1005, 2008.

3. Schwartz TH, Fraser JF, Brown S, Tabaee A, Kacker A, Anand VK: Endoscopic cranial base surgery: classification of operative approaches. Neurosurgery 62:991–1002; discussion 1002-1005, 2008.

4. Singh A, Wessell A. Surgical anatomy and physiology for the skull base surgeon. *Operative Techniques in Otolaryngology-Head and Neck Surgery.* 2011 Sep;22(3):183–252.

5. Wessell A, Singh A, Litvack Z. One-piece modified gasket seal technique. *J Neurol Surg B Skull Base.* 2013 Oct; 74(5):305:10.

6. Wessell A, Singh A, Litvack Z. Preservation of olfaction after unilateral endoscopic approach for resection of esthesioneuroblastoma. *J Neurol Surg Rep.* 2014 Aug;75(1):e149–53.

40 Endoscopic Endonasal Modified Lothrop Approach to Anterior Cranial Fossa

Yi Chen Zhao, Peter-John Wormald, and Stephen Santoreneos

40.1 Introduction

The endoscopic endonasal modified Lothrop approach is an endoscopic approach, which provides access to the frontal sinus and the anterior skull-base, through a minimally invasive trans-septal, endonasal surgical route.

It is indicated in the treatment of lesions harboring from the anterior cranial fossa, located anterior to the anterior ethmoidal artery.

40.2 Indications

- Endonasal endoscopic modified Lothrop is an access procedure to the anterior cranial fossa that is required when the pathology extends or is located anterior to the anterior ethmoidal artery.

40.3 Patient Positioning

- **Position:** The patient is positioned supine in reverse Trendelenburg position.
- **Body:** The body is placed in reverse Trendelenburg with elevation of the head to 20° to the horizontal (**Fig. 40.1**).
- **Head:** The head is positioned neutrally to keep the skull base parallel to the endoscope pathway to avoid inadvertent injury to the skull base. Head is placed on a head ring.
- **Instrument and surgeon setup:** The monitor stack should be placed at the head of the patient making a straight line

with the patient's head and the surgeon. The right-handed surgeon typically will sit on the right side of the patient with the second surgeon standing behind. The scrub nurse stands on the contralateral side to the surgeon with the tray table facing the monitor (**Figs. 40.2, 40.3**).

40.4 Nasal Preparation

- Preparation of nasal cavity with topical local anesthetic and injections is carried out.
- Half strength betadine is used to prepare the face.
- Full strength betadine is used to prepare thigh for possible tensor fascia lata harvest.
- Image guidance system is set up and calibrated.

40.5 Soft Tissue Dissection

- Key landmarks to identify intra-nasally before the start of endoscopic Lothrop procedure are as follows:
  - Nasal septum.
  - Middle turbinate.
  - Superior turbinate.
  - Frontal sinus ostium.
  - Nasal vault.
  - Skull base.
- Typically, bilateral endoscopic middle meatal antrostomy, complete spheno-ethmoidectomy, and frontal recess

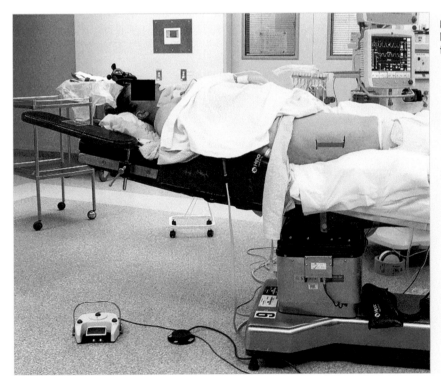

Fig. 40.1 Patient setup with reverse Trendelenburg position with lateral thigh exposed for potential tensor fascia lata harvest.

dissection is performed first to identify the skull base from the planum sphenoidale to the posterior table of the frontal sinus.

- Resection of both middle turbinates is typically required to access the anterior skull base.
- If a skull base defect is anticipated, then a unilateral Haddad nasoseptal mucoperichondrial flap based on the posterior nasal artery is raised and placed into the posterior nasal space. A bilateral flap is raised if the entire skull base is resected.
- Middle meatal antrostomy followed by anterior ethmoidectomy, posterior ethmoidectomy, and sphenoidectomy is performed.
- The sphenoid sinus is then widely opened with removal of the anterior face of the sphenoid to clearly identify the skull base.
- Care needs to be taken when performing the sphenoidectomy that the pedicle of the nasoseptal flap is not injured along the anterior wall of the sphenoid sinus.
- A superior septectomy is then performed. Specific measurements are not given for the size of the septal window, as it needs to be tailored to individual patient's anatomy (**Fig. 40.4**).
- The septal windows need to be large enough anteriorly to see the following:
  - The contralateral frontal process of the maxilla.
  - The ipsilateral middle turbinate (posteriorly).
  - The contralateral axilla of the middle turbinate (inferiorly).
  - The roof of the nasal cavity (superiorly).
- Anteriorly based lateral nasal mucosal flaps are raised bilaterally from the lateral nasal wall superior to the attachment of the middle turbinate. Posteriorly it extends 2 mm behind the axilla of the middle turbinate, superiorly to the roof of the nose, and inferiorly at the axilla of the middle turbinate.

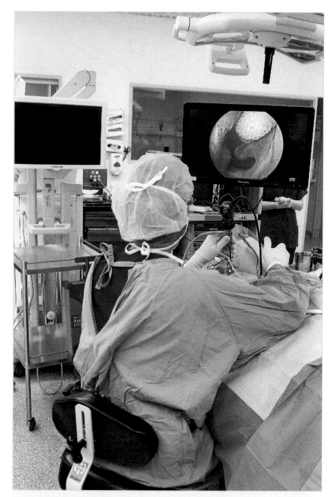

Fig. 40.2 Positioning of video monitor and patient in line with the operative position of the surgeon.

Fig. 40.3 Setup of two-surgeons approach. Scrub nurse position opposite the surgeons.

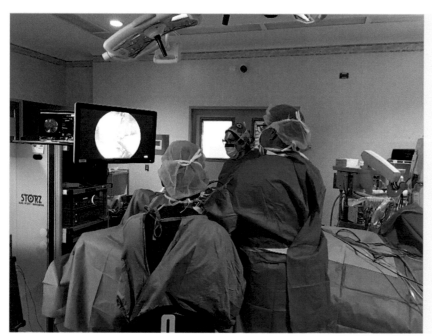

40.6 Bone Exposure

- Bone removal begins with a high-speed drill (long endonasal attachment, 40° cutting burr) by directing it across the septal window to remove the bone of the ascending process of the maxilla (**Figs. 40.4**, **40.5**).
- The bone removal is then directed superiorly from the frontal ostium into the frontal sinus. It is important to ensure that bone is removed superior-laterally first prior to moving medially to avoid inadvertent injury of the skull base (**Fig. 40.6**, **40.7**).
- The procedure is repeated on the opposite side. The floor of the frontal sinus is removed. Any septation is also removed to create a single cavity to improve drainage from the frontal sinus to the nose.
- The mucosa over the roof of the nose is reflected until the first olfactory neurons are encountered. This location can further be confirmed with image guidance. This marks the anterior limit of the skull base and the posterior limit of the bony dissection of the endoscopic modified Lothrop procedure (**Fig. 40.8**).
- The remnant of the floor of the frontal sinus ("frontal T") is lowered to the level of the skull base (**Fig. 40.9**).
- The remnant of the frontal beak of the maxilla is then removed with an angled cutting burr under 30° scope guidance until the anterior nasal skin is reached (**Fig. 40.10**).
- At the end of the bone removal, the entire skull base should be exposed from the sphenoid to the posterior table of the frontal sinus (**Fig. 40.11**).

- Anterior and posterior ethmoidal arteries are identified along the skull base or within their mesentry and are bipolar cauterized before divided with skull base scissors.

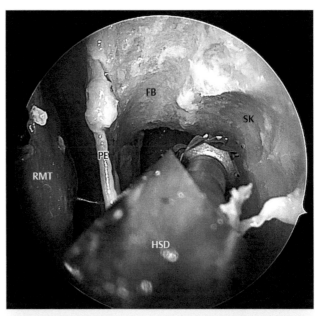

Fig. 40.5 Cadaveric dissection demonstrating initial drilling laterally to expose the subcutaneous skin marked with SK.
Abbreviations: FB = frontal beak which form the floor of the frontal sinus; HSD = high-speed drill; PE = posterior edge of septectomy; RMT = middle turbinate of the right side; SK = skin of the lateral nasal wall marking the lateral extent of the drilling.

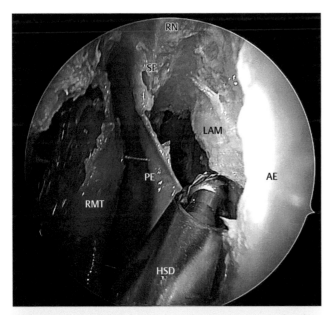

Fig. 40.4 Cadaveric dissection photo demonstrating completed septal window with drill on the ascending process of the maxilla passing through the septal window.
Abbreviations: AE = anterior edge of septectomy; HSD = high-speed drill; LAM = ascending process of maxilla of the left side; PE = posterior edge of septectomy; RMT = middle turbinate of the right side; RN = roof of nasal cavity; SE = superior edge of septectomy.

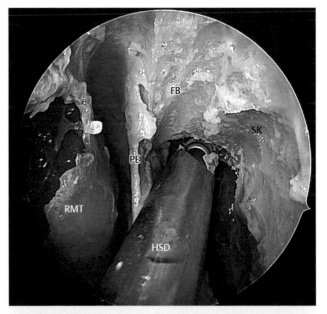

Fig. 40.6 Cadaveric dissection demonstrating drilling directed superiorly from frontal ostium toward frontal beak.
Abbreviations: FB = frontal beak which form the floor of the frontal sinus; HSD = high-speed drill; PE = posterior edge of septectomy; RMT = middle turbinate of the right side; SK = skin of the lateral nasal wall marking the lateral extent of the drilling.

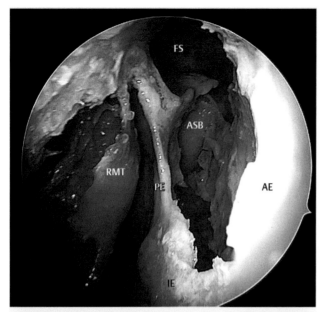

Fig. 40.7 Cadaveric dissection through the floor of the left frontal sinus. Note this is done through the septal window from the contra-lateral side.
Abbreviations: AE = anterior edge of septectomy; ASB = anterior skull base at the transitional zone between the posterior wall of the frontal sinus to the ethmoidal roof; FS = frontal sinus; IE = inferior edge of septectomy; PE = posterior edge of septectomy; RMT = middle turbinate of the right side.

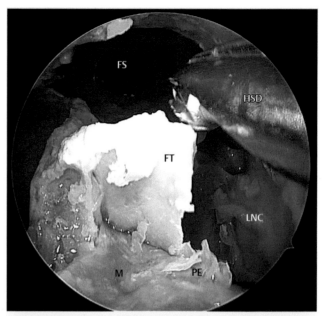

Fig. 40.9 Cadaveric dissection demonstrating lowering of the "frontal T" with straight burr. Note the frontal sinus that can be seen in the distance.
Abbreviations: FS = frontal sinus with the intersinus septum seen in the distance; FT = frontal T; HSD = high-speed drill; LNC = left nasal cavity; M = mucosa; PE = posterior edge of septectomy.

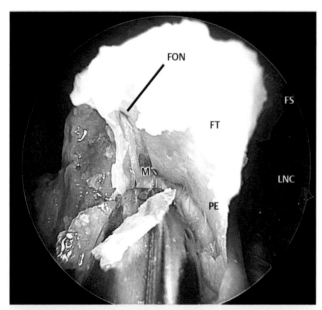

Fig. 40.8 Cadaveric dissection demonstrating mucosa of roof of nose reflected to demonstrate first olfactory neuron by the arrow.
Abbreviations: FON = first olfactory neuron; FS = frontal sinus; FT = frontal T which is formed by the raiment of the superior septum; LNC = left nasal cavity; M = mucosa; PE = posterior edge of septectomy.

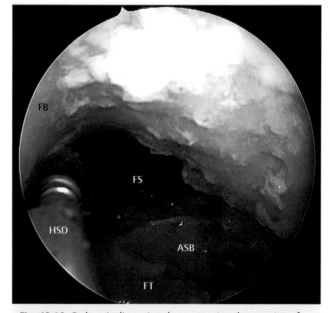

Fig. 40.10 Cadaveric dissection demonstrating the opening of the frontal sinus.
Abbreviations: ASB = anterior skull base; FB = frontal beak which forms the floor of the frontal sinus; FS = frontal sinus; FT = frontal T; HSD = high-speed drill.

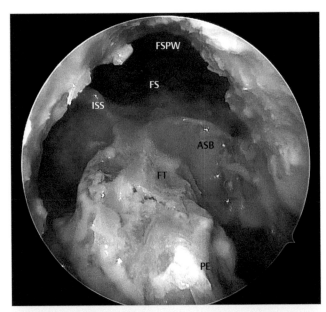

Fig. 40.11 Cadaveric dissection after completion of Lothrop procedure demonstrates view of posterior table of frontal sinus and anterior skull base.
Abbreviations: ASB = anterior skull base; FS = frontal sinus or the Lothrop cavity; FSPW = frontal sinus posterior wall; FT = frontal T already lowered; ISS = intersinus septum of frontal sinus; PE = posterior edge of septectomy.

40.7 Craniectomy/Skull Base Removal

- The specific size and location of the craniectomy depends on the location of the targeted pathology.
- Endoscopic craniectomy is frequently performed with an endoscopic 3.2 mm diamond burr, which safely thins the bone and exposes underlying dura in a controlled manner.
- A translucent and fragile layer of bone is often left on the dura and removed with Kerrison rongeurs.
- The margins of the craniectomy can be extended as required.
- Suprasellar tumors generally require an extended transphenoidal exposure, which includes the pituitary fossa, tuberculum, and planum sphenoidale. The exposure has a typical dumbbell shape with the narrowest diameter at the level of the opticocarotid recesses (OCRs). The lateral and medial OCRs are well visualized and important landmarks for the lateral exposure at the level of the tuberculum and the carotids.
- The more anterior the tumor, the larger the bone resection required. Ultimately a modified Lothrop exposure is necessary and the cribriform plate needs to be drilled sacrificing olfaction if tumors attached to the falx are approached.

40.8 Dura Opening

- Dura is opened with a size 11-scalpel blade mostly and completed with skull base scissors. Reusable dural knives of various shapes can be useful in this step particularly of the most anterior margins of the dura.

- For relatively small sellar or suprasellar tumors we prefer a cruciate incision.
  - o The vertical limb extends through the dural fold distally and coagulation is required to control the intercavernous sinus.
  - o Coagulation of the dural leaves augments exposure to define the relevant anatomical landmarks such as the pituitary stalk, optic chiasm, optic nerves and vascular anatomy.
- For large anterior skull base tumors, we prefer to use a circumferential incision of the dura.
  - o This commences on each side distally at the planum or tuberculum dura and extends along the lateral margins of the craniectomy to meet in the midline just anterior to crista galli.
  - o It allows for the very important access and division of the falx attachment, encourages the tumor to descend and generally exposes the junction of tumor and brain.
- The crista galli is frequently drilled away with the diamond burr. The attachment of the falx cerebri to the crista is then bipolar cauterized and incised with scissors or 11-blade with counter traction. There is a natural tendency to continue dividing the falx deeply following the length of the falx. It is important to direct the incision posteriorly to disconnect the attachment.
- Bridging veins draining to the falx cerebri need to be coagulated and divided carefully. Although venous anatomy can be variable, bridging draining veins from the olfactory bulbs and frontal poles are quite constant.
- Branches of the frontopolar and medial orbitofrontal arteries need to be preserved. The falx cerebri attachment must be divided to allow the anterior skull base to "drop" into the nasal cavity.

40.9 Tumor Resection

- The techniques employed in resecting a tumor endoscopically are no different to transcranial surgery. The fundamental principles of early devascularization by removing the bony and dural base followed by debulking of the tumor internally and collapsing the capsule whilst preserving the surrounding structures, remain the same.
- Often, particularly with smaller lesions, the arachnoid plane is preserved and en block resection or delivery of the capsule is relatively straightforward by sweeping arachnoid away with a regulated sucker on cottonoid or a dissector.
- Large tumors, however, in particular if the brain is edematous, as signaled by high T2 signal in the surrounding brain on MRI, inevitably may require subpial resection. The bipolar forceps, suction, and microscissors are the instruments used most commonly and interchangeably to develop the plane.
  - o It is important to achieve absolute hemostasis using direct coagulation, thorough irrigation and, often, hemostatic agents such as oxidized cellulose.
  - o Care is required not to miss a developing hematoma within the frontal lobes from a retracted divided or avulsed vessel or to leave unsecured vessels behind that are in spasm but may bleed later.
- Central debulking of the tumor is performed with an Ultrasonic Aspirator (CUSA, Integra Lifesciences, NJ,

USA) or Sonopet (Stryker, MI, USA). Not unlike transcranial procedures, the use of these instruments close to critical structures needs to be precise, extremely careful, and at appropriate settings for the consistency of tumor.

- The final step in the resection is to inspect the dural margins. If endoscopic surgery is to match the outcomes of transcranial meningioma resection, then it is important to achieve gross total dural resection, if safe. This is often limited by the internal carotids at the medial OCR as well as the extent of the tumor laterally. Margins beyond the midpoint of the orbital roof are difficult to visualize or reach.

40.10 Skull Base Reconstruction

- Once resection is completed, the skull base is reconstructed in a multi-layered fashion. The internal layer is placed as an underlay graft using tensor fascia lata or DuraGen (Integra, New Jersey, USA). In larger defects, a titanium mesh plate is also used to provide structural support.
- A second layer of fascia or DuraGen is then placed as an overlay fashion before the vascularized nasoseptal flap is placed to mucosal covering and Duraseal (Integra, Lifesciences, NJ, USA) is used to seal the area.

References

1. Alokby G, Casiano RR. Endoscopic resection of sinonasal and ventral skull base malignancies. Otolaryngol Clin North Am 2017; 50(2):273–285.
2. Hadad G, Bassagasteguy L, Carrau RL, et al. A novel reconstructive technique after endoscopic expanded endonasal approaches: vascular pedicle nasoseptal flap. Laryngoscope 2006; 116(10):1882–1886.
3. Snyderman CH, Carrau RL, Kassam AB, et al. Endoscopic skull base surgery: principles of endonasal oncological surgery. J Surg Oncol 2008; 97(8):658–664.
4. Wormald PJ. "Chapter 9 Extended Approaches to the Frontal Sinus: The Frontal Drillout or Modified endoscopic Lothrop (Draf 3) Procedure" Endoscopic sinus surgery: anatomy, three-dimensional reconstruction, and surgical technique. 4th ed. Thieme; 2017.
5. Wormald PJ. "Chapter 20 Endoscopic Resection of Anterior Cranial Fossa Tumours" Endoscopic sinus surgery: anatomy, three-dimensional reconstruction, and surgical technique. 4th ed. Thieme; 2017.
6. Zuniga MG, Turner JH, Chandra RK. Updates in anterior skull base reconstruction. Curr Opin Otolaryngol Head Neck Surg 2016; 24(1):75–82.

41 Endoscopic Endonasal Odontoidectomy

Ellina Hattar, Eleonora F. Spinazzi, Jean Anderson Eloy, Cristian Gragnaniello, and James K. Liu

41.1 Introduction

The transoral route has served as the gold-standard approach for treating pathologies of the craniocervical junction. Since its emergence, this microscopic transoral approach has been the preferred route for performing anterior odontoidectomy to decompress the craniovertebral junction.

Pathologies that have been treated with this route have included basilar invagination, platybasia with retroflexed odontoid process, rheumatoid pannus, chordomas, and chondrosarcomas.

Extended versions of the transoral approach used to increase visualization as well as the operative field have included the extended "open-door" maxillotomy, transpalatal, transmaxillary, and transmandibular approaches. In recent years, the endoscopic endonasal approach has emerged as a minimally invasive surgical alternative.

The technique is especially well suited for pathologies located above the palatine line. By avoiding the oral cavity and obviating the need for oral retraction, the endonasal route avoids complications associated with tongue swelling, prolonged intubation, tracheal swelling, velopharyngeal insufficiency, dysphonia, and dysphagia. The procedure is also associated with a shorter hospital stay and post-operative recovery. In this chapter, we describe the operative technique and surgical nuances for performing endoscopic endonasal odontoidectomy.

41.2 Indications

- Irreducible basilar invagination causing brainstem compression and myelopathy.

- Symptomatic and compressive rheumatoid pannus refractory to posterior stabilization.
- *Os odontoideum.*
- Retroflexed odontoid process associated with Type I Chiari malformation resulting in compressive myelopathy.

41.3 Patient Positioning (Figs. 41.1, 41.2)

- **Position**: The patient is positioned supine in neutral position with the head fixed with a Mayfield head holder.
- **Body**: The body is positioned horizontal.
- **Head**: The head is placed in neutral position, no flexion or extension, no head rotation are needed.
- **Anti-decubitus device**: All pressure points are adequately padded; an anti-decubital pad is placed on the sacrum.
- **The nasal tip** is the highest point in the surgical field.
- **Gentle axial traction** can be applied to the head before final fixation of the Mayfield head holder to allow for some decompression of the cervico-medullary junction.
- Use CT-based frameless stereotactic image guidance for intraoperative localization.
- Use somatosensory and motor evoked potential neurophysiologic monitoring.

41.4 Exposure and Incision

- **Goldman elevator** is used to lateralize the middle and inferior turbinates.

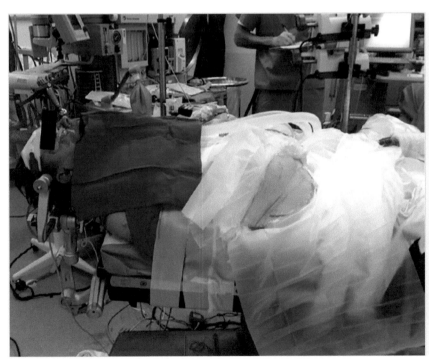

Fig. 41.1 Patient positioning. The patient is positioned supine with the head in a Mayfield head holder.

- **Pedicled Nasoseptal Flap (PNSF) (See Chapters 38 and 39)**
  - ○ Right flap is harvested with care to preserve the vascular pedicle supplied by the posterior septal branch of the sphenopalatine artery.
  - ○ Flap is elevated from the muco-perichondrium and muco-periosteum.
  - ○ Flap is tucked into the ipsilateral middle meatus until the reconstruction phase with the vascular pedicle superior to the level of the choana.
  - ○ PNSF harvesting is repeated on the contralateral side.

- **Posterior septectomy** (Fig. 41.3)
  - ○ The posterior and inferior aspect of the bony and cartilaginous septum are removed to allow triangulation of instruments using binostril access.
  - ○ The mucosal integrity of the posterior nasal septum is preserved.

41.4.1 Critical Structures

- Eustachian tubes.
- Bilateral upper cervical carotid arteries.
- Bilateral vertebral arteries.
- Sympathetic chain.

41.5 Soft Tissue Dissection

- **Mucosal incision and pharyngeal muscles** (Fig. 41.4)
  - ○ A longitudinal midline incision is made over the posterior or pharyngeal mucosal wall overlying the tubercle of the atlas (C1).
  - ○ The incision is extended vertically to expose the inferior clivus (superiorly), down to the second cervical vertebral (C2) body (inferiorly).
  - ○ The incision is extended through the mucosa along the midline raphe, between the pharyngeal muscles, and through the anterior longitudinal ligament down to the bone of C1.

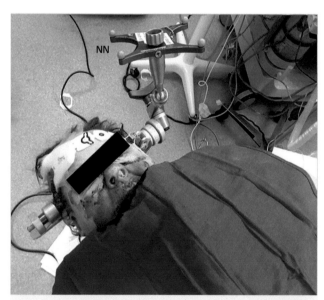

Fig. 41.2 Stereotactic frameless image guidance is used and the nose and nares are prepped with betadine.
Abbreviations: NN = neuronavigator.

- ○ The *longus colli* and *longus capitis* muscles are mobilized laterally with an extended length and protected tip Bovie monopolar cautery in a subperiosteal fashion to better expose the anterior tubercle of C1.

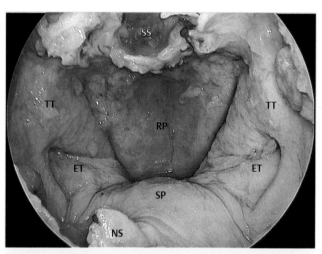

Fig. 41.3 Endoscopic endonasal exposure. A posterior septectomy has been performed at the inferior aspect of the nasal septum at the level of the hard palate to allow binostril access to the craniovertebral junction at the posterior pharyngeal wall. The soft palate is visualized in the midline posteriorly and the *torus tubarius* and Eustachian tube are visualized on each side laterally. The floor of the sphenoid sinus is exposed here to help orient the midline and the top of the lower third of the clivus.
Abbreviations: ET = Eustachian tube; NS = nasal septum; RP = rhinopharynx; SP = soft palate; SS = sphenoid sinus; TT = torus tubarius.

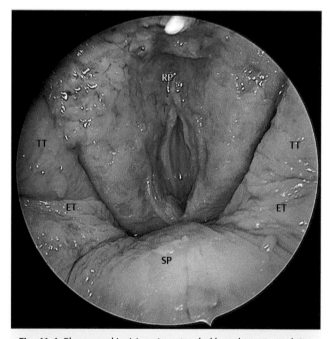

Fig. 41.4 Pharyngeal incision. An extended length, protected tip, Bovie monopolar cautery is used to make a vertical incision in the mucosa of the nasopharynx and through the pharyngeal muscles down to the arch of C1. Care is taken to stay in the midline. The soft palate is visualized in the midline here.
Abbreviations: ET = Eustachian tube; RP = rhinopharynx; SP = soft palate; TT = torus tubarius.

○ A suction-rotation microdebrider is used to debulk the overlying muscles to minimize any obstruction of line of sight to the arch of C1.

• **Bony exposure** (**Figs. 41.5, 41.6**)
○ In select cases of platybasia, a sphenoidotomy is performed and the midline mucosal incision is expanded from the floor of the sphenoid sinus down to the inferior clivus. This allows access to the lower clivus, which may need to be removed in order to access the odontoid in severe cases of basilar invagination.
○ All soft tissues are removed from the anterior arch of C1 and the odontoid process.

41.5.1 Critical Structures

• Vertebral arteries.
• Carotid arteries.
• Vidian nerves.

41.6 Endoscopic Endonasal Odontoidectomy and Decompression

• **Removal of C1 anterior arch** (**Figs. 41.7, 41.8**)
○ The anterior arch of C1 is removed with a high-speed cutting drill with a slight curve and piggy-back self-irrigation using eggshell technique.

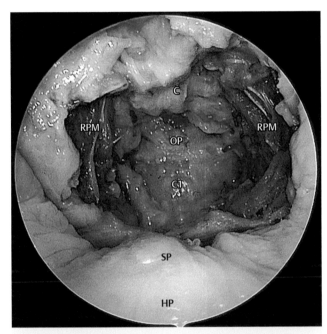

Fig. 41.5 The anterior arch of C1 is exposed sub-periosteally. The top of the odontoid process is seen behind the C1 arch and the bottom of the clivus is seen above the tip of the odontoid. The hard palate and soft palate are visualized along the floor of the nose. Abbreviations: C = clivus; C1 = anterior arch of C1; HP = hard palate; OP = odontoid process; RPM = retropharyngeal muscles; SP = soft palate.

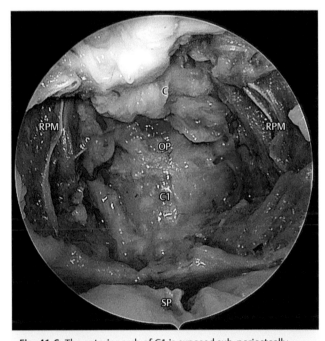

Fig. 41.6 The anterior arch of C1 is exposed sub-periosteally. View at higher magnification. Abbreviations: C = clivus; C1 = anterior arch of C1; OP = odontoid process; RPM = retropharyngeal muscles; SP = soft palate.

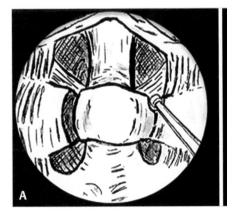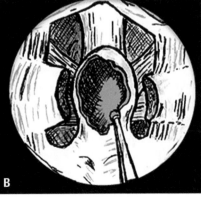

Fig. 41.7 Drawing depicting the endoscopic endonasal technique for anterior arch removal (**A**) and subsequent odontoidectomy (**B**). The anterior arch of C1 is drilled off with care not to violate the C1 lateral masses. The odontoid process is hollowed out, leaving an eggshell layer of cortical bone that is removed with curettes and rongeurs.

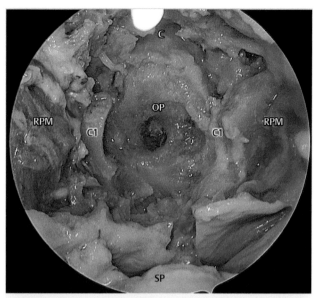

Fig. 41.8 C1 arch is drilled out to expose the odontoid process. Care is taken to preserve the C1 lateral masses laterally. Abbreviations: C = clivus; C1 = anterior arch of C1; OP = odontoid process; RPM = retropharyngeal muscles; SP = soft palate.

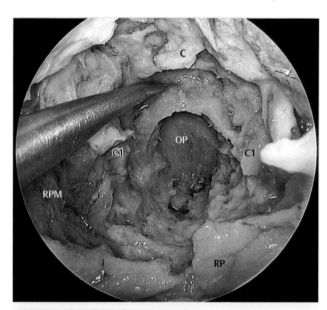

Fig. 41.9 The odontoid process is hollowed out with a high-speed drill leaving a thin cortical rim. Abbreviations: C = clivus; C1 = anterior arch of C1; OP = odontoid process; RP = rhinopharynx; RPM = retropharyngeal muscles.

- ○ Residual bone is removed with angled curettes and Kerrison rongeurs.
- ○ The width of the arch resection must allow adequate exposure of both lateral margins of the odontoid process.
- ○ Care is taken to avoid violation of the medial aspects of the lateral masses of C1.

- **Odontoid process resection** (Figs. 41.8, 41.9)
  - ○ The edges of the odontoid process are freed from the apical and alar ligaments using sharp straight and angled curettes.
  - ○ A soft-tissue pannus located in the atlanto-dental interval space may be present in patients with atlantoaxial

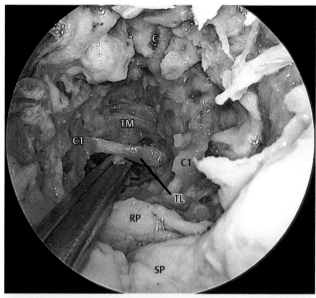

Fig. 41.10 The thin cortical shell of the odontoid process, the ligamentous structures, including the transverse ligament, is carefully dissected away from the underlying dura with an angled curette and removed with Kerrison rongeurs. Any remaining pannus and compressive fibrous tissue is removed to expose the underlying dura of the craniovertebral junction. Abbreviations: C = clivus; C1 = anterior arch of C1; RP = rhinopharynx; SP = soft palate; TL = transverse ligament; TM = tectorial membrane.

instability and should be removed with a Bovie monopolar cautery and pituitary rongeurs.
- ○ The center of the odontoid process is hollowed out with a high-speed cutting drill with a slight curve and piggy-back self-irrigation using eggshell technique.
- ○ The outer cortical layer is removed with a high-speed diamond drill to avoid iatrogenic durotomy.
- ○ Residual eggshell thin bone is out-fractured away from the spinal cord and removed with up-angled curettes and pituitary rongeurs.
- ○ In cases of severe basilar invagination, the inferior clivus is removed using eggshell technique with a high-speed diamond drill to access the retroclival odontoid.

- **Ventral decompression** (Figs. 41.10, 41.11)
  - ○ The transverse ligament, tectorial membrane, and any residual ligaments are removed to decompress dura mater overlying the craniovertebral junction.
  - ○ Any soft tissue pannus is carefully dissected off the dura with an up-angled curette and removed with pituitary and Kerrison rongeurs.
  - ○ If there is any dense adhesion to the dura, the pannus is debulked so that minimal soft tissue adhesions remain on the dura to avoid a cerebrospinal fluid (CSF) leak.
  - ○ Visualization of re-expansion of the dural tube is necessary to ensure adequate ventral decompression.

41.7 Reconstruction

- **When there is no evidence of CSF leak**
  - ○ Both PNSFs are returned to their harvest site and secured with absorbable sutures running in a quilting pattern.

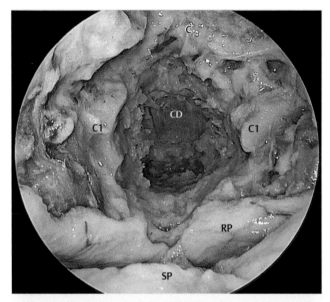

Fig. 41.11 Final view after odontoidectomy, showing the dura of the craniovertebral junction. The cut edges of C1 and the base of C2 are visualized.
Abbreviations: C = clivus; CD = clival dura; C1 = anterior arch of C1; RP = rhinopharynx; SP = soft palate.

○ Surgicel and gentamicin-soaked Gelfoam pledgets are placed into the odontoidectomy defect, with care not to compress the dural tube.

- **In the event of a CSF leak**
  ○ The durotomy is plugged with an Alloderm graft followed by a fascia lata onlay graft.
  ○ A fat graft is used to fill the odontoidectomy dead space.
  ○ One of the two previously harvested PNSFs is rotated over the defect.
  ○ The contralateral PNSF is returned to its original position and secured with absorbable sutures.
  ○ Surgicel and gentamicin-soaked Gelfoam pledgets are placed over the PNSF followed by an expandable Merocel pack which is removed on postoperative day 10 to 12.
  ○ Postoperative lumbar drainage is used for 3 to 5 days.

41.8 Surgical Corridor Landmarks

- **Laterally:** Eustachian tubes.
- **Inferiorly:** Nasal floor, soft and hard palates.
- **Superiorly:** Clivus-septum junction.

41.9 Pearls

- Use CT-based frameless stereotactic image guidance for intraoperative localization.
- Use somatosensory and motor evoked potentials neurophysiologic monitoring.
- Naso-axial line helps predict the inferior limit.
- Lateral C-arm fluoroscopy can be used to assess the extent of odontoidectomy and ventral decompression.
- Staying in the midline is critical to avoid injury to laterally based critical structures.
- Eggshell drilling technique with a high-speed drill followed by removal of thin cortical shell.
- Avoid using Kerrison rongeurs in patient with severe compressive myelopathy, as the foot plate of the Kerrison rongeur can cause increased spinal cord compression in pre-existing severe stenosis. Safer to use a 4-0 or 5-0 up-angled curette to out-fracture eggshelled cortical bone.
- Leave thin remnants of fibrous soft tissue adhesions to the dural tube to avoid durotomy and CSF leak.
- In the event of CSF leak intraoperative, use a multi-layered repair with PNSF reconstruction.

References

1. Aldana PR, Naseri I, La Corte E. The naso-axial line: a new method of accurately predicting the inferior limit of the endoscopic endonasal approach to the craniovertebral junction. Neurosurgery 2012;71(2, Suppl Operative) ons308–ons314, discussion ons314.
2. Choudhri O, Mindea SA, Feroze A, Soudry E, Chang SD, Nayak JV. Experience with intraoperative navigation and imaging during endoscopic transnasal spinal approaches to the foramen magnum and odontoid. Neurosurg Focus 2014;36(3):E4.
3. de Almeida JR, Zanation AM, Snyderman CH, et al. Defining the nasopalatine line: the limit for endonasal surgery of the spine. Laryngoscope 2009;119(2):239–244.
4. Liu JK, Patel J, Goldstein IM, Eloy JA. Endoscopic endonasal transclival transodontoid approach for ventral decompression of the craniovertebral junction: operative technique and nuances. Neurosurg Focus 2015;38(4):E17.

42 Endoscopic Transoral Approach

Edward E. Kerr, Lamia Buohliqah, Farid M. Elhefnawi, Ricardo L. Carrau, and Daniel M. Prevedello

42.1 Introduction

The endoscopic transoral approach is a midline approach to the craniocervical junction. It is suitable for surgical exposure of the clivus, as well as the anterior aspect of the magnum foramen, the atlas, and the axis (C1 and C2).

Surgical exposure can be further widened laterally through the retrostyloid approach gaining access to the jugular foramen region.

The midline approach is indicated for extradural lesions involving the anterior aspect of the craniovertebral junction. The lateral variants are instead indicated to treat lesions involving the jugular foramen, lower cranial nerves.

42.2 Indications

42.2.1 Midline Approach to the Craniovertebral Junction

- Extradural neoplasms (chordoma, chondrosarcoma) situated in the anterior midline craniovertebral junction region.

- Cord-compressive masses (such as reactive pannus secondary to trauma or rheumatoid diseases) situated anteriorly to the lower cranial nerves, at the craniovertebral junction in the setting of a contraindication to an endonasal approach.

42.2.2 Parapharyngeal Retrostyloid Approach

- Paragangliomas situated mostly or entirely caudal to the jugular foramen.
- Benign peripheral nerve tumors (schwannomas and neurofibromas) of the lower cranial nerves.
- Carotid body tumors below the foramen lacerum.

42.3 Patient Positioning (Fig. 42.1)

- **General position:** The body is positioned supine with the head on a horseshoe or cranial fixation pins.
- **Head position:** For maximum surgeon comfort, the neck should be neutral or slightly flexed. Assuming a two-surgeon team

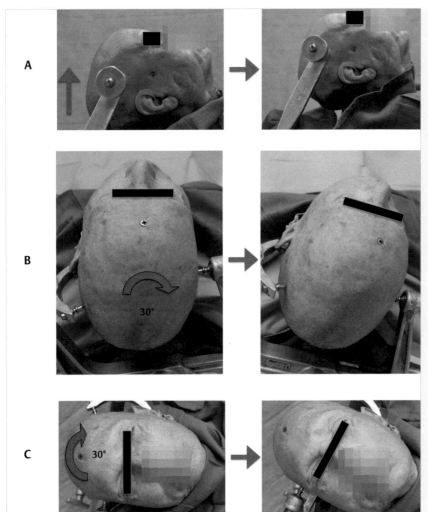

Fig. 42.1 Head positioning. **(A)** The head is translated vertically to prevent the instruments from hitting the chest, especially when the head must be placed in a flexed position. **(B)** The head is rotated approximately 30° to the right along the coronal plane of the body if both surgeons are right-handed. This may be left neutral if one member of the team is left-handed. **(C)** The head is tilted approximately 30° along the sagittal axis of the body if both surgeons are right-handed to prevent them from having to reach across the torso to operate. This may be left neutral if one member of the team is left-handed.

(typically an otolaryngologist and a neurosurgeon), a three-step process further maximizes ergonomics for the surgeons:

- o **1.** The head is elevated slightly from the body (**Fig. 42.1A**).
- o **2.** It is tilted slightly toward the left relative to the axis of the body for right-handed teams (**Fig. 42.1B**).
- o **3.** It is further turned slightly toward the right or left for surgical teams that are completely right- or left-handed, respectively or left neutral for teams of mixed handedness (**Fig. 42.1C**).

- **Anti-decubitus device:** Standard pressure point padding for dependent pressure points in the supine position, including the elbow joints, ulnar nerves if wrapping the patient and foregoing the use of arm boards, the sacral prominence, and the heels might be used.
- **Unique preparation consideration:** The periumbilical and/ or anterolateral thigh should be prepared using the surgeon's choice of antimicrobial agent and draped so that they are available for fat and/or muscle graft if needed for dural defect repair or carotid artery injury.

42.4 Oropharyngeal Access and Retraction

- No skin incision is required to access the posterior oropharyngeal mucosa.
- An oral retractor (such as a Dingman or Spetzler Sonntag retractor) is used to keep the mouth open and tongue retracted caudally throughout the case, carefully avoiding injury to the teeth and protecting the endotracheal tube behind the retractor.
- The two anatomic regions relevant to the skull base neurosurgeon via this approach are the craniovertebral junction (may require a midline transpalatal approach) and the

region of the parapharyngeal internal carotid artery (ICA), foramen lacerum, and jugular foramen (requiring a parapharyngeal retrostyloid approach).

42.4.1 Critical Structures

- Tongue.
- Teeth.
- Soft palate.
- Uvula.
- Palatoglossal arch (anterior pillar).

42.5 Midline Approach to the Craniovertebral Junction

- Once patient is under general anesthesia and the endotracheal tube is secured very laterally in the mouth, a rubber band is passed from the nostrils and it is encountered in the oropharynx. The rubber band is retracted anteriorly bringing the soft palate away from the oropharynx allowing for palate sparing transoral approach.
- In cases of high position of C2, the authors prefer a transnasal approach. However, if there is a need for transoral approach, the soft palate can be transected entirely to permit lateral retraction for oropharyngeal exposure. To accomplish this, an incision is made just lateral to the uvula on either side and curved toward midline above the uvular base. This is extended cranially to the junction with the hard palate (**Fig. 42.2**). Hooks or sutures are then used to maintain lateral retraction of the split soft palate.
- The oropharyngeal mucosa is incised at the midline (**Fig. 42.3**) and reflected laterally, exposing the horizontally-oriented

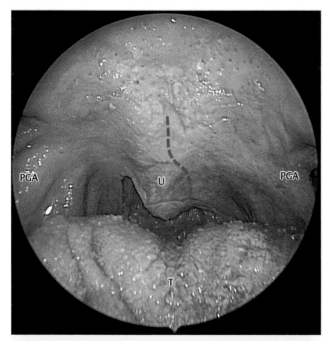

Fig. 42.2 Oral cavity with retractor in place. Red line depicts soft palate incision from the hard palate superiorly and to either side of the uvula inferiorly (left side arbitrarily selected in this figure). Abbreviations: PGA = palatoglossal arch (anterior pillar); T = tongue; U = uvula.

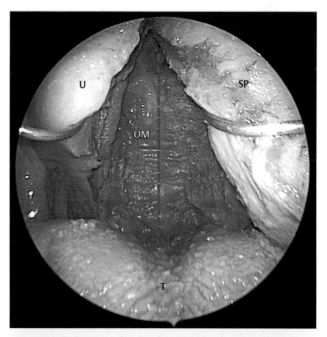

Fig. 42.3 Oral cavity with soft palate incised and retracted laterally. Red line depicts midline oropharyngeal mucosal incision, which should be limited caudally to only that which is necessary for access to pathology to minimize risk of dysphagia. Abbreviations: OM = oropharyngeal mucosa; SP = soft palate; T = tongue; U = uvula.

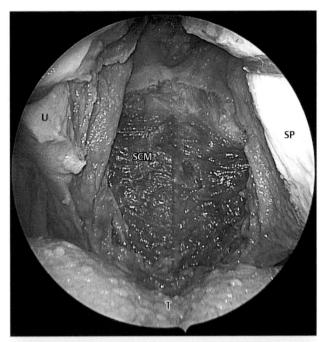

Fig. 42.4 Oral cavity with the oropharyngeal mucosa incised and reflected laterally. Red line depicts midline incision on the superior constrictor muscle, which should be limited caudally to only that which is necessary for access to pathology to minimize risk of dysphagia.
Abbreviations: SCM = superior constrictor muscle; SP = soft palate; T = tongue; U = uvula.

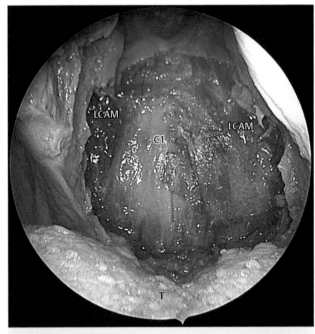

Fig. 42.5 Oral cavity with the superior constrictor muscle incised and reflected laterally. The prevertebral fascia is seen overlying the C1 anterior arch and the longus capitis muscles.
Abbreviations: C1 = C1 anterior arch; LCAM = longus capitis muscle; T = tongue.

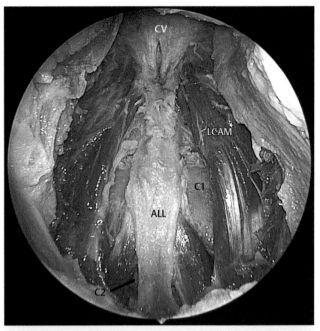

Fig. 42.6 Resection of prevertebral fascia at the craniovertebral junction, revealing the anterior longitudinal ligament, clivus, C1 anterior arch, C2 body, longus capitis muscles, and longus colli muscles.
Abbreviations: ALL = anterior longitudinal ligament; C1 = C1 anterior arch; C2 = C2 body; CV = clivus; LCAM = longus capitis muscle.

fibers of the superior constrictor muscle, which terminates at approximately the level of the superior aspect of the C1 anterior arch and the C2 body (**Fig. 42.4**). Greater tongue retraction facilitates exposure of the C3 body caudally.

- The superior constrictor muscle is divided in the midline and reflected laterally, exposing the fascia overlying the craniovertebral junction and paravertebral musculature, and C1 anterior arch (**Fig. 42.5**). This prevertebral fascia is resected, exposing the clivus, C1 anterior arch, and C2 body, as well as the anterior longitudinal ligament overlying these structures (**Fig. 42.6**).
- The anterior longitudinal ligament is removed, and the *longus colli* are detached from the caudal aspect of the C1 anterior arch (**Fig. 42.7**); C1 anterior arch is drilled out laterally to the point of the *longus capitis* bilaterally, facilitating access to the dens and exposing the apical and alar ligaments (**Fig. 42.8**).
- The dens is drilled in its entirety, exposing the transverse ligament posteriorly (**Fig. 42. 9**), which must be removed in most of the pathologic situations forming pannus in order to achieve appropriate decompression.

42.5.1 Critical Structures

- Soft palate/uvula.
- Superior constrictor muscle.
- *Longus colli.*
- *Longus capitis.*
- C1 anterior arch.
- Body of C2, dens, and apical ligament/alar ligaments.
- Transverse ligament.
- Clivus.

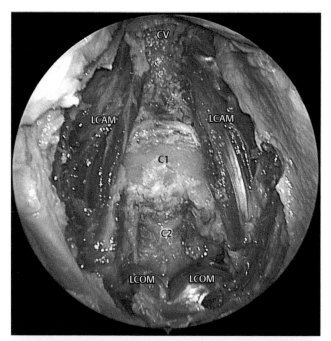

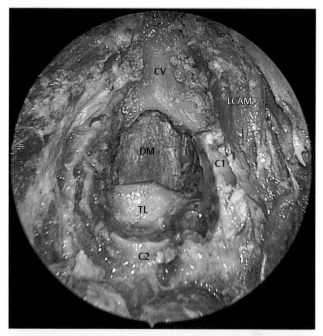

Fig. 42.7 Resection of the anterior longitudinal ligament and detachment of longus colli from C1 bilaterally, fully exposing the C1 anterior arch.
Abbreviations: C1 = C1 anterior arch; C2 = C2 body; CV = clivus; LCAM = longus capitis muscle; LCOM = longus colli muscle.

Fig. 42.9 Exposure of transverse ligament and craniocervical junction dura mater after removal of the dens with a drill.
Abbreviations: C1 = C1 anterior arch; C2 = C2 body; CV = clivus; DM = dura mater; LCAM = longus capitis muscle; TL = transverse ligament.

42.6 Parapharyngeal Retrostyloid Approach to the Jugular Foramen Region

- A vertical incision is made just lateral to the palatoglossal arch (anterior pillar) from the hard palate rostrally to the posterolateral floor of the mouth caudally through the mucosal and submucosal layers until the prestyloid space is opened (**Fig. 42.10**).
- This is bordered by the oropharynx medially and the medial pterygoid muscle laterally (**Fig. 42.11**).
- The lingual nerve is seen coursing inferiorly from just lateral to the medial pterygoid toward the tongue (**Fig. 42.12**).
- After removal of fat from the prestyloid space, the styloglossus muscle is the anterior-most muscle seen attached to the styloid process, and it courses inferomedially toward the base of the tongue.
- Lateral retraction of this reveals the stylopharyngeus muscle, which attaches more posteriorly to the styloid process and courses nearly horizontally toward the superior constrictor muscle (**Fig. 42.13**).
- Lateral retraction of the stylopharyngeus muscle reveals the glossopharyngeal nerve situated on the anterior aspect of the parapharyngeal segment of the internal carotid artery (**Fig. 42.14**).

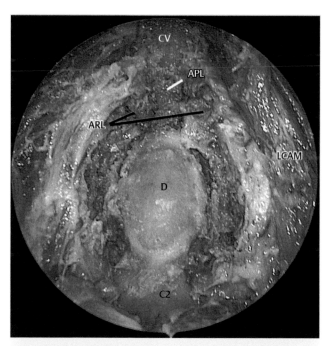

Fig. 42.8 Dens and alar ligament exposure after removal of the median portion of the C1 anterior arch with a drill.
Abbreviations: APL = apical ligament; ARL = alar ligament; C2 = C2 body; CV = clivus; D = dens; LCAM = longus capitis muscle.

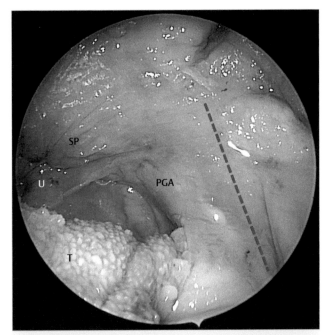

Fig. 42.10 Oral cavity with retractor in place in preparation for a left parapharyngeal retrostyloid approach. Red line depicts mucosal incision made just lateral to the palatoglossal arch (anterior pillar) from the hard palate rostrally to the posterolateral floor of the mouth caudally.
Abbreviations: PGA = palatoglossal arch; SP = soft palate; T = tongue; U = uvula.

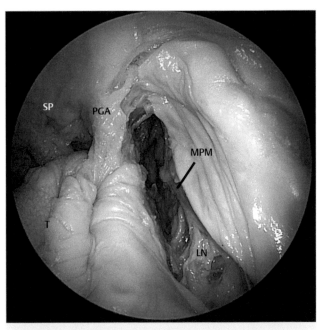

Fig. 42.12 The lingual nerve is seen coursing inferiorly from just lateral to the medial pterygoid toward the tongue.
Abbreviations: LN = lingual nerve; MPM = medial pterygoid muscle; PGA = palatoglossal arch; SP = soft palate; T = tongue.

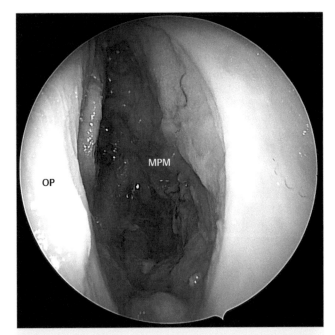

Fig. 42.11 Prestyolid space bordered by the oropharynx medially and the medial pterygoid muscle laterally.
Abbreviations: MPM = medial pterygoid muscle; OP = oropharynx.

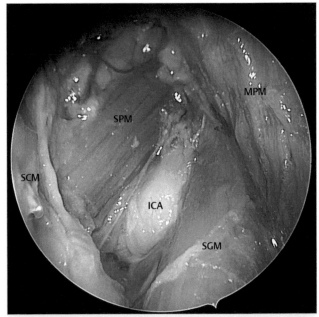

Fig. 42.13 The styloglossus muscle is the anterior-most muscle seen attached to the styloid process, and it courses inferomedially toward the base of the tongue. Lateral retraction of this reveals the stylopharyngeus muscle, which attaches more posteriorly to the styloid process and courses nearly horizontally toward the superior constrictor muscle medially.
Abbreviations: ICA = internal carotid artery; MPM = medial pterygoid muscle; SCM = superior constrictor muscle; SGM = styloglossus muscle; SPM = stylopharyngeus muscle.

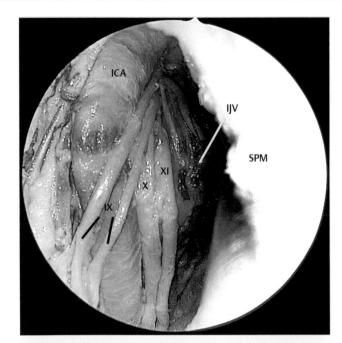

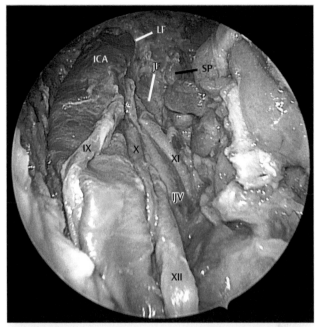

Fig. 42.14 The glossopharyngeal nerve situated on the anterior aspect of the parapharyngeal segment of the internal carotid artery, as seen with lateral retraction of the stylopharyngeus muscle. The vagus nerve is found in between the parapharyngeal segment of the internal carotid artery and the internal jugular vein, with the spinal accessory nerve located just lateral to this. Abbreviations: ICA = internal carotid artery; IJV = internal jugular vein; IX = ninth cranial nerve (glossopharyngeal); SPM = stylopharyngeus muscle; X = tenth cranial nerve (vagus); XI = eleventh cranial nerve (spinal accessory).

Fig. 42.15 Lateral retraction of both the styloglossus and stylopharyngeus muscles and reduction of the styloid process reveals all cranial nerves and major blood vessels in the posterior aspect of the parapharyngeal space. Abbreviations: ICA = internal carotid artery; IX = ninth cranial nerve (glossopharyngeal); IJV = internal jugular vein; JF = jugular foramen; LF = lacerum foramen; SP = styloid process; X = tenth cranial nerve (vagus); XI = eleventh cranial nerve (spinal accessory); XII = twelfth cranial nerve (hypoglossal nerve).

approach, lowering the risk of dysphagia, dysphonia, and infection.

• We therefore advocate reserving the use of the transoral approach for cases in which craniovertebral junction pathology extends too caudal to be fully addressed via an endonasal approach.

• Reduction or resection of the styloid process and inferior retraction of the styloglossus and stylopharyngeus muscles exposes the parapharyngeal segment of the internal carotid artery to the foramen lacerum and the jugular foramen contents from anteriorly, including the internal jugular vein, glossopharyngeal nerve, vagus nerve, spinal accessory nerve, and hypoglossal nerve (**Fig. 42.15**).

42.6.1 Critical Structures

• Palatoglossal arch (anterior pillar).
• Lingual nerve.
• Styloid process.
• Internal carotid artery.
• Jugular vein.
• Cranial nerves: ninth, tenth, eleventh, twelfth.

42.7 Pearls

• It is usually possible to address midline anterior pathology in the craniovertebral junction region via an endonasal

References

1. Dallan I, Seccia V, Muscatello L, et al. Transoral endoscopic anatomy of the parapharyngeal space: a step-by-step logical approach with surgical considerations. Head Neck 2011;33(4):557–561.
2. Seker A, Inoue K, Osawa S, Akakin A, Kilic T, Rhoton AL Jr. Comparison of endoscopic transnasal and transoral approaches to the craniovertebral junction. World Neurosurg 2010; 74(6):583–602.

43 Transmaxillary Approaches

Federico Biglioli, Luca Autelitano, Nicola Boari, Filippo Gagliardi, Fabiana Allevi, and Pietro Mortini

43.1 Introduction

Lesions involving the clival area, the middle and posterior skull base, and the upper cervical spine represent a significant challenge for neurosurgeons, ENT surgeons, and maxillofacial surgeons, due to the troublesome exposure of the surgical site.

Neoplastic, degenerative or inflammatory lesions can arise in this peculiar region, involving and compressing the cervico-medullary junction and inducing craniocervical instability. Surgical decompression and subsequent craniocervical stabilization represent the gold standard of treatment. Although aggressive surgical resection has been advised for some of these local aggressive lesions, such as chordomas and chondrosarcomas, wide exposure of this region is difficult to obtain because of the surrounding anatomy and potential neurologic morbidity.

Multiple approaches have been described to gain adequate surgical exposure. The choice of the correct surgical approach depends on several factors, such as patient's age and general health condition, tumor histopathology, extension and growth rate, and the exact location of the lesion.

Four different broad categories of surgical techniques have been proposed in literature: open-transfacial, microsurgical, endoscopic, and robotic techniques provide all good visualization of this hard-to-reach anatomical area, each one of them obviously showing definite pros and cons.

In particular, the Le Fort I transmaxillary approach and the following downward displacement of the maxilla provides a wide exposure of the posterior nasopharynx, from the sphenoid sinus to the clivus and the anterior part of the foramen magnum. This technique allows obtaining an acceptable cranio-caudal exposure of the clival and paraclival region, associated to a reduced lateral vision.

43.2 Indications

- Neoplastic, degenerative or inflammatory lesions involving the clival area, the middle and posterior skull base and the upper cervical spine.

43.3 Patient Positioning

- **Position:** The patient is positioned supine with the head fixed on a horseshoe head holder.
- **Body:** The trunk and the head are slightly elevated to facilitate the venous backflow.
- **Head:** The head is placed in neutral position.
- **Neck:** The neck is slightly extended (about 20°), to facilitate further brain relaxation after dural opening.
- **Intubation:** Submental orotracheal intubation. (**Fig. 43.1**).

43.4 Mucosal Incision (Fig. 43.2)

- Mucoperiosteal incision is performed at the superior vestibular fornix of the oral cavity.
- Incision is carried out 1 cm above the gingival reflection, along the upper alveolar margin between the bilateral first molars.

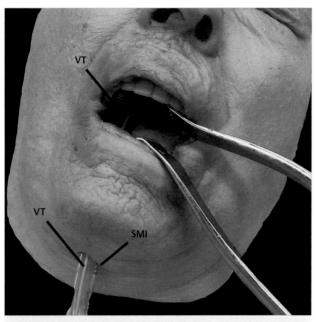

Fig. 43.1 Submental orotracheal intubation.
Abbreviations: SMI = submental incision; VT = ventilation tube.

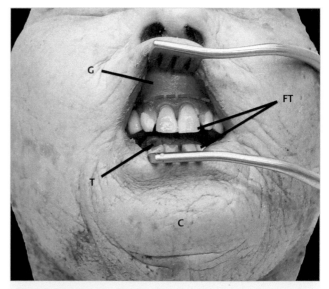

Fig. 43.2 Mucosal incision.
Abbreviations: C = chin; FT = frontal teeth; G = gingiva; T = tongue.

43.4.1 Critical Structures

• Branches of the superior alveolar artery.

43.5 Soft Tissue Dissection

• **Pericranial layer**
  ○ A subperiosteal dissection of soft tissues is carried out using an elevator instrument.
• **Bone exposure**
  ○ Bone exposure is accomplished through the exposure of the anterior wall of the maxilla, the piriform aperture, the infraorbital foramen and the infraorbital nerve at the exit of its canal.
  ○ Then, the surgeon must detach the cartilaginous portion of the nasal septum from the nasal spine and the vomer (**Figs. 42.3, 43.4**).

43.6 Osteotomy (Figs. 43.5, 43.6)

• Osteotomy has to be performed 1 cm above the teeth roots, using an oscillating saw or the piezosurgery.
• In order to avoid postoperative loss of individual occlusion, premodeling of 4 miniplates on both sides is accomplished. At the end of surgery, exact position of the maxilla is guaranteed by replacing the premodeled plates by screws insertion in the previous driven holes.

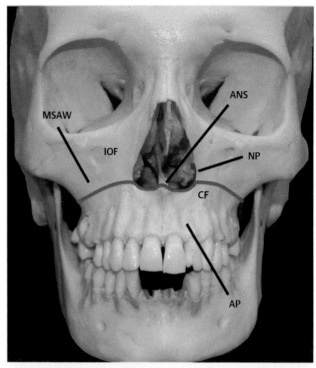

Fig. 43.4 Osteotomy, landmarks.
Abbreviations: ANS = anterior nasal spine; AP = alveolar processes; CF = canine fossa; IOF = infra-orbital foramen; MSAW = maxillary sinus anterior wall; NP = nasal piriform aperture.

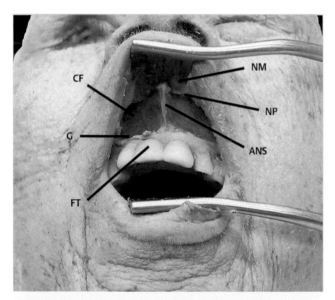

Fig. 43.3 Cartilaginous portion of the nasal septum are detached from the nasal spine and the vomer.
Abbreviations: ANS = anterior nasal spine; CF = canine fossa; FT = frontal teeth; G = gingiva; NM = nasal mucosa; NP = nasal piriform aperture.

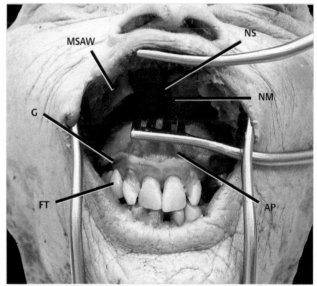

Fig. 43.5 Osteotomy, step 1.
Abbreviations: AP = alveolar processes; FT = frontal teeth; G = gingiva; MSAW = maxillary sinus anterior wall; NM = nasal mucosa; NS = nasal septum.

• Once the osteotomy has been performed, the nasal septum can be separated from the maxilla and the pterygoid-maxillary junctions divided with a curved chisel.
• The maxilla will be displaced downward, preserving the palatine vessels and nerves.
• The surgeon has now to expose and remove the nasal septum and vomer.

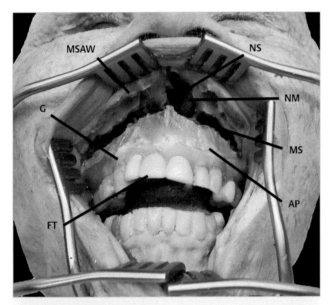

Fig. 43.6 Osteotomy, step 2.
Abbreviations: AP = alveolar processes; FT = frontal teeth; G = gingiva; MS = maxillary sinus; MSAW = maxillary sinus anterior wall; NM = nasal mucosa; NS = nasal septum.

• Once the sphenoidal rostrum is reached, the sphenoid sinus is reached.
• Incision of the pharyngeal mucosa and dissection of the pharyngeal muscles allows exposure of the clivus from the sella to the anterior border of the foramen magnum (**Fig. 43.7**).
• **Osteotomy landmarks**
Anatomical landmarks which have to be take into consideration in designing the osteotomy are as follows:
  ○ **Superiorly:** Piriform aperture, the infraorbital foramen and the infraorbital nerve at the exit of its canal.
  ○ **Inferiorly:** Alveolar processes.
  ○ **Laterally:** Maxillary tuberosity.
  ○ **Medially:** Cartilaginous portion of the nasal septum from the nasal spine and the vomer.

43.7 Variants

43.7.1 Le Fort I Transmaxillary Approach with a Transantral and Transpterygoid Approach (See Chapter 44)

• Following removal of the middle and inferior turbinates and opening of the maxillary antrum, the posterior wall of the maxillary sinus can be removed, reaching the pterygopalatine fossa, where noble neurovascular structures can be identified and mobilized.
• A further lateral exposure can be obtained with the removal of the pterygoid plates and the dissection of pterygoid muscles.

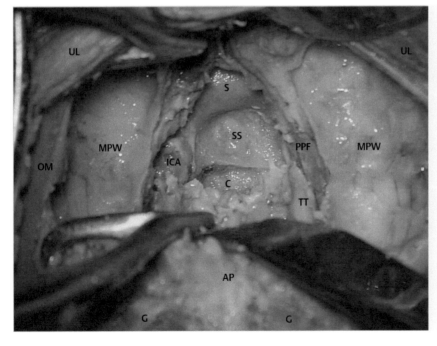

Fig. 43.7 Microscopic view of clival exposure. Abbreviations: AP = alveolar process; C = clivus; G = gingiva; ICA = internal carotid artery; MPW = maxillary posterior wall; OM = oral mucosa; PPF = pterygopalatine fossa; S = sella; SS = sphenoid sinus; TT = torus tubarius; UL = upper lip.

43.7.2 Splitting of Soft Palate and/or Tongue

Le Fort I osteotomy can be coupled with splitting of soft palate and/or tongue in order to grant further specific vertical widening of the surgical field.

- The split of the soft palate allows accessing the lower clivus, the craniocervical junction, C1 and C2.
- It must be noted that the soft palate split requires a precise reconstruction of each layer in order to avoid velo-pharyngeal incompetence.
- Splitting the tongue allows further caudal extension of the surgical field, down to C3 and C4.
- No movement alterations have been described in the literature, being the residual damage after healing even less than in cosmetic tongue splitting, the incision must be strictly kept on the median line in order to avoid peripheral neuropathies.

43.8 Pearls

- It is worth noting that submental orotracheal intubation, usually employed during cranio-maxillofacial traumas treatment, can be used as a safe technique for airway management during transfacial approaches to the cranial base.
- It avoids the complications associated with tracheostomy.
- It also permits considerable downward retraction of the maxilla after a Le Fort I osteotomy and is associated with good clival exposure.
- Furthermore, it does not interfere with maxillo-mandibular fixation at the end of the surgery.

43.9 Reconstruction

Transfacial approaches also have a distinct and useful role in the repair of large breaches of the cranial base, since they allow enough field exposure to grant the use of local and pedicled flaps.

Proactive repair of large cranial base defects directly improves patient survival and surgical success rate preventing infections, ocular functional issues and distortion of facial morphology. Since a complete coverage of cranial base defects goes beyond the scope of this book, detailed information can be found in other Thieme references.

References

1. Biglioli F, Mortini P, Goisis M, Bardazzi A, Boari N. Submental Orotracheal Intubation: An alternative to tracheotomy in transfacial cranial base surgery. Skull Base 2003; 13(4):189–195.
2. Boari N, Roberti F, Biglioli F, Caputy AJ, Mortini P. Quantification of clival and paraclival exposure in the Le Fort I transmaxillary transpterygoid approach: a microanatomical study. J Neurosurg 2010;113(5):1011–1018.
3. Hernández Altemir F. Transfacial access to the retromaxillary area. J Maxillofac Surg 1986;14(3):165–170.
4. Liu JK, Couldwell WT, Apfelbaum RI. Transoral approach and extended modifications for lesions of the ventral foramen magnum and craniovertebral junction. Skull Base 2008;18(3):151–166.
5. Williams WG, Lo LJ, Chen YR. The Le Fort I-palatal split approach for skull base tumors: efficacy, complications, and outcome. Plast Reconstr Surg 1998;102(7):2310–2319.

44 Transmaxillary Transpterygoid Approach

Nicola Boari, Federico Biglioli, Filippo Gagliardi, and Pietro Mortini

44.1 Introduction

The transmaxillary transpterygoid approach is a variant of the standard Le-Fort I transmaxillary approach, suitable for midline extradural tumors, extending from the sella turcica to the anterior rim of the foramen magnum and laterally to the internal carotid artery (ICA), invading the pterygopalatine fossa, the medial infratemporal fossa and the medial parapharyngeal space.

44.2 Indications

- Clival chordomas and chondrosarcomas.
- Other non-chordomatous lesions of the clivus.
- Esthesioneuroblastoma.
- Malignancy of the anterior skull base-sinonasal tumors.

44.3 Anesthesia And Patient Intubation

- Downward retraction of the maxilla can be improved by using tracheostomy or submental orotracheal intubation according to Hernandez-Altamir (**see Chapter 43**).
- Subsequent enhanced exposure of the lower clivus is obtained.

44.4 Patient Positioning

- **Position:** The patient is positioned supine with the head fixed to a horseshoe head holder.
- **Body:** The body is placed in neutral position with the trunk elevated of 30° to increase venous backflow and the legs elevated at the level of the heart.
- **Head:** The head is tilted back 20°and toward the left shoulder 25°. The surgeon is placed on the right side of the patient.
- **Anti-decubitus device:** Rolls are placed under the knees.
- **The zygoma** must be the highest point in the surgical field.

44.5 Mucosal Incision (See Chapter 43)

A mucoperiosteal incision is performed between the first molars, 1 cm above the gingival reflection along the upper alveolar margin, leaving a cuff of mucosa on the gingival side.

44.5.1 Critical Structures

- Superficial temporal artery.
- Facial nerve.

44.6 Soft Tissues Dissection (See Chapter 43)

- **Mucosal level**
  ○ Gingival mucosa is detached till the maxillary-malar reflection on both sides and the floor of the nasal cavity are identified.
- **Bone exposure**
  ○ The bony exposure is continued to the level of the last molar.
  ○ Subperiosteal dissection is carried out to expose the anterior maxilla and the piriform aperture, as far as the inferior rim of the infraorbital foramen is exposed.
  ○ The infraorbital nerve is identified at the exit from its canal. The cartilaginous septum is detached from the nasal spine and vomer.

44.6.1 Critical Structures

- Infraorbital nerves.

44.7 Maxillar Osteotomy (See Chapter 43)

- A Le Fort I osteotomy is performed 8-10 mm above the roots of the teeth with an oscillating saw.
- The nasal septum is then divided from the maxilla on the midline, and a curved chisel is used to divide the pterygoid-maxillary junctions.
- The hard palate is down-fractured and mobilized into the oral cavity.
- A self-retaining retractor is positioned between the maxilla and the hard palate.

44.7.1 Critical Structures

- Palatine nerves and arteries.

44.8 Clival Exposure

- The sphenoid sinus is opened and the posterior sinus wall is drilled out, exposing the sellar floor, the carotid and optic prominences (Fig. 44.1).
- A longitudinal incision is performed on the midline along the rhinopharynx mucosa and the parapharyngeal muscles, together with the mucosa, are dissected in a subperiosteal fashion from the underlying clival bony surface.
- Clival resection is completed by drilling the middle and lower clival bone until the foramen magnum.

44.8.1 Critical Structures

- Internal carotid arteries (ICA): C3, C4 and C5 segments.
- Optic nerves and chiasm.

44.9 Paraclival Exposure (Figs. 44.2–44.5)

- Lateral exposure is completed by removing the inferior and middle turbinates and by resecting the posterior wall of the maxillary sinus.
- Pterygopalatine fossa is opened, gaining access to the third segment of the maxillary artery, which is mobilized laterally by dividing the sphenopalatine artery.

- The greater palatine artery is preserved. The vidian nerve is completely skeletonized to the lacerous segment of the internal carotid artery.
- The pterygoid plates on both sides are removed, widening the paraclival dura exposure to the infratemporal segment of the mandibular branch of the trigeminal nerve (V3).
- The Eustachian tube can be divided opening the surgical access to the parapharyngeal space.

44.9.1 Critical Structures

- ICAs: C2, C3 and C4 segments.
- Maxillary arteries.
- Greater palatine nerves and arteries.
- Pterygopalatine ganglions.
- Maxillary (V2), and mandibular branch (V3) of the trigeminal nerve.
- Eustachian tubes.
- Twelfth cranial nerves (hypoglossal nerve).

44.10 Dural Opening (Fig. 44.6)

- The dura is divided longitudinally on the midline.
- Bleeding from the basilar plexus must be managed by compression and by using hemostatic agents.

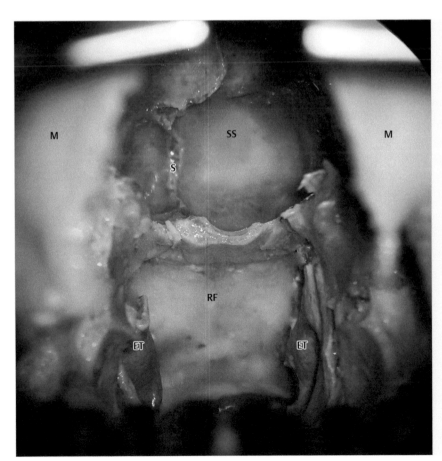

Fig. 44.1 The clivus is exposed from the sella turcica to the anterior border of the foramen magnum.
Abbreviations: ET = Eustachian tube; M = maxilla; RF = rhinopharynx; S = septum; SS = sphenoid sinus.

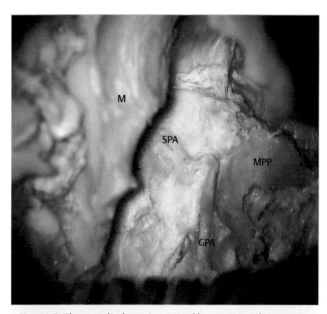

Fig. 44.2 The paraclival area is exposed by removing the posterior wall of the maxillary sinus.
Abbreviations: GPA = greater palatine artery; M = maxilla; MPP = middle pterygoid process; SPA = sphenopalatine artery.

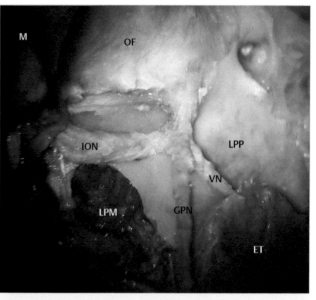

Fig. 44.4 Exposure of the lateral pterygoid process.
Abbreviations: ET = Eustachian tube; GPN = greater palatine nerve; ION = infraorbital nerve; OF = orbital floor; LPM = lateral pterygoid muscle; LPP = lateral pterygoid process; M = maxilla; VN = Vidian nerve.

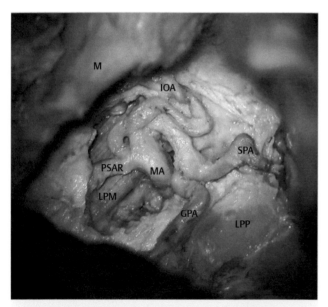

Fig. 44.3 Vascular structures of the pterygopalatine fossa.
Abbreviations: GPA = greater palatine artery; IOA = infraorbital artery; LPM = lateral pterygoid muscle; LPP = lateral pterygoid process; M = maxilla; MA = maxillary artery; PSAR = posterior superior alveolar artery; SPA = sphenopalatine artery.

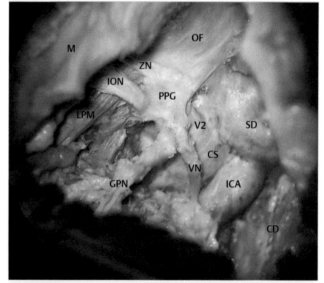

Fig. 44.5 The operative field after removal of medial and lateral pterygoid plates.
Abbreviations: CD = clival dura; CS = cavernous sinus; GPN = greater palatine nerve; ICA = internal carotid artery; ION = infraorbital nerve; OF = orbital floor; LPM = lateral pterygoid muscle; M = maxilla; PPG = pterygopalatine ganglion; SD = sellar dura; V2 = maxillary nerve; VN = Vidian nerve; ZN = zygomatic nerve.

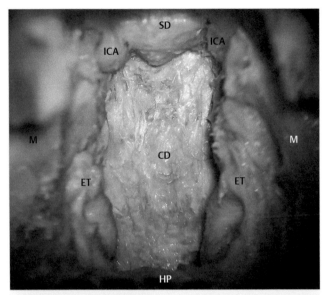

Fig. 44.6 Exposure of clival dura.
Abbreviations: CD = clival dura; ET = Eustachian tube; ICA = internal carotid artery; M = maxilla; HP = hard palate; SD = sellar dura.

44.10.1 Critical Structures

- Basilar artery.
- Brainstem.
- Sixth cranial nerves (abducens nerve).

44.11 Intradural Exposure (Fig. 44.7)

- **Parenchymal structures:** Pituitary gland, ventral aspect of the brainstem.
- **Arachnoidal layer:** Chiasmatic cistern, inter-peduncular cistern, pre-pontine cistern.
- **Cranial nerves:** Optic nerves, sixth and lower cranial nerves.
- **Arteries:** Vertebral arteries, basilar artery, posterior-inferior cerebellar artery, anterior inferior cerebellar artery, superior cerebellar artery, posterior cerebral artery.

44.12 Dural Reconstruction

- Free mucosal graft and fascia lata flap are indicated for small dural defects.
- Pedicled fascial, pericranial, galeopericranial, or mucosal flaps are necessary for the repair of larger defects.
- Nasal packing is performed.
- A lumbar drainage is positioned and left in place for 5 days is recommended.

44.13 Pearls

- Maxillary pre-plating before Le Fort I osteotomy minimizes the risk of dental malocclusion.

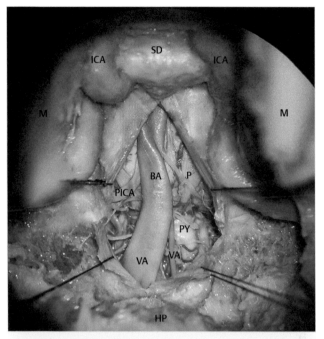

Fig. 44.7 Intradural exposure.
Abbreviations: BA = basilar artery; HP = hard palate; ICA = internal carotid artery; M = maxilla; P = pons; PICA = posterior inferior cerebellar artery; PY = pyramid; SD = sellar dura; VA = vertebral artery.

- Bilateral closure of the greater palatine arteries can increase the risk of aseptic necrosis of the maxilla.
- Identification of the optic and carotid prominences in the parasellar area is crucial to avoid neurovascular injuries.
- Onodi cell (spheno-ethmoidal air cell) must be identified when present.
- An endoscopic-assisted procedure is suggested in order to improve the visualization of paraclival anatomical structures.
- Sacrifice of the cartilaginous part of the Eustachian tube can lead to unilateral deafness; in this case, a tympanic drain should be placed to preserve adequate ventilation of the middle ear.
- Meticulous multilayer dural reconstruction is crucial in order to avoid cerebrospinal fluid (CSF) leak through the nose.
- The same clival and paraclival exposure can be obtained through an extended endoscopic endonasal approach.

References

1. Biglioli F, Mortini P, Goisis M, Bardazzi A, Boari N. Submental orotracheal intubation: an alternative to tracheostomy in transfacial cranial base surgery. Skull Base 2003;13(4):189–195.
2. Boari N, Roberti F, Biglioli F, Caputy AJ, Mortini P. Quantification of clival and paraclival exposure in the Le Fort I transmaxillary transpterygoid approach: a microanatomical study. J Neurosurg 2010;113(5):1011–1018.
3. Gagliardi F, Boari N, Mortini P. Reconstruction techniques in skull base surgery. Review J Craniofac Surg 2011;22(3):1015–1020.
4. Roberti F, Boari N, Mortini P, Caputy AJ. The pterygopalatine fossa: an anatomic report. J Craniofac Surg 2007; 18(3):586–590.

45 Endoscopic Endonasal Transclival Approach with Transcondylar Extension

Wei-Hsin Wang and Juan C. Fernandez-Miranda

45.1 Introduction

The endoscopic endonasal transclival approach is a midline endoscopic approach, which provides a great surgical exposure through a minimally invasive procedure. The approach can be tailored according to the pathology, which has to be treated.

When needed, it can provide the exposure of the whole clivus. Transcondylar extension enables the surgeon to extend the resection laterally.

The approach is suitable to treat both extra and intradural lesions, with the possibility to harvest wide mucosal reconstruction flaps.

45.2 Indications

- Extradural lesions originating from the clivus or petroclival fissure with predominant ventral extension: chordomas, chondrosarcomas.
- Intradural midline lesion ventral to pons and medulla located in between the vertebral arteries: ventral foramen magnum meningiomas, jugular tubercle meningiomas, epidermoid and neuroenteric cysts.
- Intra-axial lesions located in the ventral aspect of the medulla and ponto-medullary junction: cavernomas.

45.3 Patient Positioning

- **Position:** The patient is positioned supine with the head fixed with Mayfield holder.
- **Body:** The body is placed parallel to the horizontal.
- **Head position:** Position of the head is neutral, slightly rotated toward the surgeon.

45.4 Clival Division (Fig. 45.1)

Clivus may be classically divided into three anatomical segments.
- **Superior third of clivus (Sellar):** From the posterior clinoid and dorsum sella to the level of the floor of the sella.
- **Middle third of clivus (Sphenoidal):** From the floor of the sella to the floor of the sphenoid sinus.
- **Inferior third of clivus (Nasopharyngeal):** From the floor of the sphenoid sinus to the foramen magnum.

45.5 Approach To The Nasal Cavity (Figs. 45.2, 45.3)

- Nasal decongestion with topical oxymetazoline (0.05%).

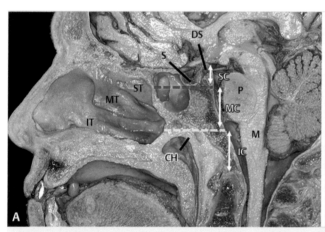
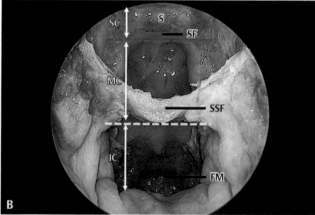

Fig. 45.1 The clivus is divided into thirds. The superior clivus is bounded inferiorly by the level of the floor of the sella (*red dotted line*). The inferior clivus extends from choana (*yellow dotted line*, the same level of the floor of the sphenoid sinus). (**A**) Sagittal view. (**B**) Endonasal endoscopic view.
Abbreviations: CH = choana; DS = dorsum sellae; FM = foramen magnum; IC = inferior clivus; IT = inferior turbinate; M = medulla; MC = middle clivus; MT = middle turbinate; P = pons; S = sella; SC = superior clivus; SF = sellar floor; SSF = sphenoid sinus floor; ST = superior turbinate.

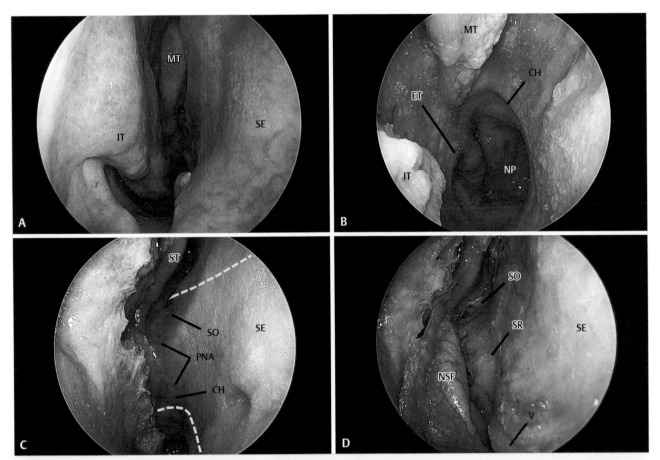

Fig. 45.2 The anatomic structures of the nasal cavity. **(A)** The superficial view of the right nostril. **(B)** The deeper view of the right nostril demonstrates the direct access to nasopharynx (corresponding to the inferior clivus). **(C)** The middle turbinate is resected to gain more space for endoscopy and better exposure. The posterior nasal artery is located approximately halfway between sphenoid ostium and choana. The yellow dotted line illustrates the incision of nasal septal flap starting from sphenoid ostium and choana. **(D)** The nasal septal flap is reflected laterally and the sphenoid rostrum can be identified.
Abbreviations: CH = choana; ET = Eustachian tube; IT = inferior turbinate; MT = middle turbinate; NP = nasopharynx; NSF = nasal septal flap; PNA = posterior nasal artery; SE = septum; SO = sphenoid ostium; SR = sphenoid rostrum; ST = superior turbinate; V = vomer.

- **Inferior turbinate**
  - The inferior turbinate is lateralized to gain a better access to the nasopharynx.
- **Middle turbinate**
  - The middle turbinate's inferior portion is resected to gain more space for endoscopy (optional).
- **Nasal septal flap**
  - The nasal septal flap is elevated at the contralateral side of the main part of the tumor or from the most favorable side if prominent septal spurs.
  - **Pedicle vessel:**
    - Posterior nasal artery (may bifurcate early in 2 branches).
    - Branch of sphenopalatine artery.
    - Halfway between sphenoid ostium and choana.
  - It is temporally stored in the sphenoid sinus or maxillary sinus.
- **Sphenoid sinus**
  - The posterior nasal septum and the vomer are detached from the sphenoid rostrum.
  - Posterior third septectomy provides binarial access.
  - A wide sphenoidotomy would benefit identification of landmarks: sella, paraclival internal carotid artery (ICA), floor of the sphenoid sinus.

- **Maxillary crest**
  - The maxillary crest is flattened to the level of the hard palate for more inferior access.

45.6 Soft Tissue Dissection (Fig. 45.4)

- **Nasopharyngeal mucosa and basopharyngeal fascia**
  - They are elevated from the floor of the sphenoid sinus, using a combination of electrocautery and blunt dissection.
  - Lateral extension is carried out up to the Eustachian tubes.
  - **Arteries:** Palatovaginal artery (*aka* palatosphenoidal or pharyngeal artery).
- **Muscular Layer**
  - **Longus capitis major**
    - Superficial layer.
    - Attached to the superior clival line.
  - **Rectus capitis anterior**
    - Deep layer.
    - Attached to the inferior clival line (same level as supracondylar groove and hypoglossal canal).
  - The two muscle layers are elevated and resected together.

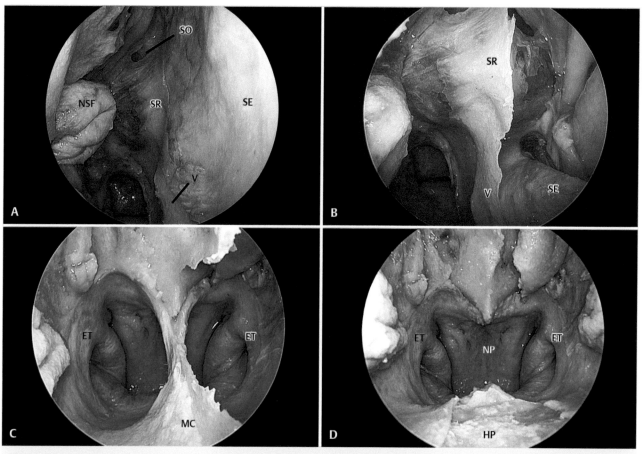

Fig. 45.3 Stepwise dissection to expose the nasopharynx. **(A)** The nasal septal flap is stored in the maxillary sinus in order not to block the access to the nasopharynx. **(B)** The posterior septum is detached from the sphenoid rostrum. **(C,D)** Maxillary crest is resected to gain more inferior access. Abbreviations: ET = Eustachian tube; HP = hard palate; MC = maxillary crest; NP = nasopharynx; NSF = nasal septal flap; SE = septum; SO = sphenoid ostium; SR = sphenoid rostrum; V = vomer.

- **Atlanto-occipital membrane**
  - It has to be resected to expose the foramen magnum and atlas (C1) anterior arch.

45.7 Bony Drilling Landmarks (Fig. 45.5)

- **Lateral limit**
  - Paraclival ICA, foramen lacerum, petroclival fissure, jugular tubercle, hypoglossal canal, occipital condyle.
- **Inferior limit**
  - Upper part of C1 anterior arch.
- **Condylectomy**
  - **Lateral limit:** An imaginary line extending inferiorly from the junction of petroclival fissure and foramen lacerum.
  - **Deep limit:** Anterior cortical bone of intracranial aspect of hypoglossal canal.

45.8 Dural Opening (Fig. 45.5)

- The basilar plexus is located between two layers of dura (hemostatic agents can easily control venous bleeding).

- Dura is incised on the midline, then it is opened like a book and resected from the inside out if needed.

45.8.1 Critical Structures

- Abducens nerve.
- Hypoglossal nerve.
- Vertebrobasilar system.

45.9 Intradural Exposure (Fig. 45.5)

- **Parenchymal structures:** Ventral medulla and ponto-medullary junction.
- **Arachnoidal layer:** Premedullary cistern.
- **Arteries:** Vertebral arteries, vertebrobasilar junction, posterior inferior cerebellar artery (PICA), anterior spinal arteries.
- **Cranial nerves:** Hypoglossal nerve and lower cranial nerves (dorsal to vertebral artery), anterior root of the first cervical nerve (C1) (ventral to vertebral artery).

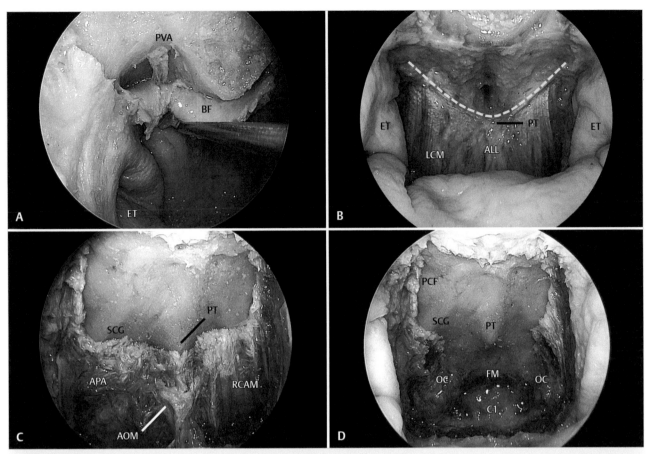

Fig. 45.4 Stepwise dissection to expose the inferior clivus and foramen magnum. **(A)** The basopharyngeal fascia is elevated from the inferior margin of the sphenoid sinus floor. The palatovaginal artery can be identified in this step. **(B)** The superficial layer of muscles attaching on the inferior clivus is the longus capitis major muscle. Its attaching points are outlined with the yellow dotted line, which is also called superior clival line. **(C)** After resecting the longus capitis major muscle, the rectus capitis anterior muscle attaching at the inferior clival line (green dotted line) is exposed. **(D)** Full exposure of the inferior clivus with extension to occipital condyle is completed. The lateral limit of medial condylectomy is an imaginary line (blue dotted line) extending inferiorly from the petroclival fissure to the occipital condyle. Abbreviations: ALL = anterior longitudinal ligament; AOM = atlo-occipital membrane; APA = anterior pharyngeal artery; BF = basopharyngeal fascia; C1 = atlas anterior arch; ET = Eustachian tube; FM = foramen magnum; LCM = longus capitis muscle; OC = occipital condyle; PCF = petroclival fissure; PT = pharyngeal tubercle; PVA = palatovaginal artery; RCAM = rectus capitis anterior muscle; SCG supracondylar groove.

45.10 Pearls

- Extended nasoseptal flap is useful for large clival defects.
- Preparation of the thigh for fascia lata harvesting and the abdomen for fat graft.
- Maxillary antrostomy is needed to store the flap during the operation away from the surgical field.
- Posterior septectomy can be minimized since most of the binarial work is done posteriorly.
- Drilling the maxillary crest is important to obtain more caudal binarial access.
- Sphenoidotomy is typically not necessary for tumors limited to the inferior clivus.
- It is key to remove the fascia and muscle layers widely to reach the petroclival fissure laterally and to identify the lower aspect of the foramen lacerum.

- Drilling should include jugular tubercle and medial aspect of the occipital condyle, following the above described landmarks.
- Ultrasonic bone curette is useful for drilling these areas.
- A well-done medial condylectomy provides access to the lateral wall of the foramen magnum, involves just a quarter of the condylar volume, and carries no risk of craniocervical instability.
- The vertebral artery enters the posterior fossa just behind the condyle and can be accessible after medial condylectomy.
- Wide dural opening is recommended for meningiomas to facilitate recognition of neurovascular structures and extracapsular dissection.
- Microsurgical-like techniques are used for extracapsular dissection.
- Angled scopes are beneficial to look around corners and identify residual tumor, specially within the hypoglossal canal.

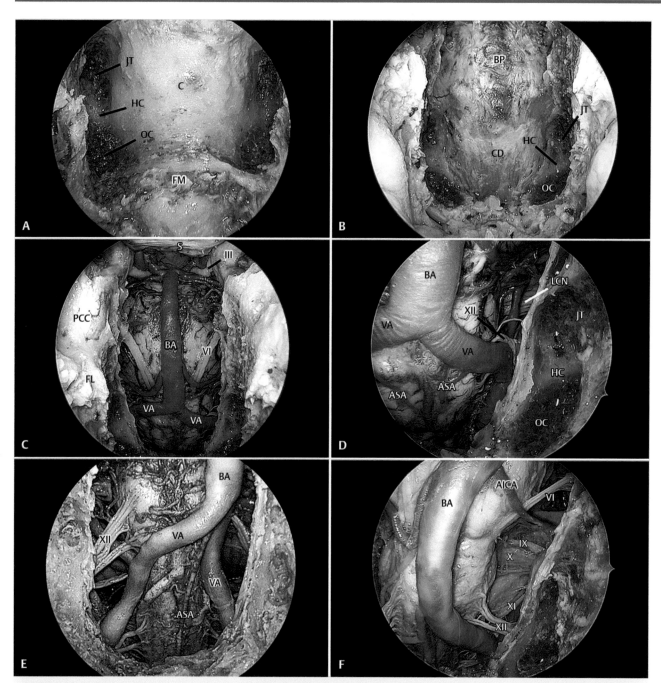

Fig. 45.5 Bone drilling and intradural exposure. (**A**) Anteromedial condylectomy is completed and the anterior cortical bone of hypoglossal canal is exposed. The jugular tubercle is above the hypoglossal canal and the occipital condyle is below the hypoglossal canal. (**B**) The clival dura is exposed after the bone drilling. (**C**) The full transclival intradural exposure extends from the sella to the foramen magnum. (**D**) Lateral intradural exposure of the foramen magnum (close view of figure 5C). Lower cranial nerves are behind the jugular tubercle. (**E**) Transclival transcondylar approach to expose the foramen magnum. (**F**) Transclival transjugular approach to expose the jugular foramen. Abbreviations: AICA = anterior inferior cerebellar artery; ASA = anterior spinal artery; BA = basilar artery; BP = basilar plexus; C = clivus; CD = clival dura; FM = foramen magnum; FL = foramen lacerus; HC = hypoglossal canal; III = oculomotor nerve; IX = glossopharyngeal nerve; JT = jugular tubercle; LCN = lower cranial nerves; OC = occipital condyle; PCC = paraclival carotid; S = sella; VA = vertebral artery; VI = abducens nerve; X = vagus nerve; XI = accessory nerve; XII = hypoglossal nerve.

- Extensive dural resection is performed for meningiomas.
- Multilayer reconstruction: inlay collagen layer, onlay fascial lata graft, fat graft reinforcement, and vascularized extended nasoseptal flap plus nasal packing and postoperative lumbar drain (3 days).

References

1. Fernandez-Miranda JC, Morera VA, Snyderman CH, Gardner P. Endoscopic endonasal transclival approach to the jugular tubercle. Neurosurgery 2012;71(1, Suppl Operative):146–158, discussion 158–159.

2. Morera VA, Fernandez-Miranda JC, Prevedello DM, et al. "Far-medial" expanded endonasal approach to the inferior third of the clivus: the transcondylar and transjugular tubercle approaches. Neurosurgery 2010;**66**(6, Suppl Operative)211–219, discussion 219–220.

3. Wang WH, Abhinav K, Wang E, et al. Endoscopic endonasal transclival transcondylar approach for foramen magnum meningiomas: anatomical considerations and technical note. Neurosurgery 2015.

4. Vaz-Guimaraes Filho F, Fernandez-Miranda JC, Wang EW. Endoscopic endonasal "far-medial" transclival approach: surgical anatomy and technique. Oper Tech Otolaryngol—Head Neck Surg 2013; 24(4):222–228.

46 Endoscopic Endonasal Transmaxillary Approach to the Vidian Canal and Meckel's Cave

Rafid Al-Mahfoudh, João Paulo Almeida, Sacit Bulent Omay, and Theodore H. Schwartz

46.1 Indications

- Tumors isolated to the Meckel's cave.
- Tumors with middle fossa–extracranial extension.
- Tumors with pure extracranial involvement along the second (V2) and third (V3) branch of the trigeminal nerve.

46.2 Patient Positioning

- **Position:** Supine with the head fixed with a Mayfield head holder.
- **Body:** The body is placed horizontal or in slight reverse Trendelenburg position (15-30°).
- **Head:** The head is slightly extended and rotated to the right.
- Abdomen and contralateral thigh are prepped and draped in a sterile fashion in case a fat graft or fascia lata are needed.

46.3 Surgical Approach (Fig. 46.1)

- Start with a rigid 0° endoscope.
- 1% lidocaine with 1:100,000 epinephrine is used to vasoconstrict the sphenopalatine artery (SPA) at the sphenopalatine foramen, in addition to infiltrating the uncinate process and vertical lamella of the ipsilateral middle turbinate.
- Resection of the posterior third of the septum allows for a binostril, 4-handed surgical technique and greater maneuverability of surgical instruments.

46.3.1 Critical Structures

- Middle turbinate
- Uncinate process

46.4 Nasal Stage (Figs. 46.2, 46.3)

- A contralateral nasoseptal flap must be harvested (**see Chapters 38 and 39**).
- Complete a septectomy by resecting the posterior nasal septum.
- Introduce the endoscope from contralateral nostril.
- Sphenoidectomy is performed.
- Uncinectomy is carried out.
- Middle turbinate is resected.
- Maxillary sinus ostium is identified.
- Ethmoidectomy is performed: the ethmoidal bulla and supra-bulla cells are both removed.
- Removing the ethmoidal bulla does facilitate the removal of the posterior wall of the medial junction of maxillary sinus.

46.4.1 Critical Structures

- Middle turbinate.
- Uncinate process.
- Ethmoidal bulla.
- Maxillary sinus ostium.

46.5 Maxillary Sinus Stage (Fig. 46.4)

- A wide maxillary antrostomy is carried out.
- The infraorbital neurovascular bundle is identified.
- Sphenopalatine artery is cauterized and divided.

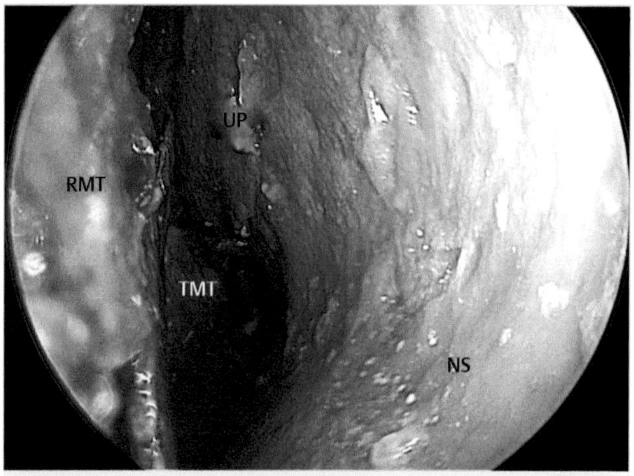

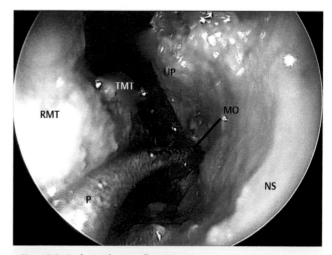

Fig. 46.1 Endoscopic view of the middle turbinate and uncinate process.
Abbreviations: NS = nasal septum; RMT = right middle turbinate; TMT = tail of the middle turbinate; UP = uncinate process.

Fig. 46.2 Probe in the maxillary sinus.
Abbreviations: MO = maxillary ostium; NS = nasal septum; P = probe; RMT = right middle turbinate; TMT = tail of the middle turbinate; UP = uncinate process.

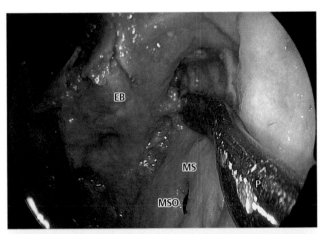

Fig. 46.3 After septectomy and uncinectomy, the maxillary sinus ostium and the ethmoidal bulla come into view.
Abbreviations: EB = ethmoidal bulla; P = probe; MS = maxillary sinus; MSO = maxillary sinus ostium.

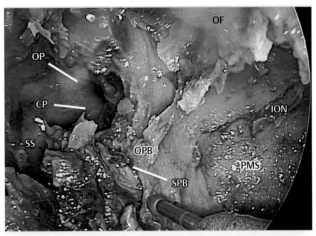

Fig. 46.5 Contents of pterygopalatine fossa: the vidian nerve, the pterygoid wedge, and V2.
Abbreviations: CP = carotid prominence; ION = infraorbital nerve; OF = orbital floor; OP = optic prominence; OPB = orbital process of the palatine bone; PMS = posterior wall of the maxillary sinus; SPB = branches of the sphenopalatine artery crossing the sphenopalatine foramen; SS = sphenoid sinus.

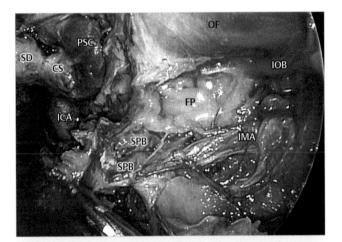

Fig. 46.4 View after maxillary osteotomy showing the sphenopalatine artery and the infraorbital neurovascular bundle.
Abbreviations: CS = cavernous sinus; FP = fat pad; ICA = internal carotid artery; IMA = internal maxillary artery; IOB = infraorbital nerve and vessels; OF = orbital floor; PSC = parasellar ICA; SD = sellar dura; SPB = sphenopalatine branches.

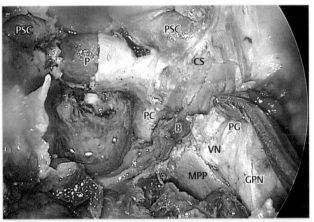

Fig. 46.6 Contents of PPF: the vidian nerve, the pterygoid wedge, and V2.
Abbreviations: B = bone over the quadrangular space; CS = lateral wall of the cavernous sinus; GPN = greater palatine nerve over the pterygoid process; MPP = medial plate of the pterygoid process; P = pituitary; PC = paraclival carotid; PG = pterygopalatine ganglion; PSC = parasellar ICA; VN = Vidian nerve.

- The posterior wall of the maxillary sinus is removed by drilling the vertical and orbital processes of the palatine bone (i.e., anterior wall of the sphenopalatine foramen).
- The periosteal layer covering the pterygopalatine fossa is opened.

46.5.1 Critical Structures

- Maxillary sinus ostium.
- Sphenopalatine artery.
- Infraorbital neurovascular bundle.
- Pterygopalatine fat and underlying blood vessels.

46.6 Exposure of the Pterygopalatine Fossa (PPF) (Figs. 46.5, 46.6)

- The contents of the pterygopalatine fossa are laterally retracted.
- The inferior portion of the medial pterygoid plate is drilled.
- The vidian nerve at the junction of the sphenoid sinus floor and medial pterygoid plate is identified.
- The pterygoid wedge (anterior junction of the medial and lateral pterygoid plates).

- The foramen rotundum and the maxillary nerve (V2) at the superior margin of the fossa are identified, by travelling laterally and superiorly toward the inferior orbital fissure.
- The maxillary nerve can be traced posteriorly to identify the foramen rotundum.

46.6.1 Critical Structures

- Vidian nerve.
- Maxillary nerve (the neural structures of the PPF lie deep to the vascular structures).

46.7 Accessing Meckel's Cave (Figs. 46.7, 46.8)

- The medial and lateral pterygoid plates are drilled back (**Fig. 46.7**).
- The vidian nerve is exposed back to the junction of the paraclival and lacerum segment of the internal carotid artery (ICA).
- The quadrangular space is exposed; it is defined by the carotid artery medially and inferiorly, by the maxillary nerve laterally and superiorly by the sixth cranial nerve and the first branch of the trigeminal nerve (V1).
- The dural opening is tailored with respect to the prominence of the tumor within Meckel's cave.

46.7.1 Critical Structures

- The ophthalmic branch of the trigeminal nerve (V1) and the abducens nerve, which both traverse along the superior aspect of the quadrangular space.

46.8 Meckel's Cave Exposure (Figs. 46.9, 46.10)

- **Parenchymal structures:** Dura of the medial middle cranial fossa.

- **Arachnoidal layer:** Trigeminal cistern.
- **Cranial nerves:** Motor and sensory roots of the trigeminal nerve, the trigeminal ganglion.
- **Arteries:** Internal carotid artery.
- **Veins:** Cavernous sinus.

46.9 Pearls

- The Vidian nerve is a crucial landmark for locating the lacerum segment of the ICA.
- Dissection should not cross the superior margin of V2 to avoid injury to the abducens nerve.

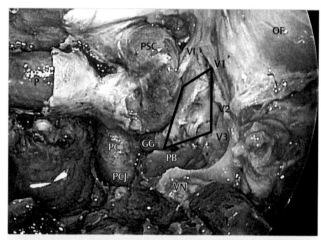

Fig. 46.8 Boundaries of the quadrangular space. The limits of the quadrangular space are shown: paraclival carotid (medially), petrous carotid and petrous bone (inferirorly), V2 and foramen rotundum (laterally), VI and V1 nerves (superiorly). Abbreviation: GG = Gasserian ganglion; OF = orbital floor; P = pituitary; PB = petrous bone over the petrous carotid; PC = paraclival carotid; PCJ = petroclival carotid junction; PSC = parasellar carotid; VI = sixth cranial nerve; VN = Vidian nerve and canal; V1 = ophthalmic nerve; V2 = maxillary nerve; V3 = mandibular nerve.

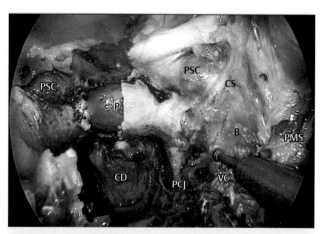

Fig. 46.7 Boundaries of the quadrangular space. Abbreviations: B = bone over the quadrangular space; CD = clival dura; CS = lateral wall of the cavernous sinus; P = pituitary; PCJ = petroclival junction of the ICA; PMS = posterior wall of the maxilla; PSC = parasellar ICA; VC = Vidian canal.

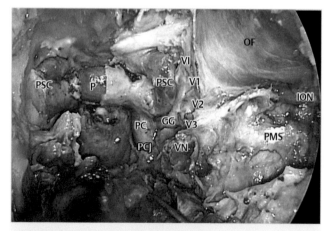

Fig. 46.9 Meckel's cave exposure (wide view). Abbreviations: GG = Gasserian ganglion; ION = infraorbital nerve; OF = orbital floor; P = pituitary; PC = paraclival carotid; PCJ = petroclival carotid junction; PMS = posterior wall of the maxilla; PSC = parasellar carotid; VI = sixth cranial nerve; VN = Vidian nerve and canal; V1 = ophthalmic nerve; V2 = maxillary nerve; V3 = mandibular nerve.

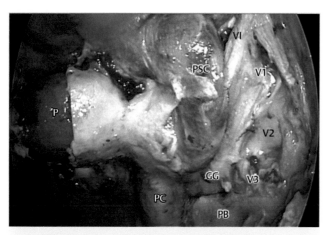

Fig. 46.10 Meckel's cave exposure (magnified view). Abbreviations: GG = Gasserian ganglion; P = pituitary; PB = petrous bone over the petrous carotid; PC = paraclival carotid; PSC = parasellar carotid; VI = sixth cranial nerve; V1 = ophthalmic nerve; V2 = maxillary nerve; V3 = mandibular nerve.

References

1. de Lara D, Ditzel Filho LF, Prevedello DM, et al. Endonasal endoscopic approaches to the paramedian skull base. World Neurosurg 2014;**82**(6, Suppl)S121–S129.
2. Hofstetter CP, Singh A, Anand VK, Kacker A, Schwartz TH. The endoscopic, endonasal, transmaxillary transpterygoid approach to the pterygopalatine fossa, infratemporal fossa, petrous apex, and the Meckel cave. J Neurosurg 2010; 113(5):967–974.
3. Raza SM, Amine MA, Anand V, Schwartz TH. Endoscopic Endonasal Resection of Trigeminal Schwannomas. Neurosurg Clin N Am 2015;26(3):473–479.
4. Simal Julián JA, Miranda Lloret P, García Piñero A, Botella Asunción C. Full endoscopic endonasal suprapetrous approach to Meckel's cave. Acta Neurochir (Wien) 2014;156(8):1623–1626.

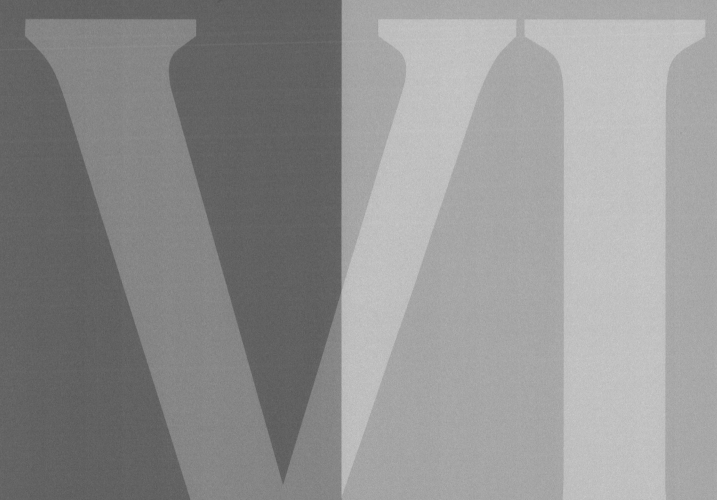

Part VI
Vascular Procedures

47 Superficial Temporal Artery – Middle Cerebral Artery Bypass

Mario Teo, Jeremiah Johnson, and Gary K. Steinberg

47.1 Indications

- Symptomatic Moya-Moya disease. To supplement cerebral blood flow due to ongoing poor cerebral perfusion.
- Complex aneurysm. To replace native cerebral blood flow when intracranial vessel sacrifice is necessary.

47.2 Patient Positioning (Fig. 47.1)

- **Position:** The patient is positioned supine with the head fixed with a Mayfield head holder.
- **Body:** A shoulder roll is placed under the ipsilateral shoulder.
- **Head:** The head is rotated 60° to the contralateral side, ensuring that venous return is not compromised due to excessive neck rotation.
- The **Sylvian fissure** has to be the highest point in the surgical field, and the operative field is parallel to the floor.

47.3 Skin Incision (Figs. 47.2, 47.3)

- From the preoperative angiogram, the most suitable superficial temporal artery (STA) branch (frontal vs parietal branch) is chosen as the donor.
- The donor STA branch is transduced using a small Doppler probe above the zygoma, and followed to the convexity for a length of about 9 cm.
- The parietal branch is preferred as it is well behind the hair line, has a straighter course, with less risk of damage to the frontal nerve during dissection.
- Minimal hair shave.

- **Linear incision**
  - A superficial skin incision is made over the STA.
  - **Starting point:** Incision starts just anterior to the tragus (posterior to the hairline).
  - **Course:** It runs along the course of the donor STA.
  - **Ending point:** The incision line ends at about 9 cm length of the STA.
- **Curvilinear incision**
  - To harvest the frontal STA branch, a curvilinear incision behind the hairline is performed.
  - **Starting point:** The incision starts just anterior to the tragus (posterior to the hairline).
  - **Course:** It runs superiorly, then curves forward to the anterior frontal line.
  - **Ending point:** Incision line ends at the mid-pupillary point at the hairline.

47.3.1 Critical Structures

- Frontal and parietal branches of STA.
- Frontal branch of the facial nerve.

47.4 Soft Tissues Dissection

- **Myofascial level**
  - The initial incision is made through the epidermis and partial thickness of dermis along the Doppler-defined projected course under microscopic examination.

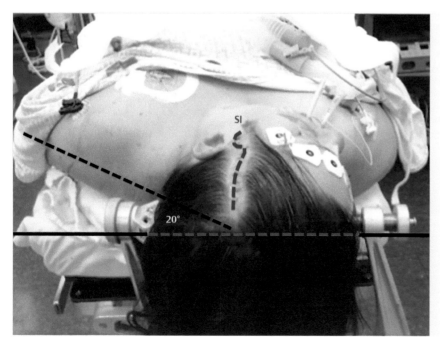

Fig. 47.1 Patient positioning. Abbreviations: SI = skin incision.

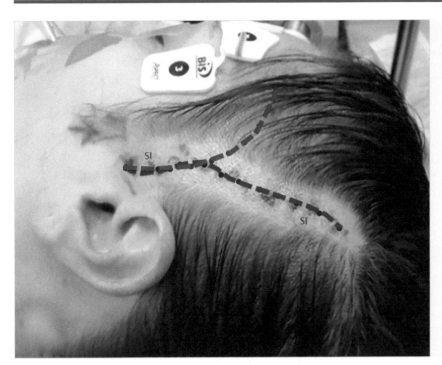

Fig. 47.2 Skin incisions are outlined. In blue over the parietal STA branch, in red a curvilinear incision to harvest frontal STA branch. Abbreviations: SI = skin incision.

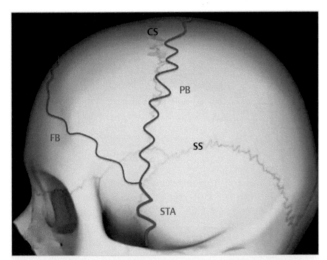

Fig. 47.3 The configuration of the frontal and parietal STA branch on a skull model.
Abbreviations: CS = coronal suture; FB = frontal branch; PB = parietal branch; SS = squamosal suture; STA = superficial temporal artery.

○ A blunt tip and fine curve scissors have to be used to perform the dissection through the remaining dermis and subcutaneous tissue to avoid damage to STA (**Fig. 47.4A**).

○ After STA vessel is visualized, dissection proceeds along the loose areolar plane around the STA vessel with a Bovie tip or microscissors (**Fig. 47.4B**), preserving a cuff of perivascular tissue, and free it from the underlying temporal fascia (**Fig. 47.4C, Fig. 47.4D**).

○ For dissection of the frontal STA branch, the vessel is dissected from the underside of the scalp flap.

• **Muscle**

○ The STA is retracted laterally, and protected with a vein retractor (**Fig. 47.5A**).

○ The temporal fascia and muscle are incised in line with the long axis of the STA, then perpendicular to this at the proximal and distal ends (in an H-shaped fashion).

○ The muscle is retracted after freeing it from the underlying bone (**Fig. 47.B**).

• **Bone exposures**

○ Subperiosteal dissection of the temporal muscle attachment is as wide anteriorly and posteriorly as allowed by the scalp incision, also from the superior temporal line superiorly to above the zygoma inferiorly.

47.5 Craniotomy (Fig. 47.6)

• **Burr holes**

○ **I**: The first burr hole is made just under the superior temporal line.

○ **II**: The second one is placed above the zygomatic process.

• **Craniotomy landmarks**

Anatomic landmarks which have to be considered in performing the craniotomy are as follows:

○ **Superiorly:** The superior temporal line.

○ **Inferiorly:** The area just above the zygomatic process.

○ **Anteriorly and posteriorly:** Anterior and posterior limit of the craniotomy are determined by the wideness of scalp exposure. A 6 cm diameter craniotomy is created to maximize the distal peri-Sylvian and recipient vessel exposure, as well to maximize the area for associated indirect revascularization to occur.

47.6 Preparing Donor Artery (Fig. 47.7)

- Donor artery preparation should be performed under microscopic guidance.
- A segment of 1–2 cm of distal STA is dissected free of all soft tissue.
- Soft tissue is also dissected off a cuff of the proximal STA for the placement of a proximal temporary clip.
- The ideal site for temporary clipping is distal to the take-off of the unused (frontal or parietal) branch of STA.

47.7 Dural Opening (Fig. 47.8)

- Dura is opened in a multiple leaflets stellate fashion.
- Dural tack-up sutures are used to obliterate epidural space.
- Large middle meningeal artery (MMA) vessels are preserved.

47.7.1 Critical Structures

- Large MMA with extensive extracranial to intracranial collateralization [determined preoperatively on the cerebral angiography, external carotid artery (ECA) injection].

47.8 Intradural Stage (Figs. 47.9–47.11)

- The arachnoid over the potential recipient middle cerebral artery (MCA) vessel is opened (**Fig. 47.9A**).

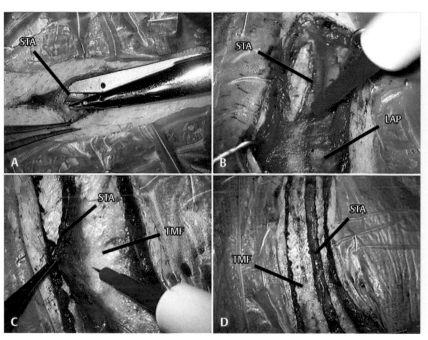

Fig. 47.4 Myofascial level. (**A**) Use a blunt tip, fine curve scissors to dissect through the remaining dermis and subcutaneous tissue to avoid damage to STA. (**B**) After the STA vessel is visualized, dissection along the loose areolar plane around the STA vessel is carried out, leaving a cuff of perivascular tissue. (**C**) STA is freed from the underlying temporal fascia. (**D**) STA is fully dissected with a thin cuff of soft tissue.
Abbreviations: LAP = loose areolar plane; STA = superficial temporal artery; TMF = temporal muscle fascia.

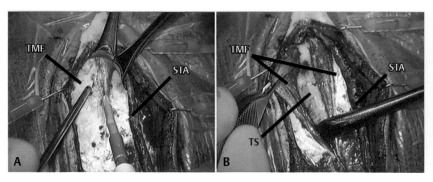

Fig. 47.5 Muscle dissection. (**A**) STA is retracted laterally, protected with a vein retractor. The temporal fascia and muscle are incised in an H-shaped fashion. (**B**) Subperiosteal muscle dissection is performed to free the temporal muscle from the underlying bone.
Abbreviations: STA = superficial temporal artery; TMF = temporal muscle fascia; TS = temporal squama.

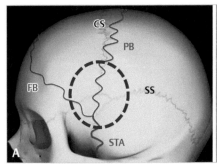
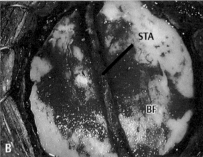

Fig. 47.6 Craniotomy. (A) The location of craniotomy on a skull model. (B) Craniotomy is performed preserving the STA. Abbreviations: BF = bone flap; CS = coronal suture; FB = frontal branch; PB = parietal branch; SS = squamosal suture; STA = superficial temporal artery.

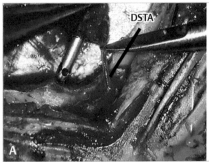
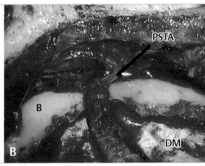

Fig. 47.7 Preparation of donor vessel. (A) Dissection of distal STA. (B) Proximal STA dissected of soft tissue for temporary clip application. Abbreviations: B = bone; DM = dura mater; DSTA = distal superficial temporal artery; PSTA = proximal superficial temporal artery.

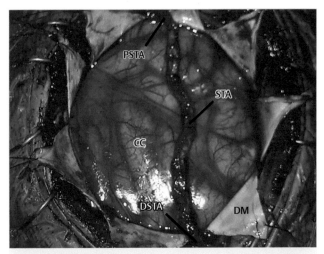

Fig. 47.8 Dural opening. Stellate dural opening, preserving the STA vessel. Abbreviations: CC = cerebral cortex; DM = dura mater; DSTA = distal superficial temporal artery; PSTA = proximal superficial temporal artery; STA = superficial temporal artery.

- A segment of 7 mm of M4 branch of MCA is prepared for temporary clipping and anastomosis.
- The minimum diameter for the recipient vessel is 0.7 mm, but ideally at least 1 mm (**Fig. 47.9B**).
- High visibility background material is passed beneath the recipient vessel.
- Before temporary clipping, blood flow is measured in the MCA branch using a Charbel Transonics ultrasonic flow probe (**Fig. 47.9C**).
- The temporary clip is applied to the proximal STA and the distal STA is divided at a 45°angle (**Fig. 47.9D**). The distal stump of the STA in the scalp is coagulated to occlude it.
- The "cut flow" in the donor artery is measured using a Charbel Transonics ultrasonic flow probe.

- The cut STA segment is flushed with heparinized saline solution (**Fig. 47.10A**).
- Prior to applying the temporary clips to the MCA vessel, MAP > 90 mmHg, hypothermia of 33–34°C and burst suppression using propofol are achieved.
- Arteriotomy is made in the recipient MCA (**Fig. 47.10B**), and the lumen is flushed with heparinized saline solution.
- The donor and recipient vessels are tinted with indigo-carmine or a sterile marking pen to better visualize the arteries during the microanastomosis.
- Monofilament sutures (10–0) are used to anchor the apices of the incision, toe stitch first (**Fig. 47.10C**), followed by the heel stitch (**Fig. 47.10D**).
- The side walls of the anastomosis are sutured in an interrupted fashion, also using 10-0 monofilament sutures.
- Sutures should be passed from outside the donor to inside the recipient or outside the recipient to inside the donor, and then tied on the outer surface of the anastomosis.
- Great care must be taken not to catch the back wall of the vessel while suturing the anastomosis.
- Once the anastomosis is complete, the temporary clips on the recipient artery are released, and then the proximal clip on the STA is removed (**Fig. 47.11A**).
- Occasionally additional sutures need to be inserted to control blood leakage at the anastomosis.
- Blood flow in the STA, proximal and distal MCA to the anastomosis is measured with a Charbel Transonics flow probe, and intraoperative indocyanine green (ICG) is performed to confirm patency and function of the bypass graft (**Fig. 47.11B**). Intraoperative Doppler of the proximal STA is also used to verify graft patency during the entire closure, including replacement of the bone flap.
- The inferior burr hole on the bone flap is enlarged appropriately to prevent compromise of the proximal STA by the replaced skull flap.

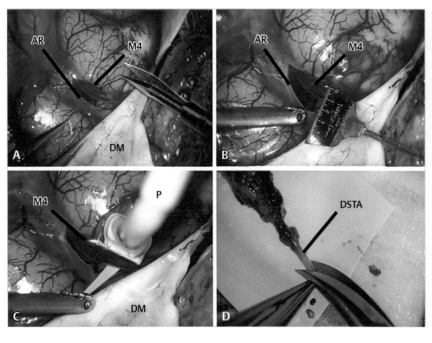

Fig. 47.9 Intradural stage. **First step.**
(**A**) Opening of the arachnoid over the potential recipient MCA vessel, exposing 7 mm of M4 branch. (**B**) Measurement of the diameter for the recipient vessel. (**C**) High visibility background material is passed beneath the recipient vessel, and blood flow is measured using a Charbel Transonics ultrasonic flow probe. (**D**) The distal STA is divided at a 45° angle. Abbreviations: AR = arachnoid; DM = dura mater; DSTA = distal superficial temporal artery; M4 = M4 branch of middle cerebral artery; P = probe.

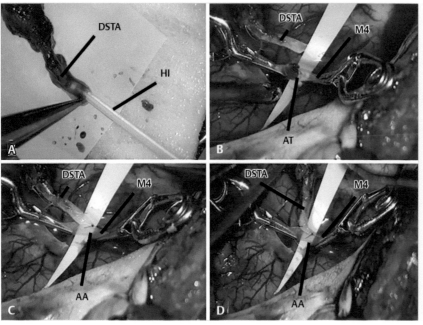

Fig. 47.10 Intradural stage. **Second step.**
(**A**) The cut STA segment flushed with heparinized saline solution. (**B**) After temporary clips are applied to MCA vessel, an arteriotomy is made and the lumen is flushed with heparinized saline solution. (**C**) The donor and recipient vessels are tinted with indigo-carmine or a marking pen to better visualize the microanastomosis. Apices of the incision are anchored with monofilament suture (10–0), toe stitch first (**C**), and heel stitch follows (**D**). Abbreviations: AA = anastomosis; AT = arteriotomy; DSTA = distal superficial temporal artery; HI = heparin injector; M4 = M4 branch of middle cerebral artery.

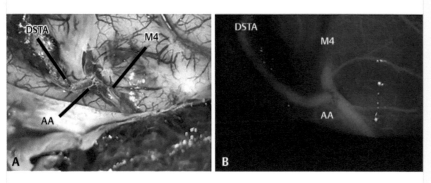

Fig. 47.11 Final view. (**A**) The side walls of the anastomosis are sutured in an interrupted fashion, also using 10–0 monofilament sutures. Once the anastomosis is complete, the temporary clips on the recipient artery are released, and then the proximal clip on the STA is removed. (**B**) Blood flow in the STA, and proximal and distal MCA to the anastomosis is measured with a flow probe, and intraoperative ICG angiogram is performed to confirm patency and function of the bypass graft. Abbreviations: AA = anastomosis; DSTA = distal superficial temporal artery; M4 = M4 branch of middle cerebral artery.

47.9 Pearls

- Successful STA-MCA bypass is a technically challenging operation, requiring operative skill, patience, and attention to detail at every stage of the operation.
- An experienced anesthetic team and specialized neurological intensive care unit (ICU) are imperative to achieve low rates of morbidity.
- For the early career neurosurgeon, laboratory microanastomosis practice and mentorship are essential for good outcomes.

References

1. Chang SD, Steinberg GK, eds. Superficial temporal artery to middle cerebral artery anastomosis. In: Techniques in Neurosurgery. Philadelphia: Lippincott Williams and Wilkins;2000; No. 6.

2. Gooderham PA, Steinberg GK, eds. Intracranial-Extracranial Bypass Surgery for Moyamoya Disease. In: Spetzler RF, Kalani Y, Nakaji P, eds. Neurovascular surgery. 2nd ed. ed: Thieme;2015.

3. Guzman R, Lee M, Achrol A, et al. Clinical outcome after 450 revascularization procedures for moyamoya disease. Clinical article. J Neurosurg 2009;111(5):927–935.

4. Miyamoto S, Yoshimoto T, Hashimoto N, et al; JAM Trial Investigators. Effects of extracranial-intracranial bypass for patients with hemorrhagic moyamoya disease: results of the Japan Adult Moyamoya Trial. Stroke 2014;45(5):1415–1421.

5. Qian C, Yu X, Li J, Chen J, Wang L, Chen G. The Efficacy of Surgical Treatment for the Secondary Prevention of Stroke in Symptomatic Moyamoya Disease: A Meta-Analysis. Medicine (Baltimore) 2015;94(49):e2218.

48 High Flow Bypass (Common Carotid Artery – Middle Cerebral Artery)

Michael Kerin Morgan

48.1 Introduction

- For the purpose of illustration, a right-sided common carotid (CCA) to middle cerebral artery (MCA) bypass with an interposition saphenous vein graft (IPSVG) is described (CCA-MCA IPSVG).
- Variations to this procedure include distal anastomosis to the internal carotid artery (ICA) and posterior cerebral artery (PCA) as well as proximal anastomosis to the external carotid artery. However, the principles of performing a CCA-ICA IPSVG can be readily applied to these variations with minor adaptation that is obvious to those once CCA-MCA IPSVG is understood. Therefore, for economy of space, the details of these variations are not included.
- Various surgical techniques, many of which are unknown to this author, can be applied to achieve the same end.
- The author owes his understanding of the technique of performing CCA-MCA IPSVG to Dr. Sundt, perhaps the greatest innovator and executor of brain revascularization surgery in history. There are minor variations that have been incorporated into the author's description from that taught by Dr. Sundt. Those ideas that you find helpful are either Dr. Sundt's or inspired by Dr. Sundt while those that you find are not helpful assume are my ideas.
- In addition to the usual preparations for major neurosurgery, aspirin commenced preoperatively is appropriate. This does create difficulty with oozing continually with the three wounds that are created during this surgery.

48.2 Indications

- The high flow bypass is rarely a choice for any specific condition. The choice of such bypass is almost always a fallback solution when no other options are available or likely to succeed.
- Replacement of major intracranial arteries. These include ICA, MCA and basilar arteries. This is most commonly due to either aneurysm treatment or resection of skull base lesions.
- In the case of aneurysm treatment, this may be combined with internal bypasses for the management of MCA aneurysms where simpler clipping procedures are deemed at high risk. CCA-MCA IPSVG to one M2 branch with rotation of the other M2 branch as an internal bypass to the bypassed M2 branch can render a bifurcation aneurysm treatable that is otherwise unclippable. For basilar artery aneurysms untreated except for trapping, CCA-PCA IPSVG to the bypass may protect the upper basilar and branch circulation.
- In an emergency, when the ICA or MCA has been inadvertently damaged during surgery and cannot be repaired.
- Augmentation of flow is rarely needed to be corrected by high flow bypass because of the danger of producing a catastrophic intracerebral hemorrhage into a region of hyperemia consequent on bypass. In such cases, low flow superficial temporal to M4 bypass is appropriate.

48.3 Patient Positioning

- **Patient position**
  - **Bypass to M2 or ICA: the patient is positioned supine**.
    - The three-point head fixation is applied with the 2 points ipsilateral to the side of cranial surgery immediately superior to the transverse sigmoid sinus and the single point placed into the superior temporal line on the frontal bone.
    - It is to be positioned so that no component of the device is in a plane above the most superior part of the skull when in the final position for surgery.
    - The table will be slightly broken with the back rotated upward 10-15° and, similarly, the lower-limbs will be rotated upward by a similar degree.
    - The table should be elevated or lowered to achieve a level in which the surgeon has his or her arms bent 90° at the elbows and the wrists are straight at level of the operating site at the head (taking into account surgical instruments at the target distal anastomosis).
  - **Bypass to the second and third part of the posterior cerebral artery (PCA), under the temporal lobe**.
    - The three-point head fixation is applied with the 2 points ipsilateral to the side of cranial surgery immediately superior to the transverse sigmoid sinus, the two-pin straddling the torcular and the single point placed into frontal bone of the forehead.
    - It is to be positioned so that no component of the device is in a plane above the most superior part of the skull when in the final position for surgery.
    - The table should be positioned at a level as for the more common bypass to the MCA.
- **Head position**
  - **Bypass to the M2 or ICA**.
    - The head is rotated 15° on its axis from the vertical, to the opposite side to the target artery, flexed 15° to the opposite shoulder in the coronal plane, rotated 15° backward in the sagittal plane and the head is lifted upward in this set position flexing the C7 on T1 and extending the skull on the cervical spine.
    - This minimal rotation facilitates easy dissection of the Sylvian fissure by ensuring that the temporal lobe can be easily supported during fissure dissection and not falling onto the temporal lobe that would result in the need for vigorous retraction.
    - In this position, the skin of the neck should be smooth and not wrinkled and the anterior border of the sternocleidomastoid muscle to be slightly tense allowing the skin incision to expose the carotid artery to be easily performed.
  - **Bypass to the PCA, under the temporal lobe**.
    - The head is rotated 60° from the vertical, to the opposite side to the target artery and tilted 10° toward the floor.
    - In this position, the neck should be similarly exposed to the above.

- After the table is put into position, the middle cranial fossa floor will be perpendicular to the room floor.
- **Shoulder position**
  - **Bypass to the M2 or ICA:** there is no role for altering the shoulders in the supine position.
  - **For bypass to the PCA under the temporal lobe:** a sandbag is placed under the shoulder to reduce any stretch on the brachial plexus but the shoulder should remain below the plane of the anterior border of the ipsilateral sternocleidomastoid muscle.
- **Lower limb position**
  - Both lower limbs are placed in a position and draped in such a way as to allow access to the entire long saphenous vein (SV) from its position immediately anterior to the medial malleolus to the inguinal ligament.
  - Mark the line of this vein prior to surgery (venous duplex ultrasound assists with this task) so that the skin incision can be made more rapidly when it comes time to harvesting vein.
  - Both lower limbs should be slightly everted so that the line of the skin incision can be readily seen. The lower limbs should be in a position that the surgeon can harvest vein below the knee by manipulating the lower limb with slight flexion of the knee to increase the ankle eversion at the time that the SV is harvested.
- **Anti-decubitus device**
  - The surgery may be prolonged, and the patient should be placed on a mat that protects pressure areas on the back.
  - Furthermore, the use of a heating blanket over the abdomen and chest is appropriate to prevent a fall in core temperature, as much of the patient will be uncovered in a cold operating room.
  - After the table is flexed into position with both the back and the lower limbs raised, the elbows and hands are placed and protected from pressure areas.
  - When the scalp flap is complete, it is critical for this scalp flap to be retracted down low over the eye and placing this flap under tension. Therefore, care needs to be made in placing pads over the eyes for protection. If these are

unduly thick, the subsequent retraction of the scalp flap over these pads may lead to excessive pressure on the eye causing blindness.
- **Anatomic structure put at highest point in the surgical field**
  - For the more commonly performed bypass to the M2 or ICA, the highest point of the surgical field is the malar eminence. For the less commonly performed bypass to the PCA, under the temporal lobe, the highest point of the surgical field is the frontal process of the zygoma.
  - For the lower limb, the medial tip of the great toe should be the highest point, slightly superior to the plane of the medial patella.

48.4 Skin Incision (Fig. 48.1)

- **Cervical incision to expose the common carotid artery (CCA) for proximal anastomosis**
  - This is the first incision performed.
  - The side selected to perform the proximal anastomosis is the ipsilateral CCA or external carotid artery (ECA) unless there is significant disease of this side and the contralateral CCA is healthy.
  - For this incision, the surgeon is standing on the right, with the assistant above the patient's head and the scrub nurse on the left.
  - The following describes the procedure from the right.
  - ***Shape:***
    - A curvilinear incision with the central stem tracking the anterior border of the sternocleidomastoid muscle (SCM) with a posteriorly directed superior limb curving toward the mastoid tip and the anteriorly directed inferior limb curving parallel to the skin crease toward the jugular notch.
    - The incision commences at the tip of the posteriorly directed superior limb.
    - It continues on the anterior border of the SMC.
    - It terminates in the anteriorly directed inferior limb curving parallel to the skin crease toward the jugular notch.

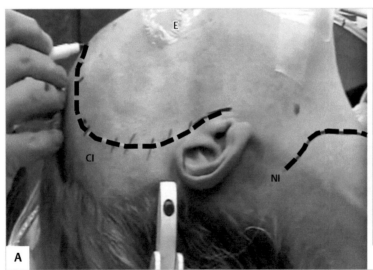
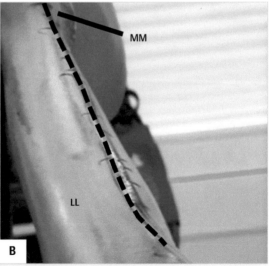

Fig. 48.1 The scalp and neck incision are marked on the right side of the head (**A**) and the left leg marking (**B**).
Abbreviations: CI = cranial incision; E = eye; LL = left leg; MM = medial malleolus; NI = neck incision.

- **Cranial incision to expose the skull for orbito-zygomatic craniotomy (for anastomosis to ICA, MCA proximal to bifurcation (M1) or M2)**
  - Curvilinear incision behind the hairline of the patient except at the inferior margin. In the case where the patient has receding hair, the incision can be placed in one of the superior forehead creases until the lateral margin of the incision where it joins the usual incision line.
  - It commences 2 cm across the midline with the knife blade penetrating to a depth through the dermis, epidermis, and just through the galea.
  - The depth to the level immediately penetrating the galea (but not through the temporalis fascia) is held constant throughout the course of the scalp incision with vascular scalp clips applied for hemostasis.
  - The inferior point is immediately anterior to ear at the level of the inferior margin of the zygomatic arch.
  - Subsequent blunt dissection with Metzenbaum scissors is performed to create the tunnel to accommodate the future introduction of the tunneler (to deliver the SV) between the craniotomy incision and the cervical incision deep to all skin layers.
  - The early establishment of this tunnel ensures sufficient time for deep and not reachable oozing within to spontaneously thrombose well before the intradural surgery to reduce the risk of run-in bleeding at the time of the anastomosis.
- **Lower limb incision to expose the long saphenous vein**
  - The site from which the SV is harvested is determined by the best and healthiest straight 23 cm length, even caliber lumen with the least number of tributaries, as determined by venous duplex ultrasound. Therefore, the site will be either left or right lower limb above or below the knee. If possible, selection of below the knee source is preferable because of the smaller diameter.
  - *Starting point, course and ending point:*
    - The incision is immediately over the vein. This is a straight line from the medial ankle to a point heading for the medial mid knee joint until two-thirds up the lower leg and then curving slightly backward and up to a point just behind the medial knee joint and then toward a point immediately medial to the femoral pulse at the inguinal ligament.
    - If commencing at the ankle, the easiest location to find the SV (as there is very little tissue between the skin and vein at this site and it can be palpated either in the standing position or the recumbent position after restricting venous flow from the ankle by compression), the place to commence the incision is immediately anterior to the medial malleolus.
    - Incision ends where 23 cm of straight, even caliber lumen, with a minimum of tributaries can be harvested. It is unusual to find such a segment included in the vein that straddles the level of the knee.

48.4.1 Critical Structures

- In the segment of the vein in the vicinity of the ankle, the saphenous nerve is immediately adjacent.
- Care in preserving the nerve will reduce the chance for bothersome paresthesia of the nearby skin.

48.5 Soft Tissue Dissection

48.5.1 Cranial Exposure

- Surgical technique of cranial soft tissue dissection is already described in **Chapter 17.**

48.5.2 Carotid Exposure

- The skin incision should be bold and include incision of the platysma with a single cut, but not penetrating the external cervical fascia (and remaining superficial to the external facial vein).
- Hemostats are placed on the platysma edge of the incision and bleeding controlled either with hemostats, clips or bipolar diathermy.
- The external cervical fascia is divided along the anterior border of the SMC, the border of which is followed deeply to the deep cervical fascia immediately superficial to the internal jugular vein (IJV).
- The dissection should be superficial to the deep cervical fascia immediately medial to the internal jugular vein. During the exposure, the common facial vein may need to be ligated and divided.
- Because of the large size of this vein and its proximity of the ligation to this venous junction with the IJV, ligation and division of the common facial vein is performed with a stitch through the vein and tie (stitch-tie) to ensure that the ligature will not subsequently slip from the divided end.
- The deep cervical fascia is opened immediately superficial to the common carotid artery (CCA) with Metzenbaum scissors inferiorly to expose the common carotid artery and carried superiorly toward the level of the hypoglossal nerve (as it crosses the external carotid artery [ECA]).
- The CCA, the intended site of the proximal anastomosis, is then dissected and mobilized from the surrounding deep cervical fascia to facilitate the placement of vascular loops around the CCA above and below the planned arteriotomy and cross clamp placement sites during the proximal anastomosis.
- During this dissection, care in preserving the more deeply placed vagus nerve (between the CCA and IJV) is essential. At the site of the intended proximal anastomosis on the CCA, the loose adventitial tissue is removed at this time to ensure that this tissue cannot be inadvertently included in the suture line of the proximal anastomosis.

48.5.3 Critical Structures

- Ansa hypoglossi, that can be seen at the time of dissection of the CCA.

48.6 Craniotomy and Orbitotomy (Fig. 48.2)

- Techniques of craniotomy and orbitotomy are already described in **Chapter 17.**

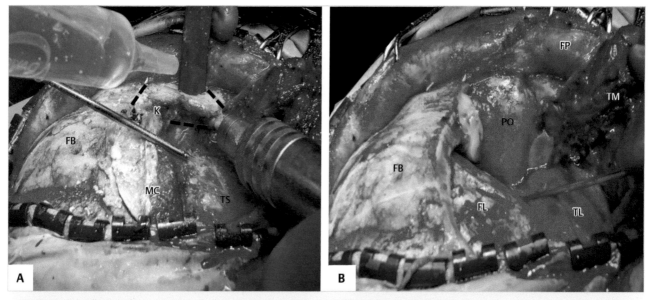

Fig. 48.2   (**A**) Following the craniotomy, the lateral orbital margin cut is performed and then the craniotome is continued under the orbital rim and exits at the keyhole burr hole. (**B**) The complete exposure before dural opening. Having removed the craniotomy flap, the dura and the periorbita are stripped from the bones of the orbit and the roof and lateral wall of the orbit are removed. The remainder of the sphenoid wing is removed allowing access to removal of the remaining orbital roof and wall to have in visual continuity the dura and the periorbita. Abbreviations: FB = frontal bone; FL = frontal lobe; FP = fat pad; K = keyhole; MC = muscle cuff; PO = periorbit; TL = temporal lobe; TM = temporal muscle; TS = temporal squama.

48.6.1 Critical Structures

- Levator palpebrae superioris.
- Frontal branch of V1.
- Lacrimal gland.
- Dissection to the floor of the middle cranial fossa with stripping of the temporalis muscle to this level risks damage to the nervous innervation, the deep temporal branch of V3.

48.7 Dural Opening (Fig. 48.3)

- The dural opening needs to be performed in a manner that reduces run-in during the distal anastomosis. This has been facilitated by the limited rotation of the head.
- The dura is opened in a curve following the free bone edge medially and posteriorly and reflected on the dural fold of the superior orbital fissure and hitched up.
- After hitching the dura, the author sutures a sucker into the inferior-posterior dura, the most dependent extradural location inside the craniotomy limits, to capture blood pooling.

48.8 Intradural Exposure

- **Parenchymal structures**
  - The frontal and temporal lobes need to be separated as much as is safely possible to facilitate the distal anastomosis. It is important during their separation that the pial margins are not violated, that significant venous drainage is not impeded and that they are not retracted with excess vigor.
- **Arachnoidal layer**
  - The Sylvian fissure is widely opened and the target and the key of the exposure. This is performed from lateral to medial. Because the patient is usually on aspirin and will

be given heparin at some stage during the surgery, it is imperative that the pial margins not be breached. By placing the external boundary of the Sylvian fissure under tension with a sucker applied to the frontal lobe (opposite where the first arachnoid incision is to be made) an incision with an 11-blade is made superior to the superficial middle cerebral vein. This incision is continued forward until access to the depths of the Sylvian fissure can be made. After this initial opening, the dissection continues deeply within the Sylvian fissure, enlarging by sharp dissection the plane that separates the superior and inferior divisions and branches of the middle cerebral artery. The arachnoid is easily divided by the 11-blade, with arachnoid made tense by judicious placement of the sucker tip and shaft, and dissected by the 11-blade and sucker, with the arachnoid tension released. The depth of the dissection should be to the deepest part of the fissure, to the deep middle cerebral vein. Once this has been achieved, dissection progresses from deep to superficial and from lateral to medial (progressively extending the division of the external barrier arachnoid membrane medially).
  - The frontal lobe is then retracted by the sucker in the left hand with the suction placing tension on the arachnoid bridging between the ipsilateral optic nerve (and chiasm) and the frontal lobe, facilitating its division with the 11-blade from medial to lateral, joining the deepest and medial opening of the Sylvian fissure.
  - The importance of a very wide opening of the Sylvian fissure is to make performing the distal anastomosis as easy as possible without the need for retraction on the brain. The latter is critical given that the arteries will have their normal flow arrested during cross-clamping.
- **Cranial nerves**
  - The optic and oculomotor nerves come into view at the medial end of the Sylvian and basal cistern exposure.

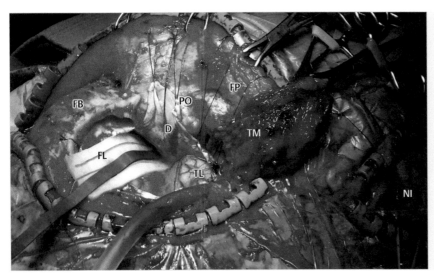

Fig. 48.3 The dural opening reflected on the superior orbital fissure creating a small degree of retraction of the periorbita. The dura is tented upward on the inferior margin to act as a gutter for blood run-in from the more superiorly placed structures. The sucker is sutured into the dura of the most dependent part of the dural opening to minimize run-in.
Abbreviations: D = dura; FB = frontal bone; FL = frontal lobe; FP = fat pad; NI = neck incision; PO = periorbit; TL = temporal lobe; TM = temporal muscle.

◦ The olfactory nerve, usually unsighted, may be placed under excess tension and damaged (as well as causing troublesome bleeding from veins at the cribriform plate end) if overly vigorous superior retraction of the frontal lobe occurs with suction placed on its orbital surface.

- **Arteries**
  ◦ The wide Sylvian fissure opening, along with the adjacent basal cisterns, allows the space between the optic tract and the oculomotor nerve to be enlarged to expose the subarachnoid course of the internal carotid and the Sylvian part of the middle cerebral arteries in its entire and continuous course and to remain on view without the need for retractor placement.

- **Veins**
  ◦ The superficial middle cerebral vein and its temporal lobe tributaries and connection with the cavernous sinus should be preserved.
  ◦ There is often a large posterior frontal vein tributary that should be preserved by marking the posterior and lateral boundary of the Sylvian fissure opening.
  ◦ More medial frontal lobe veins that bridge the developing space created by the Sylvian fissure opening are usually small and can be divided. Although, normally, one would desire complete venous preservation, these smaller bridging veins might prove slightly restrictive at the time of performing the distal anastomosis, a difficult task that should not be made slower unnecessarily.
  ◦ At the root of the medial Sylvian fissure, with the frontal lobe retracted by the dissector, a small vein bridging between the deepest part of the superficial middle cerebral vein, the anterior cerebral vein, is placed under tension and may need to be divided. Otherwise, the veins can be generally preserved.

48.9 Harvesting the Long Saphenous Vein (Fig. 48.4)

- The fascia and superficial areolar tissue immediately superficial to the long saphenous vein is divided with Metzenbaum scissors slightly opened and sliding from inferior to superior. Deviation from an immediate superficial location risks inadvertent and premature division of tributaries to the long saphenous vein. At and near the ankle, care should be made of preserving the saphenous nerve during the vein dissection.
- After the long saphenous is completely uncovered of fascia and superficial areolar tissue, the lateral adherent connective tissue, within which the tributaries can be found, is divided, at a short distance from the vein, between these tributaries by placing the vein on slight tension with a vascular loop.
- The tributaries are then sequentially ligated and divided by ligature or clip throughout the veins length on either side.
- The vein is undermined with sharp dissection to be free of all tissue connections between the long saphenous vein and the leg.
- A minimum of 23 cm of straight, consistently even diameter, is an appropriate length of vein to harvest for the required distance between the MCA (or ICA or PCA) and CCA. This allows for some potential loss of length if tributaries, valves or trauma at either end requires a very short segment to be removed.
- Each end of the dissected free long saphenous vein is ligated and divided.
- The free ankle end of vein is cannulated with a round nosed cannula and sutured into place (both to ensure the watertight closure at this point and to facilitate ensuring the correct direction of the vein is retained until the anastomoses are commenced) and quickly the vein is irrigated to clear the lumen of blood.
- Having cleared the blood, the vein is sequentially gently dilated by combining the injection of irrigation with manual manipulation of the restricted irrigand solution forcing the distension of the lumen. The dilated vein should be of even caliber throughout its length.
- The last of the vein, at the cut free end, cannot be dilated in this way and will be cut and discarded after the vein is positioned immediately before the distal anastomosis is executed.
- Leaks in the vein during irrigation distension are repaired by placing a ligaclip on the vein or, if insufficient length of tributary, by 7-0 prolene (or similar) suturing of the hole, closed in a line in the long-axis of the vein. By orienting the suture in the long-axis of the vein may slightly shorten the length but will not reduce the radius.

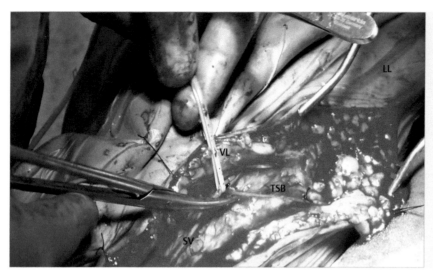

Fig. 48.4 The saphenous vein is harvested with gentle retraction of the vein with a vascular loop. The round nosed cannula is inserted and secured in the ankle end of the vein for irrigation and gentle distension. Distension is performed in very small sequential segments from the cannula upward to minimize the amount of pressure applied to cause distension.
Abbreviations: LL = left leg; VL = vascular loop; SV = saphenous vein; TSB = tied side branch.

48.10 Positioning Saphenous Vein Between Planned Proximal and Distal Anastomosis

- At all times, an untwisted orientation of the vein must be maintained. To avoid twisting the vein during placement between cervical and cranial sites, an essential safety precaution, the vein is untwisted immediately after harvest, distension and before placement into the tunneller at the cervical end.
- Distension with rapid irrigation, ensuring that the vein is free to conform to the orientation unhindered by external force, facilitates this untwisting. While untwisted and distended by irrigation, the vein is sucked into the tunneller (with a lumen wide enough not to restrict the vein from untwisting) with the suction tubing placed over the cranial end of the tunneller until the vein reaches the cranial end of the tunneller.
- Precautions against sucking the vein into the suction tubing need to be made such as being in a position to clamp the suction tubing and a firm grasp on the vein at the cervical end. The vein should be subjected to minimal trauma during this delivery.
- Once the vein is in position between the cranial and cervical openings, the tunneller is removed without rotation via the cranial end, over the vein, while the vein is being aggressively irrigated to ensure no twisting caused by removal of the tunneller.
- The vein is then pulled through until there is sufficient length to perform the distal anastomosis. This length requires slack to facilitate moving the vein around during the construction of the distal anastomosis. This slack is removed later, after the distal anastomosis is completed and before the proximal anastomosis is commenced, when the correct length is determined to minimize the chance of redundancy and consequent kinking.
- The distal vein is then prepared by cutting the end with fine scissors in a segment that is distended and excludes valves and tributaries in the immediate terminal region. Because of the large mismatch in size between vein and MCA, a fish-mouth opening is not necessary in the vein at the distal anastomosis.

- Loose adventitial tissue is removed from the last 1 cm of vein to ensure that no loose tissue could be inadvertently included in the anastomosis and that needle placement through the wall, including the endothelial layer, is accurate.

48.11 Distal Anastomosis (Fig. 48.5)

- The distal anastomosis is normally an end-to-side anastomosis on the M2 or PCA and end-to-end on the ICA. For the example of the high-flow bypass in this chapter, I will describe the M2 anastomosis. The vein has been prepared and is ready for anastomosis.
- The length of the vein within the fissure must have the appropriate redundancy at, and during, the distal anastomosis to eliminate all potential tension. It cannot be too short, as the vein will not be persuaded to oppose the arteriotomy with tightening and tying a 9-O suture. Similarly, excessive length may also pull away because of gravity. It is useful to have just enough redundancy to perform a suture on the easier side first and then, if required, pulling the vein down to gain a little extra length for the opposite side and opening up the aperture between arteriotomy and vein with a retractor very gently placed over a cottonoid on the vein to hold it in position. It is important if using this retractor that no pressure is placed on the vein or brain. The retractor is for holding the vein in place making it easier to complete the anastomosis. If this is not required then it should not be used.
- It is important that, once sutures have been placed, any attempt to shorten the vein redundancy within the Sylvian fissure must not result in tension on the suture line. Tension can occur when pulling the vein in the cervical wound to correct for length. This can cause a stretching of the vein placed within the subcutaneous tunnel between the two anastomoses sites, leading to a delayed correction of the stretched segment with sudden pulling of the vein at the distal anastomosis. This is prevented by gentle movement of the vein, back and forth, between the two openings.

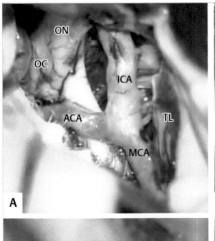

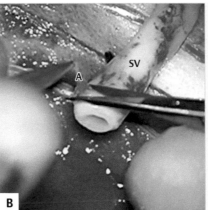

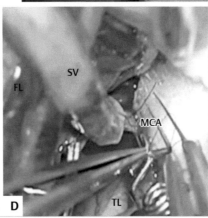

Fig. 48.5 Proximal anastomosis.
(A) Intradural view. **(B)** The saphenous vein is trimmed of loose adventitia that could interfere with the distal anastomosis construction. **(C, D)** The proximal anastomosis is being constructed with a running 7-0 prolene having first placed the double-armed suture in the heel of the fish-mouthed vein and distal arteriotomy of the common carotid artery. It is very important that the length has been appropriately set at this time. This usually means that the heel stitch is under very slight tension, anticipating the lengthening of the vein when blood is flowing within its lumen.
Abbreviations: A = adventitia; ACA = anterior cerebral artery; FL = frontal lobe; ICA = internal carotid artery; MCA = middle cerebral artery; OC = optic chiasm; ON = optic nerve; S = stich; SV = saphenous vein; TC = temporary clip; TL = temporal lobe.

- After preparing the anesthetist to increase the blood pressure and administering agents that enhance cerebral protection and awaiting the reversal of any temporary falls in blood pressure that may result from administering ischemic protection drugs (e.g., barbiturates) and placing the prepared vein into position adjacent to the planned site of anastomosis, the selected segment of artery for the distal anastomosis is cross clamped with temporary clips.
- The length of segment selected must be of sufficient to ensure the arteriotomy will accommodate the vein without a stenosis in the end of the vein (after establishing the bypass) as well as allowing the anchoring sutures to be placed at each end in the long axis of the artery without their needles coming into contact with the temporary clips. It is far more important to have the appropriate length and longest arteriotomy possible than to reduce cross clamp time by reducing the length of arteriotomy and save on suture time. Shortening of the arteriotomy is a false economy, as the mid-side walled sutures do not take very long to place.
- The segment selected for bypass should have no branches. Any back bleeding from such unintentionally included arteries will be troublesome in executing the bypass and will result in infarction to brain to which they are distributed (because there is no pressure and back bleeding will occur with reversed capillary flow).
- If such arteries are discovered after performing the arteriotomy, they should immediately have a temporary or microclip applied to stop back bleeding.
- The distal temporary clip is placed before the proximal temporary clip to increase the tension within the cross clamped segment to facilitate opening of the arteriotomy.

- The arteriotomy can be opened with an eye knife, fine needle or, by holding the adventitia, with scissors. Once the initial opening is made, the arteriotomy should be extended to the appropriate length with fine microscissors.
- The vein that has been previously positioned adjacent to the arteriotomy is then anastomosed by placing and tying an interrupted 9-0 suture at the proximal and distal end of the arteriotomy.
- The needle must be through endothelium and the vein must be slightly everted by having a needle trajectory through the thick vein wall that prevents inversion. It goes without saying that all knots must be outside the lumen of the artery and vein and therefore, each stitch must be initiated from outside the vessel. It is normally easier to commence with the needle going through the artery before the vein.
- The first throw of the tie over the knot tying forceps should be a double loop and when pulling the knot tight, should be performed with the knot flat, and therefore having the tips of the knot tying forceps at the level of the arteriotomy, pulling the sutures in opposite directions.
- The tension on tightening the first throw should be held for a few moments after the knot has been tightened. This decreases the likelihood that the artery and vein will pull away from each other and loosen the stitch.
- The second throw on the two corner anchoring stitches should be in the same direction as the first throw, allowing the knot to be slightly tightened.
- The third and final throw should be in the opposite direction to lock the tied stitch. The length of the suture thread depends upon whether the suture is to be a running stitch or the first interrupted suture.

- The amount of suture that you pull through before tying must allow for easy and minimal number of grabs to perform the tie. The length needed for a running suture needs to take into account the requirement to tie the stitch to the other anchoring point.
- The technique for running the suture requires the suture thread to be relatively loosely placed between each stitch so that the space between the vein and the arteriotomy can be visualized to ensure placement of the needle through the full vessel wall including the intima. If the suture is tightened after performing each stitch, it is difficult to place the last stitch with confidence as there will be no gap between artery and vein to be sure that the needle passes into the lumen of both artery and vein and has not passed through the full vessel wall.
- In addition, it is difficult to maintain sufficient tension in the suture thread at each stitch with continuous suturing, necessitating a requirement to ensure each stitch is tightened. Therefore, it is appropriate to do this tightening task once rather than having to repeat after each stitch as well as at the end, before tying to the anchoring stitch.
- The technique for interrupted sutures can be performed in a number of ways.
  - Each stitch can be inserted and tied in order of their insertion. However, the same problem described above can make the last stitch, adjacent to the anchoring stitch, difficult to perform with confidence that the needle has negotiated the full wall of both artery and vein.
  - Passing each stitch, but not tying them until all have been placed, can overcome this problem. This is completed on one side of the anastomosis before repeating the same on the opposite side of the anastomosis.
  - Another technique that I believe is more useful, providing the vein is not inadvertently moved significantly during stitch placement, is to insert each needle of the suture between vein and artery, but not pushing the needle all the way through. This allows a rigid scaffolding of needles holding the gap steady between vein and artery and making the next stitch placement less difficult. After all have been inserted, the needle and suture thread can be pulled through and then tied. This is completed on one side of the anastomosis before repeating the same on the opposite side of the anastomosis.
- Having completed the anastomosis, heparin is administered and allowed to circulate, followed by placing a temporary clip on the IPSVG before removing the distal temporary clip, checking for leaks, and subsequently removing the proximal temporary clip.
- If leaks occur at the suture line, this can be repaired by a single stitch placed and tied at each leaking point. Reapplying the temporary clips during this task is usually not necessary.
- The health of the anastomosis is usually readily apparent without special techniques at this time. If there is uncertainty, there may be a technical error. By inserting a number 15 needle into the MCA side of the IPSVG immediately before the temporary clip should cause a high fountain, appropriate for the blood pressure, from the IPSVG. It is wise to move the microscope from the field during this maneuver as the stream of blood may hit the microscope lens cover or the microscope drape and immediately drip back into the wound. When this occurs, a cottonoid placed over the bleeding point will almost always result in the spontaneous sealing of the leaking point.
- Immediately at the completion of the distal anastomosis, the extraneous length is removed by carefully pulling the IPSVG with fingers holding the vein on each side of the craniotomy and cervical wounds.
- It is wise to gently pull the vein in both directions for a brief distance to ensure that it has not become held up at a point within the tunnel. If this has occurred, applying tension in positioning the vein may subsequently cause stretching and a sudden retraction of the anastomosed vein toward the tunnel with potentially catastrophic consequences at the site of anastomosis. Ensuring that the IPSVG remains free (or forcing the veins release from a point of adherence) in the tunnel by moving the vein back and forth is important. Judging the correct length is difficult, because once the vein is distended with blood under arterial pressure, it does slightly lengthen. However, it is important to avoid a point of IPSVG kinking.

48.12 Proximal Anastomosis (Figs. 48.6 and 48.7)

- The proximal anastomosis is performed next.
- The vein is cut at a point where there is sufficient length to be anastomosed without tension but not long enough for kinking to occur on establishing flow. Again, it must be remembered that the IPSVG will slightly lengthen with arterial pressure on releasing the cross clamp.
- Check to see that there is no twisting of the vein. It is important to do a wide fish-mouth.
- The end of the vein is cut at 45° and then the vein opened further, extended by small Pott's scissors, by the same length again as the flattened vein opening. This provides a very large circumference and minimizes the resistance that this anastomosis will present to the subsequent flow of blood within.
- Excess loose tissue is quickly removed from the end of the vein.
- The vein opening is then placed on the common carotid artery under very slight tension to check the site and length of the subsequent arteriotomy. If this site is not clear of loose adventitial material, it is cleared at this time.
- The CCA is cross clamped with sufficient distance for the arteriotomy, including the distance on the common carotid artery proximal and distal to the intended arteriotomy, to accept needle placement without coming into contact with the carotid clamps.
- The arteriotomy is opened with a number 11 knife and a sufficient opening is cut to allow access to the Pott's scissors that subsequently enlarge the arteriotomy to the length appropriate for the vein.
- To confirm that this is sufficient, it may be necessary to juxtapose the opened vein end with the arteriotomy. With practice this is unnecessary.
- The inside of the artery is then irrigated with heparinized saline solution to flush all blood from within. The heel of the planned anastomosis (i.e., that end of the vein that is fashioned by the Pott's scissors sutured to the distal limit of the arteriotomy) is the point of commencing the running suture.

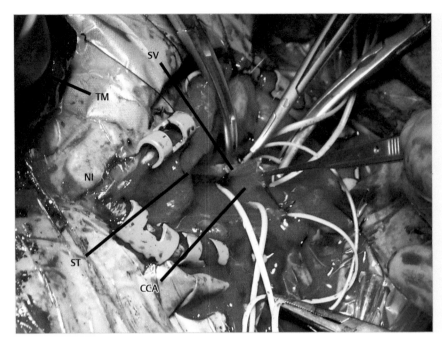

Fig. 48.6 Distal anastomosis.
Abbreviations: CCA = common carotid artery; NI = neck incision; ST = subcutaneous tunnel; SV = saphenous vein; TM = temporal muscle.

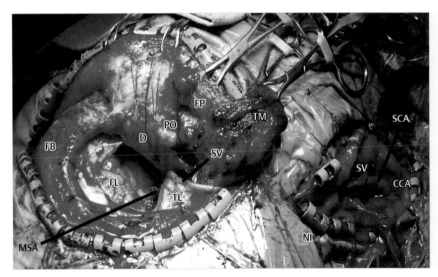

Fig. 48.7 Final view.
Abbreviations: CCA = common carotid artery; D = dura; FB = frontal bone; FL = frontal lobe; FP = fat pad; MSA = middle cerebral artery saphenous vein anastomosis; NI = neck incision; PO = periorbit; SCA = saphenous vein-common carotid artery anastomosis; SV = saphenous vein; TL = temporal lobe; TM = temporal muscle.

- The needle of the double-armed 7-O prolene is first placed in the vein from without to within followed by driving the needle through the distal point of the arteriotomy from within to without. This is then tied at the heel before running the suture.
- The first needle placements on each side and adjacent to the heel stich are slightly difficult as they need to be placed close to the heel stitch and angled at about 45° orientation to the arteriotomy edge, (halfway between the alignment of the heel stitch at 0° to the arteriotomy edge and each subsequent stich that is placed 90° to the edge of the arteriotomy).
- The suture thread needs to be held in such a way that allows tension to be maintained in the direction of suturing while running the stitch and the suture thread does not interfere with the next needle placement nor allows the suture thread to become locked when pulled through.
- Each stitch of the running sutures is placed at equal distance from each other, sufficient to be both water-tight but not too close together.

- The free edge of the vein opening must be held under tension by the needle as the needle is pushed through the arteriotomy from within. If this tension cannot be maintained at the toe (i.e., the proximal end of the arteriotomy and the apex of the free edge of the vein opening) of the anastomosis, the arteriotomy may need to be slightly extended to ensure that the size match is excellent between vein and arteriotomy.
- The needle placement at the toe end of the arteriotomy must be paced in the long axis of the artery, as was done for the heel.
- The suture is continued to be run until midway through the arteriotomy where a rubber shod mosquito forceps anchors this suture thread to a fixed point (often a retractor suture) to ensure that tension is maintained whilst running the other suture to meet and tie at this point.
- Cutting the needles and leaving a long thread of suture for a hand tie, the first throw of the knot between the two sutures is made and suture tension controlled.
- After this tension is under control of the surgeon, the distal

carotid clamp is released to allow backflow and de-airing of the carotid.

- The suture is tied with a repeat throw in the same direction as the first tie to allow tightening of the knot with added tension. The next four throws of the knot tying are each opposite the previous direction to lock the knot.
- The proximal carotid clamp is then released and the anastomosis rapidly assessed. A #15 needle then de-airs the IPSVG at the highest point. This will spontaneously seal with a cottonoid placed over the bleeding. If a stitch is needed to be placed to stop the bleeding, the needle should be directed in the long-axis of the vein to prevent narrowing of the lumen.
- The microscope is then redirected at the distal anastomosis and the blood pressure checked. The blood pressure should be neither high (challenging the integrity of the anastomosis) nor low (to have low shear that would promote thrombosis). When watching the anastomosis, the temporary clip on the IPSVG is removed. The vein is then checked by Doppler for flow.

48.13 Pearls

- The harvested vein is living tissue of which the endothelium is rendered ischemic once harvested. In this ischemic state, additional damage by overdistension or placing objects under pressure into contact with the endothelium can create damage that leads to a predisposition to thrombosis. Furthermore, the time to establish flow in the vein is important and from the time the vein is harvested from the leg, until flow is reestablished in the bypass, should be as short as possible.
- At both anastomoses, normal endothelium must be joined to normal endothelium without incorporating any other tissue on a luminal surface that comes in contact with flowing blood.
- Although a minimal suture technique with ELANA is attractive because of the ability to reduce cross-clamp time, surgeons that use these techniques must remain a master of the technique described in this chapter. It would be a mistake to assume that these new techniques make the surgery of high-flow bypass easier and that it overcomes a deficiency in surgical skills because the fallback solution, when there are technical difficulties, requires all the skills necessary to perform the high-flow bypass. Furthermore, the cost, expense and theoretical increased internal pressure on the ischemic vein endothelium (with consequent predisposition to thrombosis) may outweigh, the promised benefits of reduced cross-clamp time.
- Blood will thrombose at low flow and when in contact with foreign bodies and damaged endothelium. Having said this, although blood will thrombose at low flow, this takes some time to occur, a time beyond the usual time of establishing flow in a bypass from the time of cross-clamping. However, in the presence of damaged endothelium and foreign bodies (*e.g.* suture material) thrombus formation can occur quickly. Furthermore, there is a potential for bothersome or troublesome bleeding because of the three large wounds that have

been created, preloading with aspirin and the administration of heparin at the time of cross-clamping. Therefore, there is an advantage in minimizing and delaying the heparin administration and minimizing the potential for oozing that might prove significant (e.g., run-in during the anastomosis or the development of significant blood loss) by administering the heparin only immediately before the cross-clamps are released at the distal anastomosis. It is unnecessary to have the heparin circulating until immediately before the flowing blood is anticipated to come in contact with the suture line of the distal anastomosis. Heparin is not required when performing the proximal anastomosis as the cross-clamp time for this is very short and the circumference of the suture line of the fish-mouthed anastomosis is very large.

- The bypass after release of all clamps must stand up in a smooth arc without kinks and have good Doppler signal during diastole (as well as systole). Anything less is of major concern and requires consideration to revision.
- Bad vein ensures a short bypass life. If the bypass fails very early with thrombus formation, irrespective of the cause of the failure (e.g., technical problems with the proximal or distal anastomosis), the vein should be discarded and further vein harvested and the distal and proximal anastomosis redone from the beginning. Unless good quality vein is found, surgery should not proceed.
- Do not compromise on the quality of the vein. By selecting the vein to be used from preoperative ultrasound examination, the best segment can be harvested. Although the size mismatch may be significant between the distal recipient artery and vein selected from the thigh, it is my impression that this is of less importance than the quality of the vein selected.
- It is critical that blood flows in veins appropriate for the direction compatible with the valves. Do not assume that you have selected a segment free of valves. Therefore, ensure that no mistake can be made when harvesting vein and cannulating the ankle end of the vein. Because inserting and securing the smooth round-tipped cannula into the end of the vein may not always succeed on the first attempt, it is possible for this end to fall back into the heparinized saline contained dish near the cranial end of the vein and creating confusion if this is not managed properly by ensuring that this cannot occur.
- The segment of vein that has been damaged by tie, internal cannula or vascular forceps should not be incorporated in the IPSVG and must be discarded.
- The sutures at each end of the distal anastomosis are the two most critical sutures and need to be perfectly placed. Because the vein wall is considerably thicker than the artery wall, care must be exercised in ensuring that the endothelium is perfectly aligned between these two vessels and that the bite on the artery wall is close to the arteriotomy edge and that the bite in the vein wall does not result in inversion and exposure of the vein wall media or adventitia to the luminal surface.
- The vascular needles (round bodied and not cutting) used for the anastomosis must be large enough to be driven through the vein wall as well as small enough for the artery.
- When planning for a high flow bypass, consideration needs

to be given to the distribution of reversed flow caused by the bypass. A shear stress sufficiently high to avoid thrombosis is required in segments that have critical branch or perforating arteries. If the demand on flow distal to such segments is insufficient to avoid thrombosis, critical small perforators may be inadvertently occluded. Therefore, in planning where an artery proximal to an aneurysm may be trapped, consideration to what might occur to critical perforators needs to be taken into account.

• As an example, a basilar trunk aneurysm above the level of both AICA, for which CCA-PCA IPSVG and basilar artery occlusion below the aneurysm is contemplated, can be treated by trapping above the AICA (where it might be anticipated that the perforator containing basilar artery may thrombose) or below both AICAs (which will provide sufficient run-off to probably keep the basilar artery patent with an expected reduced likelihood of aneurysm growth or rupture but a reduced run-off from the vertebral arteries and consequent thrombosis of the proximal basilar artery) or below one AICA and above the other AICA (allowing sufficient flow in both directions).

• In addition, consideration needs to be given to the arterial segment of antegrade flow proximal to the point of trapping. The lenticulostriate arteries need to be considered in

trapping of an MCA bifurcation aneurysm. I have sometimes performed CCA-M2 IPSVG and M2 to M2 bypass and have then trapped the outflow vessels without a proximal ligation for these aneurysms, the aneurysm subsequently thromboses without M1 thrombosis and with preservation of lenticulo-striate flow.

References

1. Sia SF, Davidson AS, Assaad NN, Stoodley M, Morgan MK. Comparative patency between intracranial arterial pedicle and vein bypass surgery. Neurosurgery 2011;69(2):308–314.
2. Sia SF, Morgan MK. High flow extracranial-to-intracranial brain bypass surgery. J Clin Neurosci 2013;20(1):1–5.
3. Sia SF, Lai L, Morgan MK. Measuring competence development for performing high flow extracranial-to-intracranial bypass. J Clin Neurosci 2013;20(8):1083–1088.
4. Sundt TM Jr, Piepgras DG, Marsh WR, Fode NC. Saphenous vein bypass grafts for giant aneurysms and intracranial occlusive disease. J Neurosurg 1986;65(4):439–450.

49 Middle Cerebral Artery – Internal Maxillary Artery Bypass

Ahmed Maamoun Ashour, Katie Huynh, Joanna Kemp, Brian Kang, Nathan Cherian, Savannah Scott, Sneha Koduru, and Saleem I. Abdulrauf

49.1 Introduction

Traditional high-flow bypass procedures involve the main trunk of the external carotid, the internal carotid artery, or the common carotid artery as the inflow for the bypass. The main limitations of the aforementioned sites are the requirement for a longer graft and the need for cervical neck incision.

In this chapter, we describe our technique of using the internal maxillary artery (IMAX) as the main inflow to the bypass. This is now commonly referred to as the "Abdulrauf Bypass." This allows for a shorter graft in addition to avoiding cervical exploration and anastomosis.

49.2 Indications

- Flow preservation to maintain cerebral blood flow (CBF) in patients undergoing acute vessel sacrifice, (i.e., aneurysm trapping or artery encased by tumor).
- Some aneurysms are not amenable to direct microsurgical clipping or endovascular coiling due to extreme size, location, calcification, atherosclerosis, dissection, or the incorporation of perforators or major arteries.
- Flow augmentation to increase CBF in patients with chronic compromised CBF (chronic cerebral ischemia, Moya-Moya).

49.2.1 Patient Positioning (Fig. 49.1)

- **Position:** The patient is positioned supine with the head fixed in a Mayfield head holder.
- **Head:** The head is rotated 30° to the contralateral side. The neck is slightly extended with the vertex aimed toward the floor. It is positioned above the level of the heart.
- The malar eminence is the highest point in the operative field. This position allows the frontal lobe to fall away from the orbital roof and the temporal lobe from the middle fossa floor, without retraction.

49.3 Skin Incision

- **Pterional shaped incision**
  - **Starting point:** The starting point corresponds to the inferior margin of the root of the zygoma, 1 cm anterior to the tragus.
  - The posterior limb (parietal branch) of the superficial temporal artery (STA) should be spared in case the STA is needed for a microvascular bypass.
  - **Course**: The incision runs, encircling posteriorly just above the external auditory meatus, and then curved anteriorly and medially toward the midline just behind the hairline.

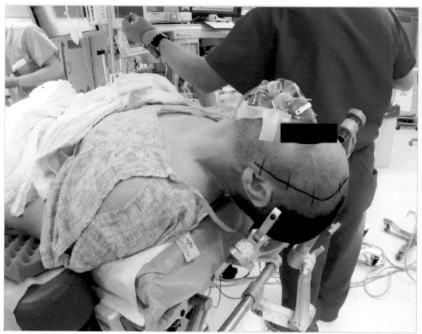

Fig. 49.1 Patient positioning. The patient is positioned supine with the head fixed in a Mayfield head holder. Head is rotated 30° to the contralateral side, neck is slightly extended with the vertex pointing down.

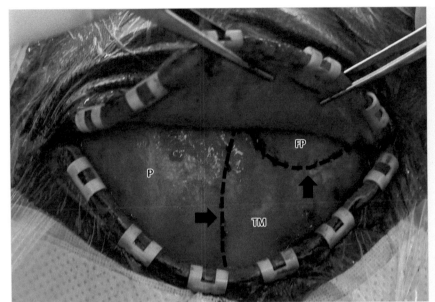

Fig. 49.2 Right side. Scalp flap is elevated from the underlying temporal fascia. Care is utilized to preserve the fat pad, which contains the frontotemporal branch of the facial nerve and the pericranium. Temporal muscle is underneath the temporal fascia. Right-pointing arrow marks the superior temporal line. Up-pointing arrow marks the C-shaped incision for interfascial dissection of the superficial and deep temporal fascia. Abbreviations: FP = fat pad; P = pericranium; TM = temporal muscle.

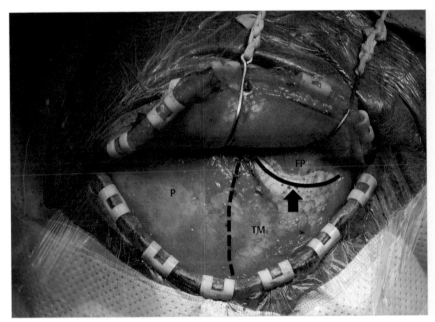

Fig. 49.3 Right side. Interfascial dissection is performed to separate the superficial and deep temporal fascia at the C-shaped incision pointed out by the black arrow to elevate the fat pad.
Abbreviations: FP = fat pad; P = pericranium; TM = temporal muscle.

49.3.1 Critical Structures

• Superficial temporal artery.

49.4 Soft Tissue Dissection

• **Fascia level**
  ○ The skin flap is separated from the underlying temporal fascia anteriorly until the superficial temporal fat pad is encountered. Care is exercised to preserve the underlying pericranium in the event it needs to be harvested in patients with large frontal sinus (**Fig. 49.2**).
  ○ A C-shaped incision is made on the temporal fascia 2 cm posterior to the zygomatic process of the frontal bone and extended from the keyhole anteriorly to the root of the zygoma inferiorly (**Fig. 49.2**).

  ○ Interfascial dissection is performed with a scalpel to separate the superficial and deep temporal fascia. This preserves the frontotemporal branches of the facial nerve (**Fig. 49.3**).
  ○ Blunt dissection is then used to elevate the superficial fascia and fat pad together from the deep temporal fascia until the lateral orbital rim and superior zygomatic arch are exposed (**Fig. 49.4**). The pericranium is harvested at this time (if indicated) (**see Chapter 17**).
• **Muscle**
  ○ The divided temporal muscle is completely elevated with the periosteal elevator before being retracted laterally and inferiorly. This provides bony exposure of the frontotemporal region (**Figs. 49.5, 49.6**).
• **Bone exposure**
  ○ The frontotemporal region, superior zygomatic arch, superior and lateral orbital rim should now be completely exposed.

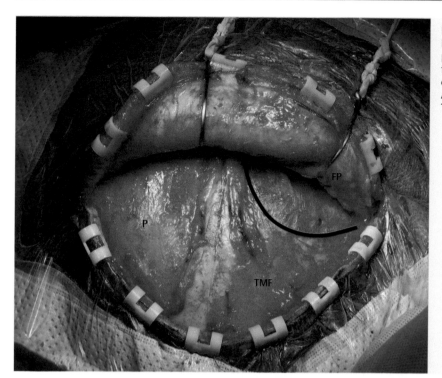

Fig. 49.4 **Right side**. Interfascial dissection is completed, the superficial fascia and fat pad are elevated from the deep temporal fascia beneath. Curved black line is the site of previous C-incision.
Abbreviations: FP = fat pad; P = pericranium; TMF = temporal muscle fascia.

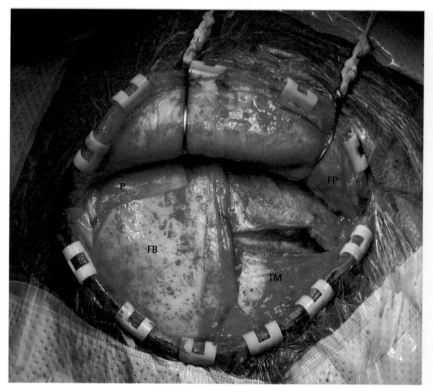

Fig. 49.5 **Right side**. In patients with thick temporal muscle, which could limit the bony window underneath, the muscle can be split a little more anterior to reduce the muscle bulk. A cuff of fascia is left on the bone to help anchor and reattach the temporal muscle during closure. The harvested pericranium is safely tucked under a moist Telfa.
Abbreviations: FB = frontal bone; FP = fat pad; P = pericranium; TM = temporal muscle.

○ The periorbit is dissected from the superior orbital rim from medial to lateral, then from the lateral orbital rim from caudal to cranial. Dissection should be performed carefully to avoid damage to the lacrimal apparatus (**Fig. 49.7**).

○ If the supraorbital nerve and vessels are in a foramen instead of a notch, they can be freed from the foramen with a small osteotome on either side of these structures to avoid injury (**see Chapter 6**).

49.4.1 Critical Structures

• Frontal branch of facial nerve.
• Lacrimal apparatus.
• Periorbit.
• Deep temporal artery.

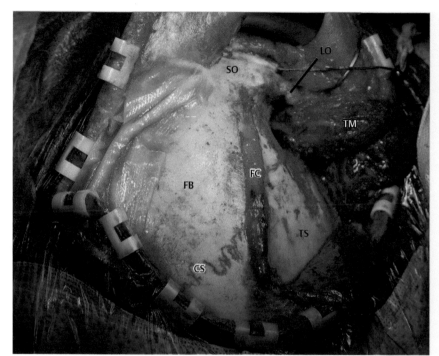

Fig. 49.6 Right side. Temporal muscle reflected anterolateral and inferiorly. Fascia cuff left on the bone to help anchor and re-attach the temporal muscle during closure.
Abbreviations: CS = coronal suture; FB = frontal bone; FC = fascia cuff; LO = lateral orbital rim; SO = superior orbital rim; TM = temporal muscle; TS = temporal squama.

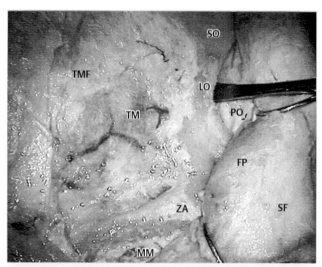

Fig. 49.7 Right side. Periorbit and lacrimal apparatus are dissected away from orbital margin starting from inferior to superior along the lateral orbital margin and from medial to lateral along the superior orbital margin, to avoid damage to the lacrimal apparatus.
Abbreviations: FP = fat pad; LO = lateral orbital rim; MM = masseter muscle; PO = periorbit; SO = superior orbital rim; TM = temporal muscle; TMF = temporal muscle fascia; SF = skin flap; ZA = zygomatic arch.

49.5 Craniotomy/Craniectomy: Cranio-Orbito-Zygomatic (Coz)

- **Burr holes**
  - ○ **Burr hole A (fronto-orbital):** Large burr hole between the

anterior aspect of the superior temporal line and the frontozygomatic suture (**Fig. 49.8**). Once done, the sphenoid ridge should be seen traversing the center of the burr hole.
  - ○ **Burr hole B:** The second burr hole is made at the most posterior extension of the superior temporal line (**Fig. 49.8**).
  - ○ **Burr hole C (inferior temporal):** The third hole is placed as close as possible to the middle fossa floor on the most inferior portion of the squamous temporal bone (**Fig. 49.8**).
- **Bone cuts**
  - ○ **L-shaped cut:** AM8 or B1 drill attachment is used to drill the lateral orbital wall (**Fig. 49.9**) and connect it with a cut at the frontozygomatic process. The orbital side has to be protected with a small dissector.
  - ○ Starting with the burr hole at the posterior aspect of the superior temporal line (**Burr hole "b," Fig. 49.8**), a footplate craniotome is used to turn a craniotomy on the frontal bone towards the orbit, cut should be kept laterally to the supraorbital foramen (**Fig. 49.10**). The craniotome will usually stop shy of the edge of the superior orbital rim and orbital roof.
  - ○ The craniotomy is connected to the orbital roof using a B1 or AM8 drill (yellow oval). The underlying periorbit is protected with a small dissector to prevent injury to the orbit (**Fig. 49.11**).
  - ○ The rest of the craniotomy is carried out with a footplate craniotome by connecting the burr holes (**Fig. 49.8**). Once the craniotomy is complete, the posterior orbital roof can be fractured off during removal of the bone flap.
  - ○ Rongeurs and high-speed electric drilling are used to remove the squamous temporal bone down to the floor of the middle fossa.
  - ○ The sphenoid process is drilled down with a diamond burr (**Fig. 49.12**).

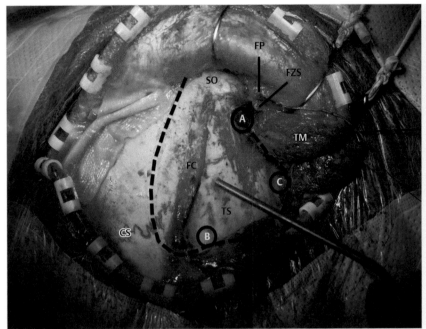

Fig. 49.8 Right side. Craniotomy. (**A**) Fronto-orbital burr hole: large burr hole between the anterior superior temporal line and the frontozygomatic suture of the external orbital process. (**B**) Burr hole at the most posterior extension of the superior temporal line. (**C**) Burr hole placed as close as possible to the middle fossa floor on the most inferior portion of the squamous temporal bone. Dashed line marks the craniotomy border to be carried out with a craniotome. Abbreviations: CS = coronal suture; FC = fascia cuff; FP = fat pad; FZS = fronto-zygomatic suture; SO = superior orbital rim; TM = temporal muscle; TS = temporal squama.

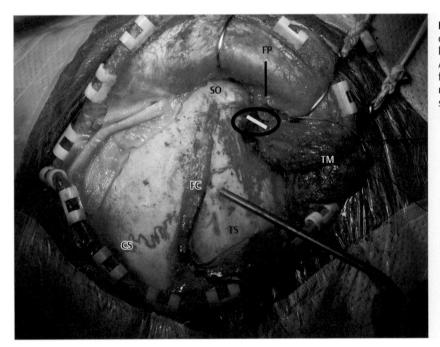

Fig. 49.9 Right Side, yellow line in the black oval is the site of the L-shaped cut at the lateral orbital wall.
Abbreviations: CS = coronal suture; FC = fascia cuff; FP = fat pad; SO = superior orbital rim; TM = temporal muscle; TS = temporal squama.

49.6 Extradural Exposure

- Standard external carotid (EC)-internal carotid (IC) bypass involves anastomosis of the M2 or M3 segment of the MCA with the internal maxillary artery (IMAX) via radial artery graft and subsequent occlusion of the internal carotid artery (ICA) or trapping of the aneurysm.
- Dissection is performed under the operative microscope.
- The middle meningeal artery is coagulated as it exits the foramen spinosum and then ligated. This will leave a short proximal stem and prevent retraction into the foramen, which may lead to subsequent uncontrolled bleeding.
- The greater superficial petrosal nerve (GSPN) is identified posteriorly. If extensive work around the petrous internal carotid artery is necessary, the GSPN is cut to avoid traction injury to the facial nerve. Inferomedial to the GSPN is the petrous internal carotid artery (ICA).
- In the majority of cases, the petrous ICA is separated from the middle fossa by only a thin fibrous layer of tissue.

• The second (V2) and third (V3) divisions of the trigeminal nerve are identified.

49.7 Extradural Drilling to Prepare for Donor Vessel

49.7.1 IMAX exposure

• Starting anterior and parallel to a line running between the foramen rotundum and ovale, bone is drill to an average depth of 4 mm into the greater wing of the sphenoid bone. This exposes an average length of 10 mm of the internal maxillary artery. The distance from the lateral edge of the foramen rotundum to the medial extent of

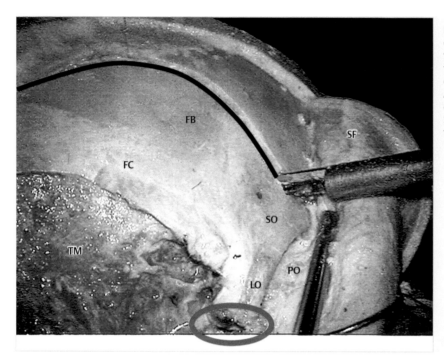

Fig. 49.10   Right side. Black line is the site of craniotomy from the posterior burr hole towards the orbital roof, staying lateral to the supraorbital foramen. Red oval is the orbital circuit.
Abbreviations: FB = frontal bone; FC = fascia cuff; LO = lateral orbital rim; PO = periorbit; SF = skin flap; SO = superior orbital rim; TM = temporal muscle.

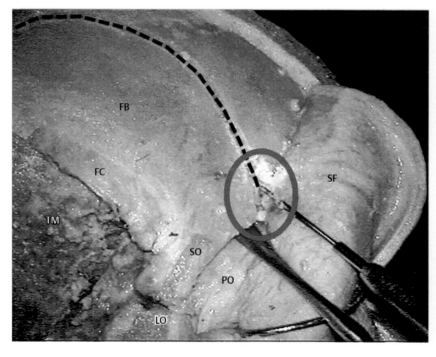

Fig. 49.11   Right side. The craniotomy is connected to the orbital roof using a B1 or AM8 drill (*red oval*). Protect the underlying periorbit with a small dissector to prevent injury to the orbit.
Abbreviations: FB = frontal bone; FC = fascia cuff; LO = lateral orbital rim; PO = periorbit; SF = skin flap; SO = superior orbital rim; TM = temporal muscle.

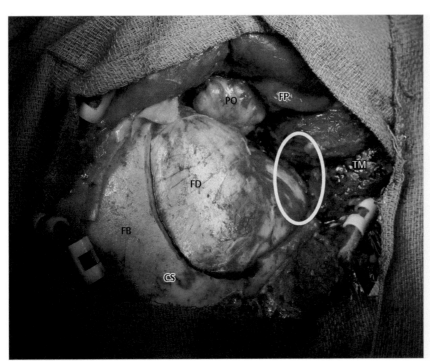

Fig. 49.12 Right side with bone flap removed. The yellow oval is the most inferior aspect of the temporal bone, at the floor of the middle fossa.
Abbreviations: CS = coronal suture; FB = frontal bone; FD = frontal dura; FP = fat pad; PO = periorbit; TM = temporal muscle.

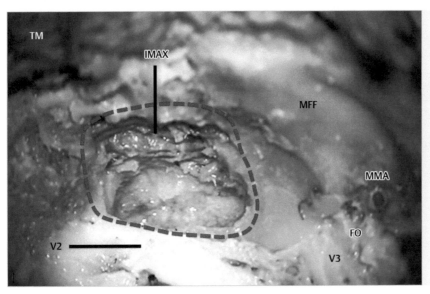

Fig. 49.13   Right Side. Starting anterior and parallel to a line running between the foramens rotundum and ovale, bone is drilled to an average depth of 4 mm into the greater wing of the sphenoid bone (marked in red). This should expose an average length of 10 mm of IMAX.
Abbreviations: FO = foramen ovale; IMAX = internal maxillary artery; MFF = middle fossa floor; MMA = middle meningeal artery; TM = temporal muscle; V2 = maxillary branch of the trigeminal nerve; V3 = mandibular branch of the trigeminal nerve.

the artery should be approximately 8 mm anteriorly (**Figs. 49.13**, **49.14**).

- In one of our previous cadaveric studies; we drew a straight line extending anteriorly from the V2/V3 apex along the inferior edge of V2. The distance from the V2/V3 apex to the lateral rotundum was 7.8 mm ± 3.033 mm. The distance from the lateral edge of the foramen rotundum to the medial extent of the IMAX was 8.6 mm ± 2.074 mm anteriorly. We then drilled to a depth of 4.2 mm ± 1.304 mm into the greater wing of the sphenoid bone, ultimately exposing an average of 7.8 mm ± 1.643 mm of the maxillary artery.

- We have now evolved to using image guidance for the identification of the IMAX and then drilling accordingly. We exposed the length of the IMAX to evaluate the ideal location for the anastomosis.

49.8 Dural Opening

- Dura is opened in a C-shaped fashion.
- Edges are reflected anteriorly toward the orbit.
- Dural flaps are reflected antero-superiorly.

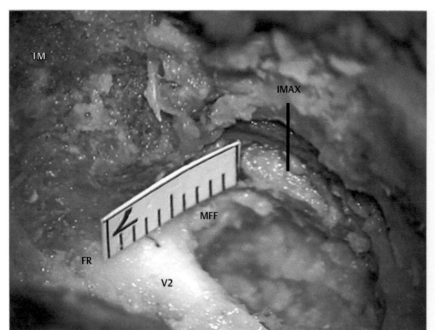

Fig. 49.14 Right side. The distance from the lateral edge of the foramen rotundum to the medial extent of the artery should be approximately 8 mm anteriorly.
Abbreviations: FR = foramen rotundum; IMAX = internal maxillary artery; MFF = middle fossa floor; TM = temporal muscle; V2 = maxillary branch of the trigeminal nerve.

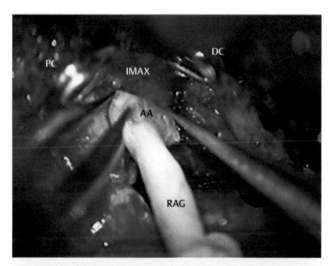

Fig. 49.15 The distal clip is applied first then the proximal clip to keep the vessel lumen distended for internal maxillary artery temporary clipping, approximating the radial artery graft to perform an end-to-side anastomosis. The two clips are placed approximately 10 mm apart.
Abbreviations: AA = anastomosis; DC = distal clip; IMAX = internal maxillary artery; PC = proximal clip; RAG = radial artery graft.

49.9 Intradural Exposure

49.9.1 Splitting the Sylvian Fissure

- The Sylvian fissure is split superficially, with dissection performed on the frontal side of the superficial Sylvian vein.
- If the superficial frontal and temporal lobes are extremely adherent, dissection should be deepened into the operculo-insular compartment of the Sylvian fissure to identify the branches of the MCA.

49.9.2 Critical Structures

- Sylvian vessels.
- Inferior frontal gyrus and posterior part of superior temporal gyrus of the dominant hemisphere.

49.9.3 MCA-IMAX End-to-Side Anastomosis Using Radial Artery Graft

- The radial artery, being comparable in caliber to common sites of cerebrovascular attachment, such as the M2 and P1 segments, facilitates anastomosis construction and prevents flow mismatch.
- Medium-sized radial arteries with a diameter of 3.5 mm and saphenous vein grafts have been used to achieve bypasses requiring higher flow rates, 40 to 70 mL/min and 100 to 200 mL/min, respectively.
- Microvascular anastomosis with an arterial graft is preferable to a venous graft due to the more rigid arterial wall allowing for easier manipulation with decreased likelihood of torsion and kinking of the graft.
- The graft should be of sufficient length to avoid being stretched too taut. Also avoid a lengthy construct that could cause torsion or kinking. This could result in strangulation and graft failure.
- Both ends of the graft are prepared by stripping the periadventitia for 1 to 1.5 cm to help facilitate a "clean" anastomosis.
- Temporary mini-clips are placed first over the distal then the proximal ends of the IMAX to occlude a 10 mm working segment for the anastomosis (**Fig. 49.15**).
- The end of the graft is cut at an angle and fish-mouthed in order to obtain an opening that is at least twice the diameter of the IMAX artery. The end is marked with ink to increase visibility under the microscope.
- A 1.0–1.5 mm longitudinal arteriotomy is made on the superior

surface of the IMAX. Anastomosis is accomplished with a 9-0 or 10-0 monofilament Nylon. It usually requires 10-14 interrupted sutures. Anastomosis could also be performed with two running sutures, with a stitch starting at each margin of the vessel.
- To check for leakage, the temporary clips of the IMAX are opened in a distal to proximal order. Minor oozing from the anastomosis site can be controlled without compressing the anastomosis by using absorbable hemostatic sponges locally.

49.9.4 Pearls

- It is possible to perform an end-to-end anastomosis, with the advantage of providing increased IMAX length after the take-off of the inferior orbital artery.
- However, this is not preferable due to the occlusion of the distal IMAX.
- The advantage of an end-to-side anastomosis over an end-to-end anastomosis is the ability to better match the size of donor and recipient vessels.

49.9.5 Micro-anastomosis to the Recipient M2/M3 Vessel

- Find an M2 or M3 cortical artery with a minimal diameter of 1 mm. Expose a 1 cm length of this recipient vessel. Make sure to coagulate and detach any tiny branches.
- A rubber dam is inserted between the cortical surface and the dissected segment of the cortical artery.
- Section off a 1 cm working segment of the MCA with temporary mini-clips first at the distal then at the proximal end. Perform an arteriotomy as described above.
- This end of the radial artery graft is cut straight. Perform an end-to-side anastomosis from the radial artery graft to the MCA using the same technique mentioned above.
- Check for leakage by releasing the temporary clips in the following order: proximal MCA, distal MCA, radial graft side.
- On completion of the anastomosis and removal of all temporary clips, the patency of the construct is checked by micro-Doppler sonography or fluorescence angiography with Indocyanine green (ICG) (**Fig. 49.16**).
- Post-operative angiogram is performed in 2-3 months to assess the patency of the anastomosis (**Fig. 49.17**).

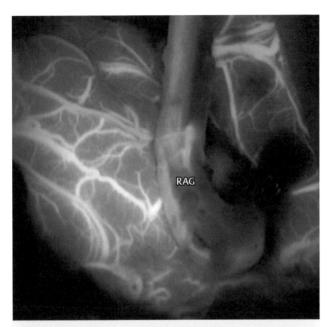

Fig. 49.16 Injection of indocyanine green (ICG) after the radial arterial graft, anastomosing middle cerebellar artery "M2" to internal maxillary artery. On completion of the anastomosis and removal of all temporary clips, the patency of the construct is checked by fluorescence angiography with ICG.
Abbreviations: RAG = radial artery graft.

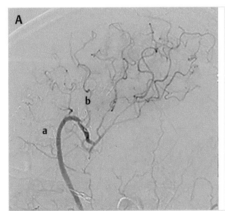
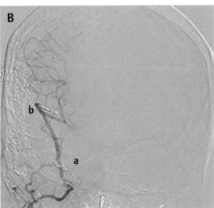
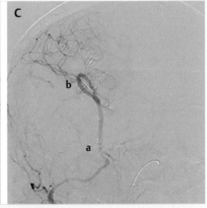

Fig. 49.17 Postoperative angiography.(**A**) Lateral view of the bypass anastomosing internal maxillary artery to middle cerebellar artery "M2." (**B**) Anterior-posterior view. (**C**) oblique view.
Abbreviations: a = internal maxillary artery; b = middle cerebral artery.

References

1. Abdulrauf SI, Sweeney JM, Mohan YS, Palejwala SK. Short segment internal maxillary artery to middle cerebral artery bypass: a novel technique for extracranial-to-intracranial bypass. Neurosurgery 2011; 68(3):804–808, discussion 808–809. doi: 10.1227/NEU.0b013e3182093355.

2. Abdulrauf SI, Ashour AM, Marvin E, et al. Proposed clinical internal carotid artery classification system. J Craniovertebr Junction Spine 2016; 7(3):161–170 . doi: 10.4103/0974-8237.188412.

3. Abdulrauf SI, Urquiaga JF, Patel R, et al. Awake High-Flow Extracranial to Intracranial Bypass for Complex Cerebral Aneurysms: Institutional Clinical Trial Results. World Neurosurg 2017;105:557–567. Epub 2017 Apr 14. doi: 10.1016/j.wneu.2017.04.016.

4. Eller JL, Sasaki-Adams D, Sweeney JM, Abdulrauf SI. Localization of the Internal Maxillary Artery for Extracranial-to-Intracranial Bypass through the Middle Cranial Fossa: A Cadaveric Study. J Neurol Surg B Skull Base 2012; 73(1):48–53. doi: 10.1055/s-0032-1304556.

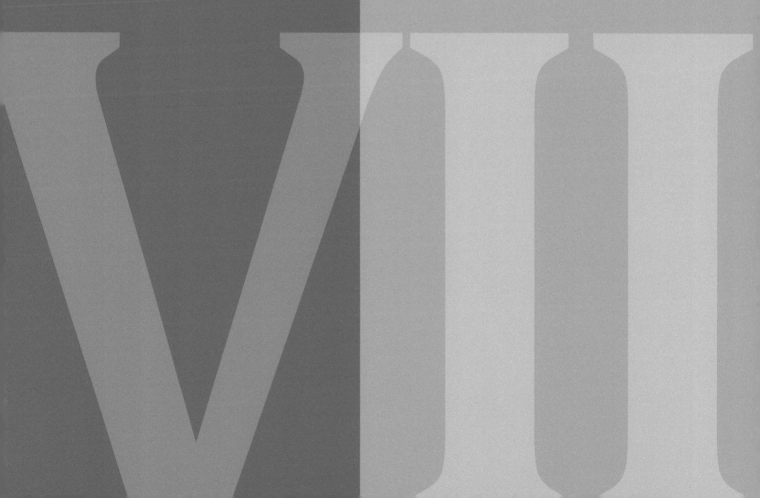

**Part VII
Ventricular Shunts
Procedures**

50 Anthropometry for Ventricular Puncture

Michele Bailo, Filippo Gagliardi, Alfio Spina, Cristian Gragnaniello, Anthony J. Caputy, and Pietro Mortini

50.1 Indications

- Acute hydrocephalus.
- Intracranial hypertension:
  - Cerebrospinal fluid (CSF) drainage.
  - Direct measurement of intracranial pressure.
- Subarachnoid/intraventricular hemorrhage.
- Intraoperative brain relaxation.
- CSF infection.

50.2 Frontal Horn (Kocher's Point) (Fig. 50.1)

50.2.1 Patient Positioning

- **Position**: The patient is positioned supine.
- **Head**: The head is slightly flexed (30°), in neutral position.

50.2.2 Skin Incision

- **Side**: The side is usually the nondominant (unless clinically indicated).
- **Starting point**: Incision starts about 3 cm lateral to midline, over the coronal suture (usually located 11–13 cm along the nasion-to-inion line) or just posterior to it.
- **Course**: It runs straight anteriorly, parallel to the midline.
- **Ending point**: It ends about 2 cm anterior to the coronal suture.

50.2.3 Craniectomy

- **Burr hole**
  - The burr hole is made about 2.5–3 cm lateral to the midline, 1 cm anterior to the coronal suture.

Critical Structures

- Arachnoid granulations.
- Dural venous lakes.
- Underlying brain parenchyma.

50.2.4 Dural Opening

- The dura is opened in a cruciate fashion.
- Bipolar electrocautery is used for dural opening.

Critical Structures

- Venous lakes and bridging veins.

50.2.5 Intradural Exposure and Catheter Insertion

- The cortical surface is coagulated with bipolar electrocautery.
- The catheter is directed perpendicularly to the cortical surface by aiming in the coronal plane, toward the medial

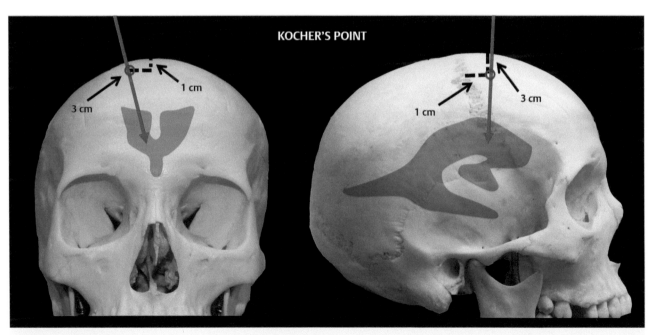

Fig. 50.1 Kocher's point.

canthus of the ipsilateral eye and in the antero-posterior plane toward the tragus.

- The catheter is advanced with the stylet until CSF comes out (5-6 cm in depth; it might be less with markedly dilated ventricles).
- The catheter is further advanced without stylet for about 1 cm.

50.2.6 Critical Issues

- The stylet has not to be advanced for more than 7 cm.
- If CSF does not come out, following aspects have to be taken into consideration:
  - Wrong site of burr hole or incorrect direction of catheter insertion.
  - Slit ventricles.
  - Brain shift.
  - Air entrance in ventricles.
  - Catheter obstruction by brain tissue, blood clot, or air lock.
- Intra-cerebral hematomas along catheter's path.
- Intraventricular bleeding from choroid plexus.

50.3 Alternative Access To The Frontal Horn

50.3.1 Kaufman's Point (Supraorbital) (Fig. 50.2)

- **Entry point**: Catheter entry point is 4 cm above the orbital rim and 3 cm lateral to the midline.
- **Direction**: The stylet is directed toward the midline.
- **Depth**: The stylet must be advanced for 6-7 cm.
- **Ventricular target**: Ventricular target corresponds to the frontal horn. Occipital horn can be reached by the same trajectory.

- **Advantage**: Accuracy rate might exceed that of Kocher access.
- **Critical issues**: Minimal cosmetic deficit.

50.3.2 Transorbital (Fig. 50.3)

- **Technique:**
  - Superior eyelid has to be retracted forward and upward.
  - Ocular globe is displaced downward.
- **Entry point**: A 18-gauge spinal needle is placed in the rostral third of the orbital roof (1 cm behind the supra-ciliary arch), just medial to the mid-pupillary line.
- **Direction**: The stylet is directed 45° according to the axial plane (orbito-meatal line) and 15–20° medial to a vertical line (cranio-caudal line).
- **Depth**: The stylet must be advanced from 3 to 8.5 cm, according to the ventricular size.
- **Ventricular target**: Ventricular target corresponds to the frontal horn (1–2 cm superior to the foramen of Monro).
- **Critical issues**:
  - Risk of damage at supraorbital neurovascular bundle, or frontal lobe vessels.
  - Intra-orbital CSF leakage.

50.4 Occipital Horn

50.4.1 Patient Positioning

- **Supine position**
  - **Head:** The head is flexed 15-20°, rotated as much as possible to the contralateral side.
  - Possible positioning of a roll under the ipsilateral shoulder.
- **Prone position**
  - The patient is prone, in neutral position.

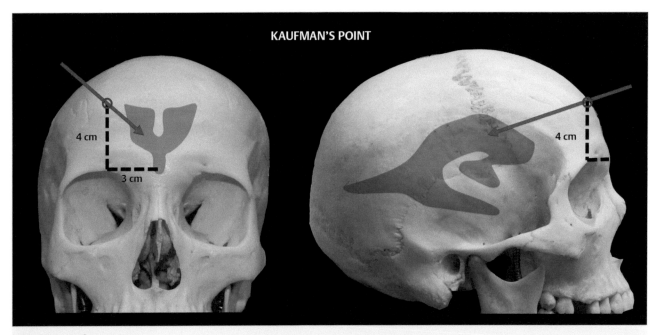

Fig. 50.2 Kaufman's point.

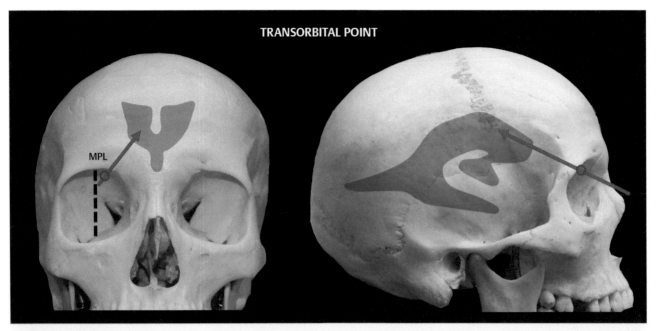

Fig. 50.3 Transorbital point.
Abbreviations: MPL = mid-pupillary line.

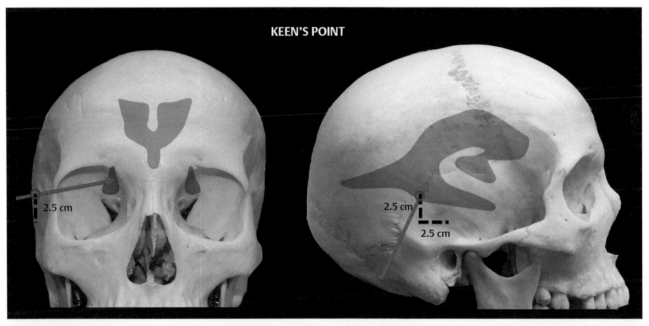

Fig. 50.4 Keen's point.

50.5 Alternative Access to the Occipital Horn and Trigone

50.5.1 Keen's Point (Posterior Parietal) (Fig. 50.4)

- **Entry point**: Catheter entry point is 2.5–3 cm posterior and 2.5–3 cm superior to the top of the pinna.
- **Direction**: The stylet is directed perpendicular to the cerebral cortex.

- **Depth**: The stylet must be advanced 4-5 cm.
- **Ventricular target**: Ventricular target corresponds to the atrium.

50.5.2 Dandy's Point (Occipital) (Fig. 50.5)

- **Entry point**: Catheter entry point is 3 cm above the inion and 2 cm lateral to the midline; it is placed on the occipital side of the lambdoid suture (in infants usually matches with lambdoid suture at intersection with mid-pupillary line).

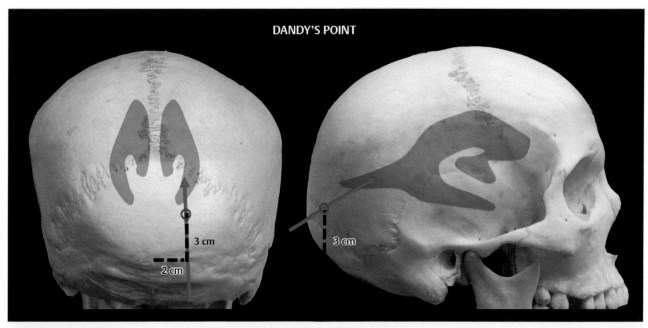

Fig. 50.5 Dandy's point.

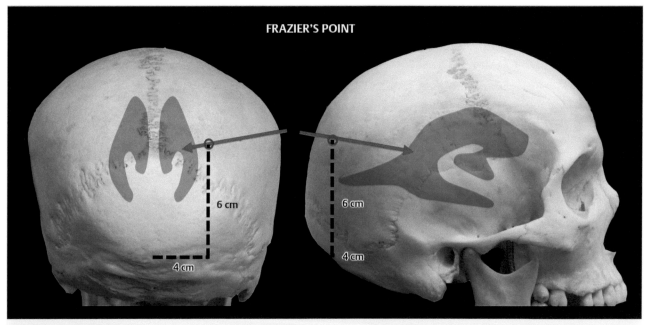

Fig. 50.6 Frazier's point.

- **Direction**: The stylet is directed perpendicular to the cortex.
- **Depth**: The stylet must be advanced 4-5 cm.
- **Ventricular target**: Ventricular target corresponds to the occipital horn.
- **Critical issues**: Significant risk of damaging visual pathways.

50.5.3 Frazier's Point (Occipital) (Fig. 50.6)

- **Entry point**: Catheter entry point is 3-4 cm from the midline and 6-7 above the inion; it is placed at the parietal side of the lambdoid suture.

- **Direction**: The stylet is directed perpendicular to the cortex, toward the omolateral medial canthus.
- **Depth**: The stylet has to be advanced 4-5 cm.
- **Ventricular target**: Ventricular target corresponds to the atrium.

50.5.4 Targeted Procedures

- Stereotactic (frame-based) placement
- Endoscopic placement
- Ultrasound-guided procedure
- Neuronavigation-guided (frameless) procedure

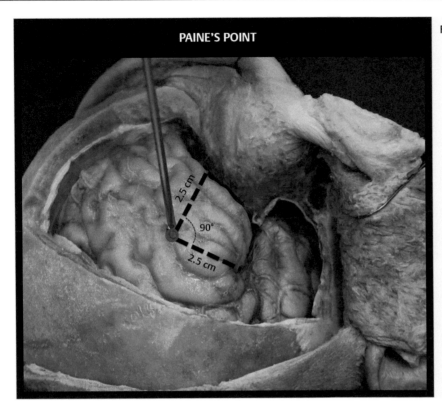

PAINE'S POINT

2.5 cm

90°

2.5 cm

Fig. 50.7 Paine's point.

50.6 Intraoperative Positioning of Ventricular Shunts

50.6.1 Paine's Point (Fig. 50.7)

- **Entry point**: Catheter entry point is inserted at the right angle formed by the intersection of the lines measuring 2.5 cm superior from the floor of the anterior cranial fossa (lateral orbital roof) and 2.5 cm anterior to the Sylvian fissure (marked by the Sylvian veins).
- **Direction**: The stylet is directed perpendicular to the cortex.
- **Depth**: The stylet must be advanced 4–5 cm.
- **Ventricular target**: Ventricular target corresponds to the frontal horn.
- **Critical issues**:
  ○ Proximity to the Broca's area in the dominant hemisphere.
  ○ Violation of the head of the caudate nucleus.

References

1. Connolly ES, McKhann GM II, Huang J. Fundamentals of operative techniques in neurosurgery. New York: Thieme Medical Publishers;2011.

2. Greenberg MS. Handbook of neurosurgery. New York: Thieme Medical Publishers;2010.

3. Madrazo Navarro I, Garcia Renteria JA, Rosas Peralta VH, Dei Castilli MA. Transorbital ventricular puncture for emergency ventricular decompression. Technical note. J Neurosurg 1981; 54(2):273–274.

4. Mortazavi MM, Adeeb N, Griessenauer CJ, et al. The ventricular system of the brain: a comprehensive review of its history, anatomy, histology, embryology, and surgical considerations. Childs Nerv Syst 2014; 30(1):19–35.

5. Park J, Hamm IS. Revision of Paine's technique for intraoperative ventricular puncture. Surg Neurol 2008; 70(5):503–508, discussion 508.

6. Schmidek HH, Sweet WH. Operative Neurosurgical Techniques. 6th ed. Vol. 2. Philadelphia: Elsevier/Saunders;2012.

7. Sekhar LN, Fessler RG. Atlas of neurosurgical techniques. Brain. Vol. 1. New York: Thieme Medical Publishers;2016.

8. Tubbs RS, Loukas M, Shoja MM, Cohen-Gadol AA. Emergency transorbital ventricular puncture: refinement of external landmarks. J Neurosurg 2009; 111(6):1191–1192.

51 Ventricular-Peritoneal Shunt

Elena V. Colombo, Filippo Gagliardi, Michele Bailo, Alfio Spina, Cristian Gragnaniello, Anthony J. Caputy, and Pietro Mortini

51.1 Indications

- Communicating hydrocephalus.
- Non-communicating (obstructive) hydrocephalus.

51.2 Patient Positioning (Fig. 51.1)

- **Position:** The patient is positioned supine, with the head placed on the bed headboard.
- **Body:** The body is placed in neutral position.
- **Head:** The head has to be free to rotate over the headboard; a rubber ring could be used to support it.
- **Shoulders:** Shoulders are placed in neutral position.
- **Upper limbs**: Upper limbs should be kept parallel to the trunk.

51.2.1 Suggestions

- If the neck lateral curvature is wide, the head can be angled downward in order to open that angle and make tunneling maneuvers easier.
- Abdomen and thorax must be kept in neutral position, free from any device (e.g., electrocardiographic leads, patches, and bandages).

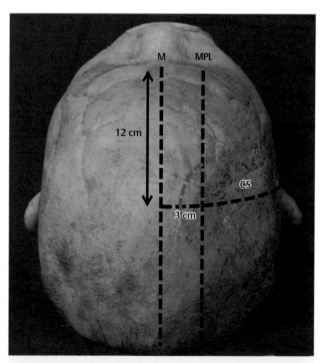

Fig. 51.1 Patient positioning and landmarks. Coronal suture crosses midline 12 cm behind the nasion. Mid-pupillary line is 2.5–3 cm lateral from the midline. Skin incision (*red dotted line*) runs around the intersection of mid-pupillary line and coronal suture line. Abbreviations: CS = projection line of coronal suture; M = midline; MPL = mid-pupillary line.

51.3 Skin Incisions

- **Head: C-shaped incision** (**Figs. 51.1, 51.2**)
  - **Anatomical landmarks:** Coronal suture can be palpated 12 cm behind the nasion on the midline. From this point, the center of the incision should be marked 3 cm laterally (at the mid-pupillary line) and 1 cm ahead.
  - **Side:** Preferably right (nondominant) side.
  - **Starting point:** Incision starts 2 cm ahead the central point, on the mid-pupillary line.
  - **Course:** Incision curves medially around the central point.
  - **Ending point:** It ends 2 cm behind the central point, on the mid-pupillary line.
- **Abdomen: linear incision** (**Fig. 51.3**)
  - **Anatomical landmarks**: Umbilicus.
  - **Starting point**: Incision starts 1 cm lateral to the umbilicus.
  - **Course**: It runs straight laterally for 5 cm.
- **Other incisions: Small linear incisions**

Adjunctive small linear incisions can be made in the supra-clavicular and/or retro-auricular areas.

- **Starting and ending points:** Starting and ending points are placed over the tunneler.
- **Course:** Incision runs 2 cm, perpendicular to the major axis of the tunneler.

51.3.1 Critical Structures

- None.

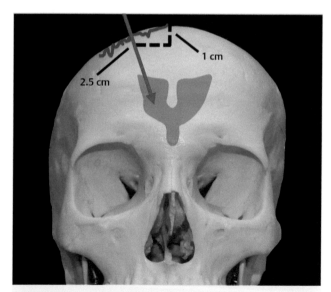

Fig. 51.2 Cranial landmarks for ventricular puncture. Burr hole must be performed 2–3 cm lateral from the midline and 1 cm anterior to the coronal suture (*blue line*).

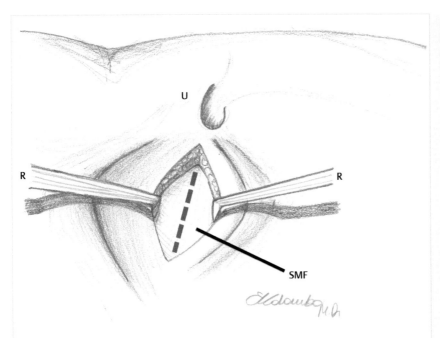

Fig. 51.3 Para-umbilical skin incision with exposure of the superficial muscle fascia. Abbreviations: R = retractor; SMF = superficial muscle fascia; U = umbilicus.

51.4 Soft Tissue Dissection

- **Myofascial level**
  - **Abdomen:** Incision runs transversally, 2 to 3 cm in length.
- **Muscles**
  - **Retro-auricular incision:** Sternocleidomastoid tendon could be crossed during tunneling, performing a small incision.
  - **Abdomen:** Rectus abdominis fibers are smoothly dissected.
- **Bone exposure**
  - Subgaleal dissection of extra-cranial soft tissues is performed to expose the coronal suture.
  - Further dissection is carried out, starting from the skin incision to the parietal bone to create a pouch for positioning the valve.
- **Tunneling (Figs. 51.4, 51.5)**
  - Head is turned laterally to flatten the angle between the neck and clavicle.
  - Starting from the abdominal incision, a tunneler is inserted in the subcutaneous layer.
  - The tunneler is pushed straight up over the rib cage and the clavicle.
  - An incision is made above the clavicle and/or behind the ear to retrieve the tunneler tip.
  - The distal catheter is then tunneled from here toward the cranial incision.

51.4.1 Critical Structures

- Superficial jugular vein in the neck.

51.5 Craniectomy (See Chapter 50)

- **Burr hole (Kocher's point) (Fig. 51.2)**
  - Burr hole is placed 2.5-3 cm lateral to the midline, on the mid-pupillary line.
  - In sagittal projection it corresponds to a point located 1 cm anterior to the coronal suture.
- **Variants (See Chapter 50)**
  - **Frazier's point (parieto-occipital).** It is located 6-7 cm above the inion and 3-4 cm lateral to midline.
  - **Keen's point (posterior parietal).** It is located 2.5-3 cm posteriorly and 2.5-3 cm superiorly to the pinna.

51.6 Dural Opening

- Dura is opened in a X-shaped fashion.
- Care must be taken not to cut underlying vessels.

51.7 Intradural Procedure

- Cortical surface is gently cauterized.
- Ventricular catheter is placed in the frontal horn of the lateral ventricle.
- **Trajectory to the frontal horn of the lateral ventricle (Fig. 51.2)**
  - Stylet trajectory is perpendicular to the bone surface.
  - Catheter is directed toward the ipsilateral medial cantus on the coronal plane and toward the external auditory meatus on the sagittal plane.
  - Using this trajectory, the tip of the catheter is directed to the Monro foramen.

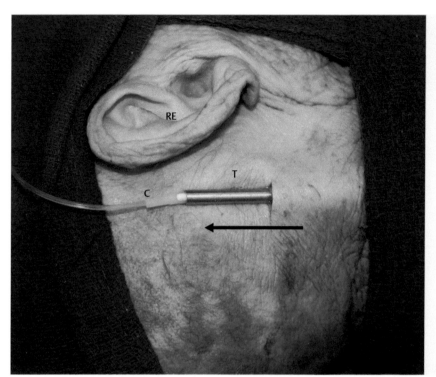

Fig. 51.4 The tunneler with an internal guide for the catheter is inserted in the subcutaneous layer from the abdominal incision toward the retroauricular zone.
Abbreviations: C = catheter; RE = right ear; T = tunneler.

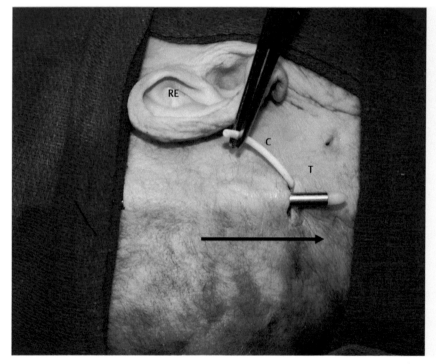

Fig. 51.5 The distal catheter emerges from the retroauricular incision after removing the tunneler from the abdomen. A short tunneler is inserted through the cranial incision to the retroauricular one. After removing the internal guide, catheter is inserted in the tunneler for the length needed to reach the cranial incision.
Abbreviations: C = catheter; RE = right ear; T = tunneler.

   ○ Stylet should be advanced for 5-7 cm.
• **Trajectory to the occipital horn of the lateral ventricle**
   ○ Catheter is directed parallel to skull base, toward the ipsilateral medial cantus.
   ○ Stylet should be advanced for 8-10 cm.

51.8 Valve Connection (Fig. 51.6)

• Cranial (proximal) catheter should be cut almost 3 cm distal to the burr hole and connected to the programmable valve.
• Valve is connected to the distal catheter, which has been previously tunneled from abdomen to the cranial incision.

- Valve is positioned in the subcutaneous pouch.
- Abdominal (distal) catheter is gently pulled down while the valve is located in the pouch.

51.9 Abdominal Procedure (Figs. 51.7–51.9)

- Smooth dissection of rectus abdominis fibers is carried out.

- Deep fascia is pinched in two points maintaining a distance of 1-2 cm between them and then incised in the center with a scissor or a knife.
- Deep fascia opening should be 2-3 mm in length.
- Parietal peritoneum (recognizable as a thin transparent membrane) should be opened in the same fashion as the deep fascia. Since the deep fascia is often coated by the peritoneum, the two structures are usually opened together.

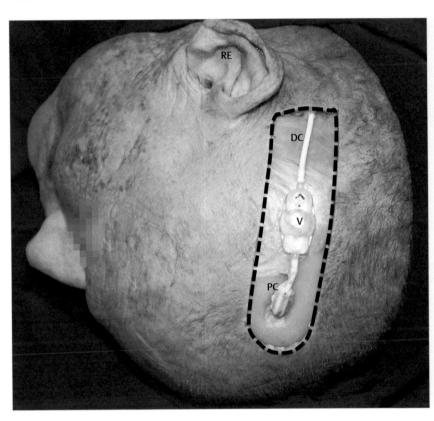

Fig. 51.6 Explicative section showing the system positioning. The distal catheter and valve are positioned in the subcutaneous space and over the temporalis fascia. The extra-cranial part of the ventricular catheter must be positioned avoiding stretching or kinking.
Abbreviations: DC = distal catheter; PC = proximal catheter; RE = right ear; V = valve.

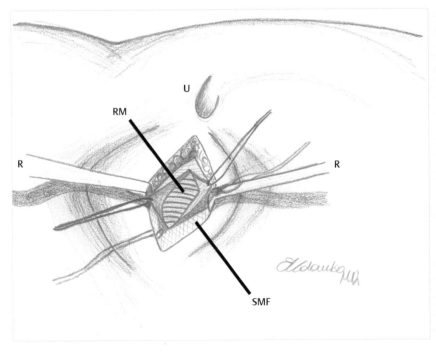

Fig. 51.7 Abdominal soft tissue dissection with exposure of rectus muscle fibers. Abbreviations: R = retractor; RM = rectus muscle; SMF = superficial muscle fascia; U = umbilicus.

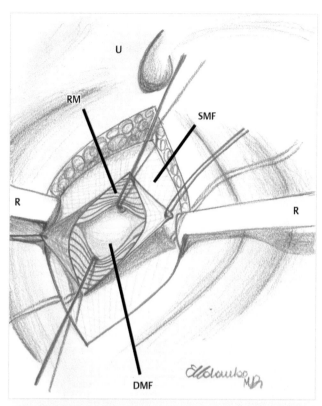

Fig. 51.8 Abdominal soft tissue dissection with exposure of the deep muscle fascia.
Abbreviations: DMF = deep muscle fascia; R = retractor; RM = rectus muscle; SMF = superficial muscle fascia; U = umbilicus.

- At this point the intra-peritoneal fat is exposed and the distal catheter could be inserted into the peritoneal cavity.
- A rounded suture is used to close the peritoneum incision and to reduce the risk of catheter's dislocation.

51.10 Variants of Ventricular Diversion

- **Ventricular-atrial shunt**
  - Distal catheter is inserted into the right cardiac atrium through the right jugular vein.
  - Jugular vein puncture must be performed by using an ultrasound guide.
  - **Indications:** in case of ventricular-peritoneal shunt contraindication, as in previous abdomen surgery or peritoneal infection.

References

1. Greenberg MS. Hydrocephalus. In: Greenberg MS, ed. Handbook of Neurosurgery. New York: Thieme Medical Publishers; 2006:619–621.
2. McComb JG. Techniques for CSF diversion. In: Scott RM, ed. Hydrocephalus. Baltimore: Williams and Wilkins;1990: 47–65.

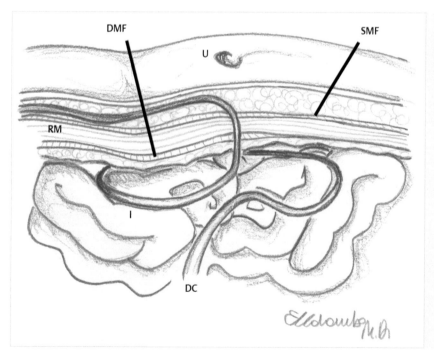

Fig. 51.9 Cross-section of abdominal catheter positioning.
Abbreviations: DC = distal catheter; DMF = deep muscle fascia; I = intestine; RM = rectus muscle; SMF = superficial muscle fascia; U = umbilicus.

52 Endoscopic Septostomy

Stefania Acerno, Filippo Gagliardi, Elena V. Colombo, Cristian Gragnaniello, Anthony J. Caputy, and Pietro Mortini

52.1 Introduction

The endoscopic septostomy is a minimally invasive, intraventricular endoscopic procedure. It allows creating a communication between both the lateral ventricles by opening the septum pellucidum. It is indicated in case of obstructive mono-ventricular hydrocephalus.

Surgical access to the lateral ventricle is just lateral as compared to the standard approach for the placement of an external ventricular shunt.

52.2 Indications

- Mono-ventricular hydrocephalus due to tumoral or membranous (inflammatory, post-hemorrhagic) obstruction in the region of foramina of Monro or fornix.
- Cysts of the septum pellucidum.
- Multi-loculated cystic hydrocephalus.

52.3 Patient Positioning (Fig. 52.1)

- **Position:** The patient is positioned supine with the head fixed to a three pins Mayfield head-holder.

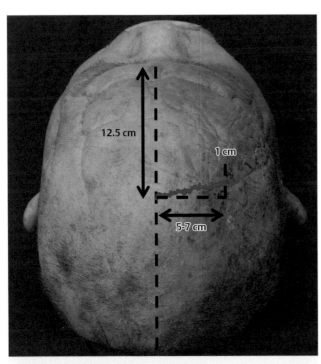

Fig. 52.1 Patient positioning and landmarks.
Abbreviations: Coronal suture (*blue line*).

- **Body:** The body is placed parallel to the horizontal plane in neutral position.
- **Head:** The head is flexed 30° and the neck is kept in straight position.

52.4 Skin Incision (Fig. 52.1)

- **Linear incision**
  - Incision is located just in front of the coronal suture, according to the selected entry point (see burr hole).
  - The incision is 3 cm long.
- **C-shaped incision**
  - The C-shaped incision is based toward the superficial temporal artery.
  - It is preferred if a cerebro-spinal fluid (CSF) reservoir needs to be implanted.

52.4.1 Critical Structures

- None

52.5 Soft Tissue Dissection

- **Galea capitis and periosteum**
  - The galea capitis and periosteum are cut according to the shape of the skin incision.

52.5.1 Critical Structures

- None

52.6 Craniotomy/ Craniectomy (See Chapter 50)

- **Single burr hole**
  - Burr hole is usually 10 mm wide.
  - It is placed 5 to 7 cm away from the midline, on the side of the dilated ventricle, just anterior to the coronal suture according to the procedure:
    - **Pure septostomy:** Hole is placed 5-7 cm paramedian in order to achieve the more perpendicular route to the septum pellucidum.
    - **Septostomy and endoscopic tumor procedures** (biopsy or endoscopic excision) in the area of the foramina of Monro: burr hole is placed 5 cm paramedian.
    - **Septostomy and endoscopic third ventriculostomy:** Hole is performed 4 cm away from the midline.

52.6.1 Critical Structures

- None

52.7 Dural Opening

- **Cross-shaped fashion**
  - A cortical exposure of 5-7 mm is needed to put the endoscope in place.

52.7.1 Critical Structures

- None

52.8 Intradural Procedure

- Intradural procedure comprises the following steps:
  - Leptomeningeal and cortex bipolar coagulation and incision.
  - Ventricle tap with a standard catheter to verify accuracy of the planned trajectory and to sample CSF when needed for laboratory testing.
  - Peel away or endoscopic sheath freehand positioning (with a dynamic reference frame on it, if neuro-navigation tools are used) and fixation on a pneumatic/mechanic holder covered by a sterile drape (**see Chapter 27**).
  - Endoscope placement through the sheath.
  - Inspection of the ventricular cavity and identification of the local anatomy and landmarks (**Fig. 52.2**).
  - Pulsated manual irrigation with lactate Ringer's solution 36-37°C (always check that there is always one irrigation port unlocked to prevent dangerous spikes of intracranial pressure).

52.9 Septosotomy

- Identification of the adequate site of the septostomy (any area of the septum, according to each case, can be fenestrated).
- "Ideal" zone to prevent injury to the fornix is the area 5 to 10 mm posterior to the foramen of Monro, midway between the corpus callosum and the fornix, carefully avoiding contact with the septal veins (**Fig. 52.3**).
- Bipolar/monopolar coagulation of the interest area in circumferential way.
- Cutting residual septum tissue with endoscopic scissors and grabbing the flap away with endoscopic forceps.
- Dilatation of the fenestration with a Fogarthy balloon (3 French) until the size of 7 to 10 mm at least in diameter, to decrease chances of occlusion of the opening by scar formation (**Fig. 52.4**).
- Endoscopic inspection of contralateral ventricular camera to ensure the size is adequate and no bleeding problem in the opposite ventricle is ongoing (**Fig. 52.5**).

52.9.1 Suggestions

- When minor bleeding occurs, simple and continuous irrigation, for a few minutes, usually clears up the view.
- Bipolar diathermy can also be used to coagulate the vessel.
- In cases of sustained hemorrhage forced irrigation or CSF aspiration, in order to create a "dry field," can help in identifying the bleeding source and obtain hemostasis.
- Major bleeding problem can induce abortion of the procedure leaving in place a ventricular catheter to allow CSF to clear.

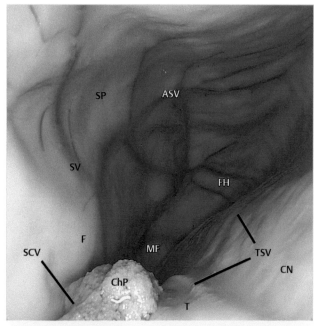

Fig. 52.2 Anatomic view.
Abbreviations. ASV = anterior septal vein; ChP = choroid plexus; CN = caudate nucleus; F = fornix; FH = frontal horn; MF = Monro foramen; SCV = superior choroidal vein; SP = septum pellucidum; SV = septal vein; T = thalamus; TSV = thalamostriate vein.

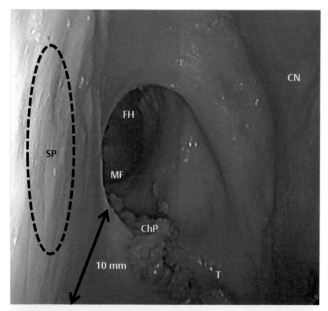

Fig. 52.3 Identification of landmarks in the ventricular cavity for septostomy.
Abbreviations: ChP = choroid plexus; CN = caudate nucleus; FH = frontal horn; MF = Monro foramen; SP = septum pellucidum; T = thalamus.

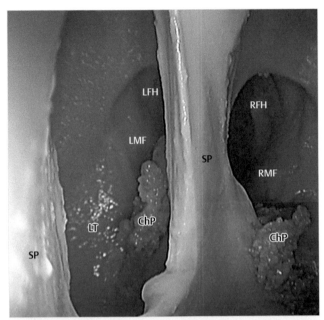

Fig. 52.4 Endoscopic view after septostomy.
Abbreviations: ChP = choroid plexus; LFH = left frontal horn; LMF = left Monro foramen; LT = left thalamus; RFH = right frontal horn; RMF = right Monro foramen; SP = septum pellucidum.

52.9.2 Critical Structures

- Septal vein.
- Fornix.
- Contralateral thalamus.

52.10 Pearls

- Endoscopic septostomy should be performed only if the anatomy of the region of interest is clearly identifiable both preoperatively by the neuroimaging and during the surgical procedure.
- Frameless neuro-navigation could be crucial to obtain the optimal entry point according to the procedure/s.
- When a simultaneous endoscopic tumor procedure is planned it is better to start with septostomy to prevent that bleeding from the tumor bed precludes the fenestration.
- In acute/subacute hydrocephalus the septum pellucidum is thick and highly flexible and could be difficult to coagulate and perforate; intermittent forced irrigation helps in identifying the thinnest part to perform safe and bloodless stomy.

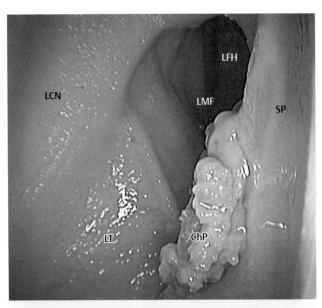

Fig. 52.5 Endoscopic view of the controlateral ventricle.
Abbreviations: ChP = choroid plexus; LCN = left caudate nucleus; LFH = left frontal horn; LMF = left Monro foramen; LT = left thalamus; SP = septum pellucidum.

- Water-jet dissection and endoscopic ultrasound probes, when available, could be an interesting variant in performing septostomy.
- The surgical field should always be prepared and draped to allow a rapid switch to micro-neurosurgery in case of major hemorrhagic complication.

References

1   Aldana PR, Kestle JR, Brockmeyer DL, Walker ML. Results of endoscopic septal fenestration in the treatment of isolated ventricular hydrocephalus. Pediatr Neurosurg 2003; 38(6):286–294.

2   Miki T, Wada J, Nakajima N, Inaji T, Akimoto J, Haraoka J. Operative indications and neuroendoscopic management of symptomatic cysts of the septum pellucidum. Childs Nerv Syst 2005;21(5):372–381.

3   Oertel JM, Schroeder HW, Gaab MR. Endoscopic stomy of the septum pellucidum: indications, technique, and results. Neurosurgery 2009;64(3):482–491, discussion 491–493.

4   Schroeder HW. General principles and intraventricular neuroendoscopy: endoscopic techniques. World Neurosurg 2013;79(2, Suppl):S14.e23–14.e28.

53 Endoscopic Third Ventriculostomy and Biopsy of Pineal Region

Joanna Kemp, Elena V. Colombo, and Samer K. Elbabaa

53.1 Indications

- **Endoscopic third ventriculostomy (ETV)**
  - Symptomatic obstructive hydrocephalus.
  - Patent subarachnoid spaces with adequate space between the clivus and the brainstem.
  - Thinned/bowed floor of the third ventricle on sagittal MRI:
    - Indicates likelihood of safe fenestration of the floor.
    - Absence of this finding is not an absolute contraindication.
- **Pineal region biopsy**
  - Presence of a lesion in the pineal region or posterior third ventricle where pathologic diagnosis will significantly impact treatment options.
  - Confirmation of absence of vascular lesion that would make biopsy contraindicated.

53.2 Patient Positioning

- **Position:** The patient is positioned supine with the head placed on a gel donut or Mayfield horseshoe headrest.
- **Body:** The body is placed supine with the arm boards or arms tucked at the side; a bilateral shoulder roll has to be used if head extension is desired for pineal region biopsy.
- **Head:** The head is kept neutral or with a slight flexion.
- The operating table is rotated 90 or 180° from anesthesia.
- Monitors are placed at the foot of the bed for the operating surgeon and assistant.
- A connection to the operating table for a pneumatic arm for the endoscope may be made.

53.3 Skin Incision

- **Desired entry points are identified**
  - **Laterality:** Right side is preferred in most cases; though if one lateral ventricle is larger than the other, the larger ventricle is utilized.
  - **ETV:** 1 cm anterior to the coronal suture at the mid-pupillary line. In infants with a patent anterior fontanelle, this can be marked at the junction of the fontanelle and the ipsilateral coronal suture
  - **Pineal region biopsy:** Depending on the anatomy of the third ventricle and location of the lesion, a more anterior entry may be required. Simultaneous ETV and pineal region biopsy may require multiple burr holes or a single hole midway between both trajectories
  - **Neuronavigation:** Particularly useful in pineal region biopsy to identify target intraoperatively and define entry, or to plan trajectory in patients with small ventricles or abnormal ventricular morphology. It can be used in any case for optimization of entry point

- C-shaped or linear incision large enough to accommodate one or multiple burr holes is made **(Fig. 53.1)**.

53.3.1 Critical Structures

- Identification of the midline.
- Coronal suture.
- Anterior fontanelle.

53.4 Soft Tissue Dissection

- Skin is opened sharply.
- Subcutaneous fat and galea may be opened sharply or with monopolar electrocautery.
- Pericranium is opened with monopolar in the location of the entry point.
- Care is taken to avoid injury to the anterior fontanelle when present.
- Skin flap is retracted with suture or a self-retaining retractor.

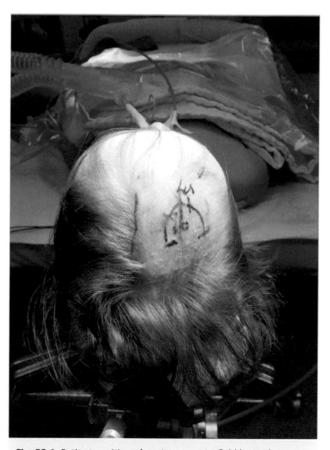

Fig. 53.1 Patient positioned supine on a Mayfield horseshoe head holder. Note the marking of midline and the C-shaped incision at the mid pupillary line.

53.4.1 Critical Structures

- Coronal suture.
- Anterior fontanelle.

53.5 Craniotomy

- **Entry point identification**
  - Repeat identification and update entry with neuronavigation, if utilized.
  - Entry point is always identified anterior to the coronal suture.
- **Burr holes**
  - With patent anterior fontanelle, the entry point can be created using Kerrison punches at the anterolateral edge of the fontanelle.
  - Without patent anterior fontanelle, the entry point is created with a pneumatic drill, Hudson brace, or hand twist drill with hole large enough to accommodate peel away sheath and endoscope.

53.6 Dural Opening

- Dura is opened in a cruciate fashion.
- Bipolar electrocautery is used to coagulate dural edges
  - Good hemostasis is important to prevent run down of blood products that would obscure view with endoscope.

53.7 Intradural Exposure

- **Cannulation of ventricle (Fig. 53.2)**
  - The determination of depth is based on the measurement of cortical mantle on MRI preoperatively.
  - Peel away sheath is inserted to depth adequate to just enter the ependyma of the lateral ventricle.
  - The inner cannula is removed to confirm cerebrospinal fluid (CSF) flow.
    - CSF is sampled if a specimen is desired.
    - Endoscope is inserted for initial confirmation of ventricular access.
    - Sheath is peeled away to the appropriate depth and stapled to skin and/or drapes.
  - Confirmation of side of entry.
    - Neuronavigation.
    - Anatomic landmarks.
- **Navigation of endoscope**
  - Identification of landmarks within the lateral ventricle **(Fig. 53.3).**
    - Foramen of Monro
    - Fornix
    - Choroid plexus
    - Septum pellucidum
    - Veins: Septal and thalamostriate
  - Identification of landmarks within the third ventricle **(Fig. 53.4)**
    - **Neural structures:** Optic chiasm, tuber cinereum, hypothalamus, thalamus, inter-thalamic adhesion, habenular commissure, posterior commissure.
    - **Arteries:** Basilar artery, perforating branches.

- **Veins:** Internal cerebral veins.
- **Recesses:** Optic, infundibular, pineal, prepontine cistern.
- Clivus.
- Cerebral aqueduct.

53.8 Pearls

- **ETV (Fig. 53.5–53.7)**
  - 0° Rigid endoscope is the most often utilized.
    - 30° Endoscope should be available if visualization is inadequate with the 0° scope.
    - Flexible scopes may be useful in cases of difficult trajectory, though optics are lower quality.
  - Fenestration is performed anterior to the mammillary bodies and basilar apex at the midline.
  - Basilar apex can be identified through thinned floor (tuber cinereum).
  - If the floor is opaque, attempts at hydrodissection or endoscopic coring of the floor may still allow visualization and safe fenestration.
  - Endoscope, blunt forceps, monopolar, laser, and Fogarty balloon have all been described as instruments used to make initial fenestration.
    - Use of monopolar and laser must be used cautiously due to risk of thermal injury to the underlying basilar artery.
  - Widening of the fenestration can be done with inflation of a Fogarty balloon or spreading of blunt forceps.

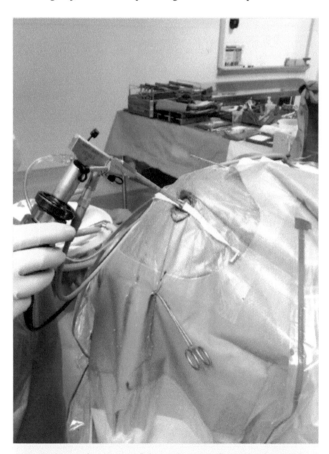

Fig. 53.2 Initial insertion of the endoscope after cannulation of the ventricle through a peel away sheath.

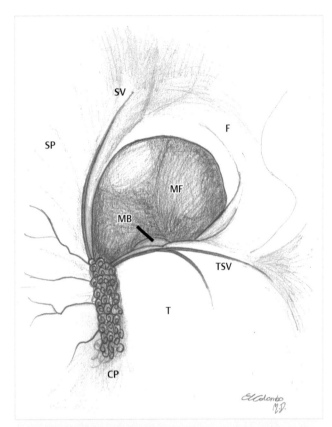

Fig. 53.3 View from the endoscope after cannulation of the right lateral ventricle.
Abbreviations: CP = choroid plexus; F = fornix; MB = mammillary body; MF = Monro foramen; SP = septum pellucidum; SV = septal vein; T = thalamus; TSV = thalamostriate vein.

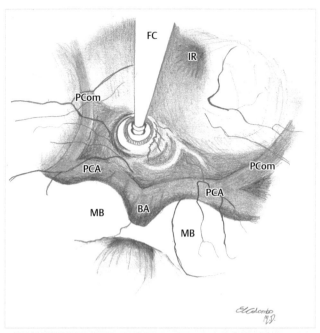

Fig. 53.5 Fenestration of the floor of the third ventricle using a Fogarty balloon anterior to the basilar apex and posterior to the infundibular recess.
Abbreviations: BA = basilar artery; FC = Fogarty catheter; IR = infundibular recess; MB = mammillary body; PCA = posterior cerebral artery; PCom = posterior communicating artery.

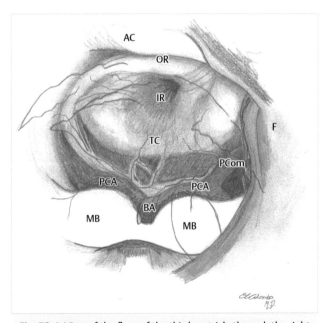

Fig. 53.4 View of the floor of the third ventricle through the right foramen of Monro.
Abbreviations: AC = anterior commissure; BA = basilar artery; F = fornix; IR = infundibular recess; MB = mammillary body; OR = optic recess; PCA = posterior cerebral artery; PCom = posterior communicating artery; TC = tuber cinereum.

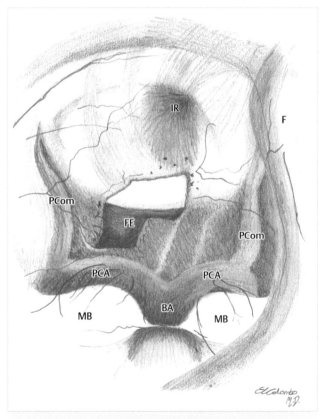

Fig. 53.6 Floor of the third ventricle after the fenestration.
Abbreviations: BA = basilar artery; F = fornix; FE = fenestration; IR = infundibular recess; MB = mammillary body; PCA = posterior cerebral artery; PCom = posterior communicating artery.

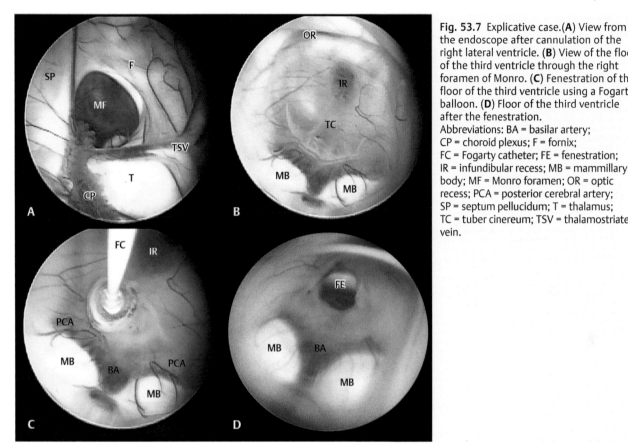

Fig. 53.7 Explicative case.**(A)** View from the endoscope after cannulation of the right lateral ventricle. **(B)** View of the floor of the third ventricle through the right foramen of Monro. **(C)** Fenestration of the floor of the third ventricle using a Fogarty balloon. **(D)** Floor of the third ventricle after the fenestration.
Abbreviations: BA = basilar artery; CP = choroid plexus; F = fornix; FC = Fogarty catheter; FE = fenestration; IR = infundibular recess; MB = mammillary body; MF = Monro foramen; OR = optic recess; PCA = posterior cerebral artery; SP = septum pellucidum; T = thalamus; TC = tuber cinereum; TSV = thalamostriate vein.

- Inspection of the cistern is required to ensure adequate opening of arachnoid adhesions or the membrane of Liliequist which may be present deep to the tuber cinereum.
- **Pineal region biopsy**
  - If ETV and pineal biopsy are planned in the same setting, the ETV should be performed first to ensure treatment of hydrocephalus prior to the added potential for bleeding or decreased visualization that may come along with biopsy.
  - May require the use of rigid 0 or 30° endoscopes, or flexible endoscope depending on ventricular size, trajectory, and entry point.
  - Neuronavigation is helpful to identify the most appropriate site for biopsy, particularly in cases when the lesion does not clearly breach the ependyma.
  - Minimization of cautery aids in improving likelihood of achieving pathologic diagnosis.
  - Samples are taken with a blunt cup forceps through the working channel of the endoscope.
  - Small venous hemorrhages from the capsule or tumor can be controlled with irrigation, Fogarty balloon tamponade, or electrocautery.
- **Complication management and avoidance**
  - Trajectory and entry point should be chosen to reduce the risk of traction on the fornix.
  - Sweeping motions of the endoscope are more likely to produce traction and pressure on the fornix and cause injury.

- Venous bleeding can most often be controlled with irrigation, balloon tamponade, or cautery.
- In cases where bleeding makes visualization impossible, the surgeon must be prepared to abort and leave behind an external ventricular drain (EVD).
- Communication with the anesthesia team is necessary during fenestration, as the patient can experience bradycardia.
- Arterial hemorrhage or basilar injury is rare but best avoided with good identification of landmarks prior to proceeding with fenestration.

References

1. Bouramas D, Paidakakos N, Sotiriou F, Kouzounias K, Sklavounou M, Gekas N. Endoscopic third ventriculostomy in obstructive hydrocephalus: surgical technique and pitfalls. Acta Neurochir Suppl (Wien) 2012;113:135–139.
2. Chibbaro S, Di Rocco F, Makiese O, et al. Neuroendoscopic management of posterior third ventricle and pineal region tumors: technique, limitation, and possible complication avoidance. Neurosurg Rev 2012;35(3):331–338, discussion 338–340.
3. Constantini S, Mohanty A, Zymberg S, et al. Safety and diagnostic accuracy of neuroendoscopic biopsies: an international multicenter study. J Neurosurg Pediatr 2013; 11(6):704–709.

4. Hermann EJ, Esmaeilzadeh M, Ertl P, Polemikos M, Raab P, Krauss JK. Endoscopic intracranial surgery enhanced by electromagnetic-guided neuronavigation in children. Childs Nerv Syst 2015;31(8):1327–1333.

5. Jallo GI, Kothbauer KF, Abbott IR. Endoscopic third ventriculostomy. Neurosurg Focus 2005;19(6):e11.

6. Limbrick DD Jr, Baird LC, Klimo P Jr, Riva-Cambrin J, Flannery AM; Pediatric Hydrocephalus Systematic Review and Evidence-Based Guidelines Task Force. Pediatric hydrocephalus: systematic literature review and evidence-based guidelines. Part 4: Cerebrospinal fluid shunt or endoscopic third ventriculostomy for the treatment of hydrocephalus in children. J Neurosurg Pediatr 2014;14(suppl 1):30–34.

7. Navarro R, Gil-Parra R, Reitman AJ, Olavarria G, Grant JA, Tomita T. Endoscopic third ventriculostomy in children: early and late complications and their avoidance. Childs Nerv Syst 2006;22(5):506–513.

Index

A

Abducens nerve
- in endoscopic endonasal transclival approach with transcondylar extension, 278f
- in retrosigmoid approach, 160f
Aboud's model, 6
Accessory nerve
- in endoscopic endonasal transclival approach with transcondylar extension, 278f
- in petrous bone anatomy, 193f
- in retrosigmoid approach, 160f
-- endoscopic, 166f
Agger nasi, 226
Alar ligament, in endoscopic transoral approach, 263f
Alveolar process, in transmaxillary approaches, 267f, 268f
Anatomical landmarks, cranial, 13, 13f
Angiography. *See* Digital subtraction angiography; Magnetic resonance angiography
Anterior cerebral artery
- in common carotid artery-middle cerebral artery bypass, 299f
- in frontotemporal and pterional approach, 98, 98f
- in nasal surgery, 226f
- in orbito-zygomatic approach, 112f
- in precaruncular approach, 80f
- in supraorbital approach, 70f
Anterior choroidal artery, in transbasal and extended subfrontal bilateral approach, 185f
Anterior clinoid process
- in extradural subtemporal transzygomatic approach, 131f, 132f
- in supraorbital approach, 75f
- in trans-ciliar approach, 80f
Anterior communicating artery, 70f
- in expanded endoscopic endonasal approach, 247f
- in frontal and bifrontal approach, 92f
Anterior cranial fossa
- endoscopic endonasal modified Lothrop approach to
-- bone exposure in, 251, 251f–253f
-- craniectomy. in, 253
-- dural opening in, 253
-- indications for, 249
-- nasal preparation in, 249
-- patient positioning for, 249, 249f
-- skull base reconstruction in, 254
-- skull base removal in, 253
-- soft tissue dissection in, 249–250, 250f, 251f
-- tumor resection in, 253–254
- presurgical imaging of, 19, 20f
Anterior ethmoidal artery
- in expanded endoscopic endonasal approach, 245f, 246f
- in precaruncular approach, 68f
Anterior ethmoidal complex, 222–223, 224f
Anterior inferior cerebellar artery
- in endoscopic endonasal transclival approach with transcondylar extension, 277f
- in far lateral approach, 170
- in petrous bone anatomy, 193f, 196f, 197f, 198f
- in precaruncular approach, 71f
- in retrosigmoid approach, 160f
- in translabyrinthine and transcochlear transpetrosal approaches, 218f
Anterior intercavernous sinus, in transbasal and extended subfrontal bilateral approach, 184f

Anterior longitudinal ligament
- in endoscopic endonasal transclival approach with transcondylar extension, 277f
- in endoscopic transoral approach, 262f
Anterior medial frontal artery, in midline interhemispheric approach, 116f, 117f
Anterior nasal spine, in transmaxillary approaches, 267f
Anterior petrosectomy
- cochlea in, 203f, 204–205, 204f
- craniotomy in, 201–202, 202f
- dural opening in, 205–206, 205f, 206f
- greater superficial petrosal nerve in, 202, 203f, 204f
- internal carotid artery in, 202–203, 203f, 204–205, 204f
- middle fossa dissection in, 202–205, 203f–206f
- patient positioning for, 201, 201f
- petrous apex in, 203–204, 203f, 204f
- skin incision for, 201, 201f, 202f
Anterior pharyngeal artery, in endoscopic endonasal transclival approach with transcondylar extension, 277f
Anterior spinal artery, in endoscopic endonasal transclival approach with transcondylar extension, 278f
Anterior squamous point, 14, 15f
Anterior sylvian point, 14, 15f
Anthropometry, cranial, 13–14, 14f
- for ventricular puncture
-- Dandy's point in, 319–320, 320f
-- Frazier's point in, 320, 320f
-- in frontal horn, 317–318, 317f
-- indications for, 317
-- Kaufman's point in, 318, 318f
-- Keen's point in, 319, 319f
-- in occipital horn, 318
-- Paine's point in, 321, 321f
-- transorbital, 318, 319f
-- in frontal horn, alternative access in, 318, 318f
Apical ligament, in endoscopic transoral approach, 263f
Asterion, 13, 13f, 207f
Atlanto-occipital joint, in retrosigmoid approach, 157f, 158f
Augmented virtual reality systems, 3

B

Basal vein of Rosenthal
- in pineal region endoscopic approach, 149f
- in supracerebellar infratentorial approach, 143f, 144f
Basilar artery
- in endoscopic endonasal transclival approach with transcondylar extension, 278f
- in endoscopic third ventriculostomy, 332f, 333f
- in orbito-zygomatic approach, 112f
- in precaruncular approach, 71f
- in supraorbital approach, 75f
- in transmaxillary transpterygoid approach, 273f
Basilar plexus, in endoscopic endonasal transclival approach with transcondylar extension, 278f
Basopharyngeal fascia, in endoscopic endonasal transclival approach with transcondylar extension, 277f
Bicoronal incision, 46, 46f
Bifrontal approach
- craniotomy in, 88–90, 88f–90f

- dural opening in, 90
- intradural exposure in, 90, 91f, 92f
- patient positioning for, 86
- skin incision for, 86, 86f
- soft tissue dissection in, 86–88, 87f
- temporal muscle dissection in, 53
Bilateral frontal craniectomy, 187, 190f
Biopsy, pineal region, 330–333, 330f–333f
Bony nasal septum, in microscopic endonasal and sublabial approach, 231f, 232f
Bovine placental vessels, 4
Brachial artery, chicken wing, 3f, 4
Brain convexity, presurgical imaging of, 23, 25, 27f, 28f
Bregma, 13, 13f, 14, 14f, 16, 16f
Bulla ethmoidalis, in nasal surgery, 222f, 223f, 224f
Burr hole placement
- in bilateral frontal craniectomy, 190f
- in endoscopic septostomy, 327
- in extradural subtemporal transzygomatic approach, 129
- in frontal horn ventricular puncture, 317
- in frontotemporal and pterional approach, 96
- in Mayfield head holder positioning, 41–42, 41f
- in middle cerebral artery-internal maxillary artery bypass, 307, 308f
- in midline interhemispheric approach, 114, 114f
- in midline suboccipital approach, 153f
- in mini-pterional approach, 101
- in occipital approach, 135, 135f
- in orbito-zygomatic approach, 107, 108f
- in retrosigmoid approach, 156, 157f
- in superficial temporal artery-middle cerebral artery bypass, 288
- in supracerebellar infratentorial approach, 139, 140f
- in temporal approaches, 120, 121f
- in transbasal and extended subfrontal bilateral approach, 178–179, 178f
- in unilateral craniectomy, 187, 188f
- in ventricular-peritoneal shunt, 322f, 323

C

Calcarine sulcus, 14, 14f, 17f, 18, 136f
Callosomarginal artery, in midline interhemispheric approach, 116f, 117f
Canine fossa, in transmaxillary approaches, 267f
Canthal ligament, in trans-frontal-sinus subcranial approach, 173f
Cavernous carotid artery, in transbasal and extended subfrontal bilateral approach, 185f
Cavernous carotid siphon, in transbasal and extended subfrontal bilateral approach, 184f
Cavernous malformation, in magnetic resonance imaging, in posterior cranial fossa, 22, 24f
Cavernous sinus
- in expanded endoscopic endonasal approach, 247f
- in extradural subtemporal transzygomatic approach, 132f
Central sulcus, 14, 14f

Cerebellar tonsils, in midline suboccipital approach, 154f
Cerebello-pontine angle, 20, 193f
Cerebral peduncle, in intradural subtemporal approach, 126f, 127f
Chicken wing artery, 3f, 4
Choana, in endoscopic endonasal transclival approach with transcondylar extension, 274f, 275f
Chorda tympani
- in petrous bone anatomy, 195f
- in presigmoid retrolabyrinthine approach, 212f
- in translabyrinthine and transcochlear transpetrosal approaches, 216f
Choroid plexus
- in endoscopic septostomy, 328f, 329f
- in endoscopic third ventriculostomy, 332f, 333f
Cingulate gyrus, 17, 116f, 117f
Clival bone
- in endoscopic endonasal odontoidectomy, 257f, 258f, 259f
- in endoscopic endonasal transclival approach with transcondylar extension, 274f, 278f
- in endoscopic transoral approach, 262f, 263f
- in expanded endoscopic endonasal approach, 245f, 246f
- in trans-frontal-sinus subcranial approach, 175f
- in transmaxillary approaches, 268f
Cochlea, in anterior petrosectomy, 203f, 204–205, 204f
Cochlear nerve, in petrous bone anatomy, 194f
Common carotid artery-middle cerebral artery bypass
- craniotomy in, 295–296, 296f
- distal anastomosis in, 298–300, 299f
- dural opening in, 296, 297f
- indications for, 293
- intradural exposure in, 296–297
- long saphenous vein in, 297, 298, 298f
- patient positioning for, 293–294
- proximal anastomosis in, 300–302, 301f
- skin incision for, 294–295, 294f
- soft tissue dissection in, 295
Computed tomography, in presurgical imaging
- anterior cranial fossa in, 19, 20f
- meningioma in, 19, 20f
- parasellar region in, 20
- pineal region in, 23, 26f
- posterior cranial fossa in, 22
-- lateral approach, 21, 22f
- schwannoma in, posterior cranial fossa, 21, 22f
- sellar region in, 20
Coronal suture, 13, 13f, 15, 15f, 88f, 91f, 114f, 179f, 187f, 188f, 288f, 290f, 307f
Corpus callosum, 17
- in frontal and bifrontal approach, 92f
- in midline interhemispheric approach, 116f, 117f
- in supracerebellar infratentorial approach, 142f
Cranial anthropometry, 13–14, 14f
Cranial landmarks, 13, 13f
Craniopharyngioma, in magnetic resonance imaging, 19–20, 21f
Craniotomy
- in anterior petrosectomy, 201–202, 202f